Structural Bodywork

This book is dedicated to

Dr Jack Haer, who showed me another path,
Robert Schleip and Pedro Prado, who guided my first steps,
and Dr David Lake, who helped me over the first potholes.

Commissioned illustrations by:
Robert Britton
Graeme Chambers
Mandy Miller
Phil West

For Elsevier:
Publishing Director, Health Professions: Mary Law/Sarena Wolfaard
Project Development Manager: Mairi McCubbin
Project Manager: Morven Dean
Designer: Judith Wright
Illustrations Manager: Bruce Hogarth

Structural Bodywork

An Introduction for Students and Practitioners

John Smith

Bachelor of Education (Syd)
Diploma Remedial Massage (NatureCare)
Certified Rolfing Practitioner
Certified Feldenkrais Practitioner
Certified Cranio-Sacral Practitioner
Certified Trager Practitioner

Somatic Therapist, Sydney, Australia

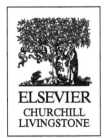

ELSEVIER
CHURCHILL
LIVINGSTONE

Edinburgh London New York Oxford Philadelphia St Louis Sydney Toronto 2005

ELSEVIER
CHURCHILL
LIVINGSTONE

First published 2005

ISBN 0 443 10010 1

British Library Cataloguing in Publication Data
A catalogue record for this book is available from the British Library

Library of Congress Cataloging in Publication Data
A catalog record for this book is available from the Library of Congress

Notice
Knowledge and best practice in this field are constantly changing. As new research and experience broaden our knowledge, changes in practice, treatment and drug therapy may become necessary or appropriate. Readers are advised to check the most current information provided on procedures featured or by manufacturer of each product to be administered to verify the recommended dose or formula, the method and duration of administration, and contraindications. It is the responsibility of the practitioner, relying on their own experience and knowledge of the patient, to make diagnoses, to determine dosages and the best treatment for each individual patient, and to take all appropriate safety precautions. To the fullest extent of the law, neither the publisher nor the author assume any liability for any injury and/or damage to persons or property arising from this publication.

The Publisher

 your source for books, journals and multimedia in the health sciences

www.elsevierhealth.com

Transferred to digital printing in 2009.

The Publisher's policy is to use paper manufactured from sustainable forests

CONTENTS

FOREWORDS

The orthodox helping professions of medicine and psychology have neglected almost completely the body's role in functional wellness. We all see the same people, but most practitioners will see only what we 'expect' to see in our frame or model of illness, and will tend to ignore the rest of the information. Nevertheless, I think that all helping professions are heading towards a confluence in the future with the active help of practitioners like the author, John Smith. His unusual ability both to collate and teach effectively in this complex field is demonstrated here, particularly when it comes to the 'how' and 'where' of intervening to enhance function.

Somatic therapists work with the body, but the body is not so easily understood. Only in the West do we so easily separate the body from the mind and the world. Yet somatic therapists will not be restricted by such concepts and are led naturally towards enquiry and exploration – hence the intellectual ferment today within fields such as Rolfing and the somatic treatment of trauma. It is imperative that creative concepts are tempered by intellectual rigour. John Smith's clear thinking and creative mind are not constrained by impractical dogmatism or orthodoxy in any field – hence this book.

By far the best part of working as a medical practitioner who uses 'alternative' techniques is meeting original thinkers. John Smith's book introduces you to him as much as to his thoughtful grasp of complex concepts. Naturally, a good practitioner will allow the client's body or mind to integrate at a higher level of function without intruding too much. I am always conscious when talking with John that 'the practitioner is the medicine' – that you are the cure as much as any technique that you use. But of course, John has provided a wealth of professional material to assimilate.

The Three Core Complementary Practices (in Chapter 3) of Constitutional, Psychological and Somatic practices include the labels of kinesiology, meridian stimulation and cognitive techniques that together are known as E.F.T. (Emotional Freedom Techniques). I am an E.F.T. practitioner. The main tenet of this 'psychological acupressure' technique is the radical concept that negative or toxic emotion is caused by a disruption in the body's energy system. My E.F.T. experience in the world of counseling and therapy in recent years has led me back to working with the body, since E.F.T. is a body energy technique mainly (with beneficial psychological consequences). I thus have a new respect for those who have always known the depth of the body's involvement in any emotional problem – especially trauma. The concept of the 'inner world', beloved of those working in the field of psychotherapy, needs to expand further to incorporate the body – and to allow it to 'be'.

This book serves as a bridge between the world of inhabiting the body, and the work of harmonizing and balancing the body. The illustrations alone provide an example of a striking translation from thought to understanding without the intervening cognitive interruption that words so often cause. There is sufficient background and history for a basic work, and the references are generous.

There is much in this book to expand your awareness of basic somatic methodologies and interventions. John has made the rich concepts of bodywork freely available. The very expansiveness of these words and notions about the body is inviting, for instance, 'structure that can be reorganized', 'the plasticity of the musculoskeletal system', 'the fascial web', 'tensegrity structure', 'body shaping', and from Ida Rolf (the source of many such concepts): 'Gravity is the therapist'.

It is a poetry of the body.

Ida Rolf stated that a lengthened and aligned body not only fostered physical health but psychological, emotional and spiritual health as well. If I may extend this idea – this book represents a symbolic intellectual 'lengthening' and 'aligning' for the interested practitioner. The book's very functional suggestions and interventions will then allow and invite a balanced perspective on somatic work to emerge. Conceptual integration occurs at a deeper level of understanding.

The book is far more than an elegant and practical introduction to a complex field. It is a passport to the world of lifelong learning about our inner world – which must include the body. There is really no room for rigid thinking or concepts – or rigid bodies (!) in this field.

John is pointing the way toward the future of bodywork with his clean, integrative framework that is informed by the pursuit of excellence.

Newport, 2004   David Lake MD

The book you hold in your hand provides the most comprehensive mapping of the world of Structural Integration to date. As such, it serves two purposes: (1) as an introduction to the wider field of discussion within the field for the 'heirs of Ida Rolf', especially those just setting out on the long and rewarding journey into practice; and (2) as a survey of Structural Integration for the interested outsider, be they a practitioner or even the interested consumer.

Dr Ida Pauline Rolf PhD, the pioneer of Structural Integration, was an extraordinary person. Known as the 'face that launched a thousand elbows', she did more to establish the field of fascial manipulation than anyone else in the modern Renaissance of natural therapies. Tireless, iconoclastic, generous, curious, and courageous (as well as difficult and peremptory), her life ranged over wide territories of both geography and intellect, always boiling what she learned down to a practical application. The practical application that emerged is a progressive system of fascial and myofascial manipulation designed to balance and lengthen the body in the field of gravity, and restore to it its natural moving and righting functions.

Aside from the practitioners whose elbows she launched, Ida Rolf left two legacies, the 'recipe' (explained herein) by which she taught her students, and her book (Rolf 1977). These were and are valuable maps, but the system requires filling in with both theoretical underpinnings and new applications, as well as adaptation to new findings and new models. This book fills that role.

Over the years since her death in 1979, in the dozen or so schools that follow her work, we have seen Structural Integration trainings with a more spiritual intent or a more osteopathic slant, each school with its unique emphasis on psychosomatic material, movement orientation, clinical bias, or preservationist fervor. It is a testament to her work that its shoulders are broad enough to bear all these interpretations and emphases easily. This book takes a wide and contextual view of these differing emphases.

One day, in one of the last classes she gave before her death, I came up to her at the beginning of a break to ask if she would like tea. Since the others had left and we were alone, I ventured a question: 'How does it feel,' I asked, "knowing that you have invented this fine thing, and established it so that it will go on after you leave?" Her answer: 'I was just getting going and my body gave out.'

Freezing her concepts as they were when she died would not honor that indomitable spirit. We must continue our explorations both at the center and out to the edges of what might be called 'Spatial Medicine' – the art and science of transforming inner shape. Osteopaths, chiropractors, physiotherapists, dance and Pilates teachers, Feldenkrais workers and Alexander teachers, yoga adepts and martial artists, as well as teachers of movement and bodyworkers of all stripes – all these, and especially the teachers of movement to children, work with Spatial Medicine. In fact, this is not a bad list of those who will be interested in this book.

We began by saying that this book is a map of the territory, and this is true at many levels. Rolfer® John Smith – careful to draw the distinction between map and territory right from the beginning – is a man with an affinity for mapping, and he guides us clearly through the plains, mountains, and riverbeds of Structural Integration.

First he maps out the context in which Structural Integration exists, and giving us its history, relation to other therapies. Along the way, his maps expand to include his own overview of complementary therapies as a whole, and quite detailed and to my eye new, diagrams of the process of getting 'stuck' and unstuck in particular. In the second section, he charts the organization within the standing and moving human body, and how it can be affected by manual work. In the third section, the practical application of structural bodywork is given a full menu, from conceptual models through bodyreading (visual assessment) basics to actual strategies for resolution of common postural dysfunctions.

Along the way, other maps emerge of the various models that are developing within the Structural Integration community over the years since Dr Rolf's death, and these sections will be of great interest to the practitioner, both within and without the actual Structural Integration community, as the exposition and comparative analysis of these theoretical models gives a sense of the scope of inquiry within this work. As far as I am aware, this is the first place in which these various models have been brought together and placed in context.

This book is the result of a lot of analysis, synthesis, and plain old hard work on the part of the author. The result, like all good maps, is easy on the reader, easy to navigate, and contains the essential information for understanding this interesting and unique approach to the soma.

Clarks Cove, 2004   Thomas Myers

Can one become a good bodywork practitioner solely by reading a book without any personal hands-on instruction? Of course not. This would be as difficult as becoming a good musician or dancer just by studying books. Personal experience and personalized coaching cannot be replaced. Yet for keen and serious students an excellent text book such as this can be an invaluable aid in understanding some of the deeper concepts behind their art. If you are a bodywork or movement practitioner of a different modality who has already experienced this profound work yourself, and you are interested in exploring some of our concepts in more depth, you will like this book; it is what many of you have been waiting for. And for those of you who have already started a professional training in this powerful work – because you have been infected by our insiders' passion and excitement for this wonderful art – you won't have a choice: this is a must have book.

The field of structural integration encompasses fascial manipulation and related movement techniques around the basic ideas of the Dr Ida Rolf (1896–1979). Since Ida Rolf's era, practitioners have been educated in this approach mostly in a semi-mystery school-like manner, i.e. student applicants are screened and chosen for personal maturity by senior practitioners, classes are small and expensive, most of the informational teaching is done in oral form, and practitioners are reminded not to pass out relevant information to outsiders. Inspired by some of the guilds of master craftsmen of former times, this is how Ida Rolf felt that learning the complexity and transformational depth of this work could be best achieved. While being criticized by some as elitist or old-fashioned, this approach is reflected by Ida Rolf's female emphasis on quality rather than quantity reproduction of her seeds.

There is a beautiful quote from German poet Rainer Maria Rilke, which exemplifies some of the qualities of this traditional learning approach and which often has been read to students by their Rolfing instructors around the middle or towards the end of their training: *'I want to beg you as much as I can, to be patient toward all that is unsolved in your heart and try to love the questions themselves like locked rooms and like books written in a very foreign tongue. Do not seek the answers which cannot be given to you because you would not be able to live them. And the point is to live everything. Live the questions now. Perhaps you will then gradually, without noticing it, live along some distant day into the answer.'* As profound and wise as Rilke's reminder is, it has been also tempting for us senior instructors to simply disguise our own ignorance about aspects which we don't understand ourselves, be it because of our personal imperfections or because current knowledge about it is still insufficient.

When John Smith, the author of this book, went through his basic training in Structural Integration (SI) more than a decade ago, he was one of the few students whose hunger for detailed understanding we could not sedate with this quote. As one of his instructors at that time, I do remember his enormous mental curiosity combined with an almost Buddhist like peaceful humbleness. *'Would it be possible, dear instructor, to read more about this or to even get a hold of the original paper?'* Little did we know at that time – yet not unsurprisingly – that he would be working for the next 10 years to publish the first comprehensive textbook on the theories of SI. Some may criticize that John Smith currently does not belong to the inner most circle of senior instructors that were chosen originally by Dr Rolf, or who are authorized as such by the current international schools. Others I am sure will find details in this book which they themselves would have described differently. Yet I doubt this book – if it had been written by any of us official instructors – would have ever become as clear and understandable for outsiders as well as comprehensive and relatively unbiased. The author's accomplishment is impressive, as he manages to not only include more of the many important aspects of this field than have been ever put into a single book before, yet also does it with a high level of detail, accuracy and in an excellent didactic manner.

The foremost highlight of this book, in my opinion, is the theoretical part, as practically all the relevant theoretical models as they are currently taught in SI classes are described. The author has spent years contacting the founders of various concepts to get their latest details and their approval for his descriptions. If several alternative models or explanations exist, he often chooses not to take sides himself, but accurately describes their basic assumptions to include some of the main pro and contra discussions. His review of the physiological basis is the best I have seen so far. Another aspect that adds great value to this book is the author's wider perspective within the somatic fields. While focusing on SI as it is currently taught, he also introduces relevant aspects of the wider field of somatic practices such as the Feldenkrais Method® and Alexander Technique as welcome adjuncts to structural bodywork. Hopefully this will trigger an indepth discussion between practitioners of structural bodywork and somatic educators/therapists, beyond the still prevalent mutual misconceptions. Rather than only summarizing the work of others – which he does extremely well – he also includes some of his own contributions, creative charts and comparative overviews, as well as his practical manual with a simple and clear working protocol at the end.

It is nevertheless with mixed feelings that I endorse this book. Together with the recent publication of the more practical manual of deep tissue techniques by his colleague and countryman Michael Stanborough, it looks like most of the informational contents of our basic trainings are being spilled out. Will this be the end for our nice and almost tribal community of passionate practitioners of this work? Will it speed up the development of cheap weekend courses and E-learning classes by average level PT or massage schools that will try to teach this work? It surely will, and the nostalgic part in me would prefer to turn the wheels backwards or at least stop them from turning so rapidly. Yet there is also a lot of fresh air of rejuvenation and inspiration, which this new area of opening and the increasing dialog with other somatic practices is already creating. If we can keep some of the profound transformational qualities of learning this work and mix them with more transparent, academic and practical teaching methods of modern times, a lot will be gained. The mature and wise reader, I am sure, will recognize in John Smith's excellent book how much more complexity and subtleties are involved that can only be learned in a personalized learning process over a longer time period.

Munich, 2004   Robert Schleip

PREFACE

Rochester: 'I once had a kind of rude tenderness of heart. When I was as old as you, I had a feeling fellow enough; partial to the unfledged, unfostered, and unlucky; but fortune has knocked me about since; she has even kneaded me with her knuckles, and now I flatter myself that I am hard and tough as an India-rubber ball; pervious, though, through a chink or two still, and with one sentient point in the middle of the lump. Yes: does that leave hope for me?'
Jane Eyre: 'Hope of what, sir?'
Rochester: 'Of my final transformation from India-rubber back to flesh?'

From 'Jane Eyre' by Charlotte Bronte

This book is a practical introduction to a growing field of somatic enquiry: structural bodywork. Structural bodywork is a 'hands-on' approach that has the fundamental aim of alleviating the structural imbalances that afflict so many of us today. It was brought to the world as a fully fledged discipline in the 1960s by Dr Ida P. Rolf, although its historical roots go much deeper. Since its inception, structural bodywork has evolved further into a complex discipline with a refined body of praxis and a rich conceptual background. This book is an attempt to clarify this conceptual background, drawing together various strands that can currently only be found within separate disciplines. It will explore the history and background of the field, sketch the anatomy and kinesiology of structure, discuss the maps and concepts that structural bodywork shares with other approaches, and it will explore the unique perspective brought by this bodywork tradition to important concepts such as 'structure', 'integration' and 'holism'; it will offer some useful models for understanding, evaluating and working with structural dysfunctions, and will provide a selection of effective techniques for structural intervention.

Structural Bodywork was written with a diverse range of practitioners in mind: somatic therapists, massage therapists and other bodyworkers who are looking to move beyond their present forms; physiotherapists who are interested in exploring new ways of working with the body; students who are undertaking a formal training program in structural bodywork, and for those who are simply interested in gaining a new or deeper understanding of their own structure. For bodyworkers, it provides a broad introduction to this exciting,

specialized field. Physiotherapists should find here some fresh strategies for dealing with postural dysfunctions, taking a more holistic view of their clients' progress; they will also find some potent techniques which may not be familiar. Students of structural integration will be orientated towards a structural way of thinking and will find here much of the theoretical background of their chosen discipline. Hence this book should be used as a reference, as a means of getting acquainted with a new discipline, and as a means of enriching the body of ideas presented during the course of formal training; although, of course, it cannot hope to supplant the ambience, the intensity and the unique learning environment that evolves during the course of a training.

My initial somatic training was in Rolfing® Structural Integration. This was a process of deep immersion. Our teachers surrounded us with an ocean of ideas, and as students we were encouraged to plunge into that ocean, to breast the waves and to play with these ideas like bright and elusive sea creatures. We were tantalized with the latest ideas emerging from anatomical, physiological and kinesiological research, confronted with the deeply challenging concepts surrounding the principles of structural bodywork and were initiated into the unique perspective of human structure that has evolved within the structural bodywork field. We explored different movement approaches, plumbing the relationship between structure and function, and undertook the perceptual challenge of looking deep into the human body to glean structural patterns hidden within the flesh.

I hope that this book will reflect something of the richness of this training; that it will provide a pool of ideas (if not an ocean!), or perhaps it may provide something to dip into in a more leisurely fashion. Any book about this fascinating field of enquiry could not even attempt to be comprehensive, but I hope it will give a broad and practical introduction to the field, sketch the conceptual background of the discipline, offer some techniques to augment your own manual skills and perhaps encourage you to think in a more structural way about your clients; taking a longer view of their process rather than always attempting to alleviate their most pressing and immediate problems.

We live in a world in which people are becoming more and more divorced from their own bodies. We see disorders like body dysmorphism and anorexia nervosa increasing disorders in which there is a complete mismatch between actual and perceived body image. The rising incidence of repetitive strain injuries is yet another indication that people are simply failing to listen to their bodies; they are not sensing themselves as fully as they might; they lack a complete, accurate internal map of their own bodies. This all highlights the great need for any practice that can put people more in touch with their own bodies. Fortunately, there is a countervailing trend unfolding; an exciting historical convergence is occurring right now in which many seeming disparate disciplines are all pointing to the stark fact that we need to live more *embodied* lives. Vastly diverse practices from many different cultural milieus are all telling us to live more fully in the body, to live a rich, sensual, embodied life: practices such as Buddhist Vipassana, Feldenkrais *Awareness Through Movement*, Yoga Nidra, Autogenic training, Hakomi Integrative Somatics, Mind Body Centering and Continuum. And the structural bodywork tradition, too, has a unique place within this movement. In undertaking to explore the structural bodywork approach, you too will be part of this movement, because this somatic discipline is an enormously powerful means, among others, that can help people live more balanced, authentic and embodied lives.

Sydney, 2003   John Smith

ACKNOWLEDGEMENTS

I am greatly indebted to the many people who have assisted me in this enterprise. I am deeply grateful for the constructive comments of those who have reviewed sections of the manuscript; Leonie Waks, Merry Pearson, Gilbert Schultz and Amber Cameron assisted greatly in the early stages, helping me to clarify my intentions, organize my thinking and making many useful suggestions on points of expression and style.

A number of Rolfers reviewed sections of this book from a Rolfing perspective, and I would especially like to express my gratitude to the Australian Rolfers Nicholas Barbousos and Chris Eyles, who have provided invaluable advice, challenged a number of unsupported ideas, and corrected some errors.

I was privileged in having Michael Ridge review the first two sections of the book. Michael, somatic therapist and long-time assistant of Bonnie Bainbridge-Cohen, was in a unique position to observe the growth of the somatic movement over many years in the United States. Having witnessed its dramatic evolution and having met and worked with many of its key players, Michael was wonderfully qualified to provide real insight into the core concepts of this tradition and in clarifying its historical context for me.

My thanks to Shirley Norwood who helped with the Hellerwork section, to Michael Trembath who helped with the Zentherapy section, to Jack Painter who reviewed the Postural Integration section, to Lee Marquette, graphic artist, who helped me with the layout of the practical section, to Josephine Hardy, librarian, for her assistance in finding a number of key research articles, to Sol Peterson, somatic educator, whose conversations helped me clarify my views on the place of structural bodywork in the context of the complementary therapy movement, to Robert Schleip, Rolfing teacher, who provided the extraordinary quotations from von Bertalanffy and Dr Andrew Taylor Still, and to Michael Stanborough, Rolfing teacher who inspired many of the myofascial releases shown in this book.

My thanks also to Kit Laughlin who inspired many of the contract–relax stretches shown in the practical section of this book and gave me free rein to make use of the stretches that he and his assistants have developed over many years, and to Peter Robinson, the model in the practical section who is a talented bodyworker and stretch-coach in his own right.

I would also like to thank the editorial staff at Elsevier who made this book possible: Mary Law, Mairi McCubbin, Morven Dean and Ceinwen Sinclair.

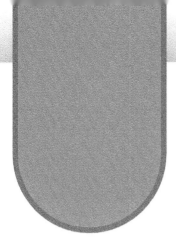

INTRODUCTION

When I undertook to write this book, my foremost aim was to produce the kind of book that I needed when I began my own studies in this field. Then, there were no published works written specifically for structural body-workers. The available texts were often dryly scientific or, on the other extreme, written for 'fringe' complementary therapists and pervaded with the pop-psychology of the 'New Age'. I believe this book steers a middle course and presents a balanced perspective that will be accessible to all somatic therapists; those with and those without a scientific background.

Having once tried to learn the guitar from a book, I understand the insuperable difficulties involved in learning any practical skill by the printed word alone. Practical skills are best learned practically: through demonstration, imitation and supervised practice. Why then this book? Practice must be informed by theory, so Sections 1 and 2 are concerned with sketching the rich conceptual milieu of this field of bodywork. They will examine the structural and functional aspects of anatomy and kinesiology, the maps you will need to negotiate this field, and will present an analysis of the relationship between structure and function. Section 3, however, is a practical introduction to the field and assumes some prior, basic experience in a manual therapy such as massage. This section will offer ways of looking at the structure of your clients; it presents some guidelines for strategizing a bodywork session and structuring a series of sessions, and offers some effective techniques with which to address structural dysfunctions.

Although this book will not make you a structural bodyworker, it may help you to experiment with a more holistic way of working and allow you to perform small-scale structural interventions with your clients. This is not the ideal approach, and without the guiding rationale of a holistic framework, it is unlikely to result in a major structural rebalancing for your clients. If used with discretion, however, it can lead you to work that may relieve your clients' problems for longer periods, certainly much longer than by just 'rubbing where it hurts'. These successes may thereby alert you to the need for a fuller training into the principles behind effective structural bodywork, principles that quite possibly can only be picked up through the kind of 'apprenticeship' offered by formal training, through observing experienced 'elders' of this work and trying to grasp just what they are seeing when they look at a body.

The kernel of this book is based on a workbook I developed for a 3-day workshop entitled 'A Holistic Approach to Working with Posture'. I taught this workshop for several years at the University of Sydney's School of Health Science, within the Continuing and Professional Education Unit. This workshop was offered to a wide range of health professionals: physiotherapists, occupational therapists, massage therapists, yoga teachers, counsellors, psychologists, nurses and Feldenkrais practitioners. It was interesting to note that, despite the considerable combined experience and the varied training of these practitioners, a number of the concepts I presented were completely novel to many of them. Even though structural bodywork in its present form has been around for about 50 years, many of its key concepts are not yet 'in circulation', ideas such as the following:

- human beings have a structure that can be reorganized
- the *connective tissue network* has structural significance
- postural dynamics can vary markedly between individuals.

Most current postural models think only in terms of muscle length and skeletal alignment, and will either advocate the 'stretch and strengthen' protocol, or will casually suggest that clients adopt and maintain certain postural habits, such as 'You need to pull those shoulders back', 'Keep your tail tucked under' or 'Tighten your tummy muscles'. Such postural advice rarely works.

Central to the structural bodywork approach is the premise that it is the fascial network that unifies and organizes the entire musculoskeletal system; which network itself is modified and organized by the functional movement patterns that our bodies experience in daily life. It is the plasticity of this network in responding to the usual stresses of life that allows us to become unbalanced in the first place, and this very plasticity that allows us, with some intelligent input, to restore some order and balance to the system. The job of structural bodyworkers then is to provide that intelligent input; to uncover the structural imbalances of their clients and to use their manual skills to resolve them.

This approach is recommended for therapists who are dissatisfied with merely helping their clients cope, and who wish to help them achieve real and lasting structural improvement. Central to this approach is the idea that the body has many levels of somatic organization, and that real and lasting changes can only take place if we work with as many of these levels as possible. We must not only reorganize soft tissue; we must also help our clients to sense, feel and embody these changes; to integrate them fully into the movement patterns of their daily life. *We must work both structurally and functionally to achieve enduring change.*

In practical terms, structural improvement means relieving areas of shortness within the connective tissue network, *of giving more length and resilience to the tissue precisely where it is needed*, whether the tissue has adaptively shortened through unbalanced usage or as part of a life-long pattern of structural imbalance. This kind of work can make upright posture easier to maintain and less stressful to the body; it removes some of the muscular strain that is required to maintain unbalanced, inefficient structures against the ceaseless influence of gravity. Structural improvements, however, can only be maintained in the longer term if clients deeply sense the structural changes taking place within them, and integrate new options into their repertoire of movement and postural patterns. This means that some form of proprioceptive education must accompany the structural interventions.

But where exactly do we lengthen? A toolbag of techniques is of no help if we do not know what to do, where to lengthen, and in what sequence – if we have no guiding rationale for our work. We need some ways

of inquiring into our client's structure and some means of assessing it: of discovering the complex patterns of adaptive shortening that can develop within the human organism. Some structural models are needed for this purpose. Dr Ida P. Rolf, the founder of Rolfing, provided some useful tools in this regard, and since her death there has been a great deal of creative thinking within the Rolfing community, resulting in the *internal–external model,* a powerful means of evaluating our client's structural tendencies and of showing what needs to be done in order to 'normalize' that structure. Several variants of this model have been developed and some of them will be examined in this book.

The approach in this book is an eclectic one, embracing aspects of Rolfing, Feldenkrais, neuromuscular techniques and scientific stretching. It is deeply influenced and informed by the Rolfing approach, *but makes no attempt at teaching structural integration.* It does not teach Rolfing or any of its variants from other schools of structural integration. It has the more modest objective of serving as a practical introduction to the field. To this end it will outline a simplified three-level approach that will be accessible to any experienced therapist, and will allow you to encourage stable and balanced structural change in your clients.

In this three-level approach, soft-tissue fixations are initially addressed using techniques of soft tissue mobilization. Then, new and isolated movement options are explored using neuromuscular techniques, generally with the intention of increasing the range of motion, improving the quality of movement around specific articulations, or of bringing about a more efficient coordination between antagonist groups. Finally, these changes have to be integrated into whole-body movement patterns of the client; otherwise they will merely provide a short-term benefit. Therefore integrative techniques are included as an indispensable ingredient of this approach.

A variety of techniques are offered in Section 3. A direct form of *myofascial release* will be introduced as an effective means of giving more length and resilience to tissue that has adaptively shortened. *Contract–relax stretching* will be shown as a means of imprinting new movement possibilities on the sensory-motor cortex; of providing an expanded range of movement, though not necessarily in creating new patterns of coordination. An array of both *passive and active stretches* will also be offered as 'homeplay' for your clients. A general protocol will be given for all these techniques, but once the principles are known, you can be as creative as you wish in applying them, and in finding your own unique variations.

These techniques are not exhaustive; they are certainly not the only ones that are effective in structural work, and they do not invalidate any other techniques and approaches that you have found to be useful. Both myofascial release and contract–relax stretching are generally useful techniques in the hands of all somatic therapists. Their use is not limited to working with posture and structure; they will prove useful wherever soft-tissue restrictions exist.

A limited selection of *movement and postural educational approaches* will be demonstrated in Section 3. An introductory book such as this cannot hope to present a comprehensive approach to teaching movement integration; the Feldenkrais training, for instance, takes 8 full months over 4 years, so only a taste, a representative offering, can be given here. The book will not explore the full range of movement possibilities that can be enhanced by this work. Instead it will focus on one of the most important human moving functions of all: walking. Observing how our clients walk is a powerful way of seeing their structural and functional fixations. Walking is a function that can be readily enhanced by structural bodywork, and is therefore a convenient starting point for this approach. The text focuses on the three main kinds of pelvic undulation that are inherent in efficient walking:

- a rocking in the sagittal plane
- the lateral sway of the pelvis in the frontal plane
- the counter-rotation of the shoulder and pelvic girdles in the transverse plane; a slight twisting and untwisting through the longitudinal axis of the body.

and will show how these movements can be enhanced through appropriately applied myofascial release and stretching, and then how these more efficient patterns can then be integrated into full body movement.

A simplified approach to postural analysis will also be outlined in Section 3. It will focus on postural deviations in the sagittal and frontal planes: front–back and left–right imbalances, and will look only cursorily at rotatory patterns in the transverse plane. However, when looking at the total pattern of muscle fibre orientations in the body, the direction of the 'grain' as it were, it is quite apparent that *the human body is designed to support spiral or helical movement patterns*, movement in the transverse plane, so a left–right and front–back analysis is obviously bound to be partial and limited. This limited perspective is, however, an extremely practical way to begin to explore structure, while resolving the front–back, left–right imbalances is a highly effective way of achieving a 'first approximation' in balancing the structure of a client.

This book talks unashamedly about how structure may be modified. It acknowledges that emotional and psychosomatic influences do have a profound impact on our bodies and often create the habits of tension and muscular armouring that lead directly to much of the structural imbalance we see in others and experience within ourselves. This book, however, touches only tangentially upon emotional and psychological issues. It is my belief that somatic therapy and psychotherapy *can* be combined, however only in a relatively limited way. When you consider the rigour of the apprenticeship necessary in both of the modalities, and the amount of experience required to be really effective in either of them, then it is a wonder that anyone would try to combine the approaches at all! What so often happens is that psychotherapists learn a little bit of somatic practice and incorporate it into their work, or else bodyworkers try to 'psychologize' their clients, naively believing that they can do it all. Both of these approaches can be useful so long as we realize our limitations and are prepared to refer our clients on when we feel we are getting out of our depth. Indeed, some of the early offshoots from the Rolfing tradition work very effectively, both psychologically and emotionally, in this relatively limited way. Occasionally, one finds rare practitioners who are extensively cross-trained in both disciplines and who do extraordinary work, but for anyone starting in this field this is only a future possibility. I believe that if you wish to be a structural bodyworker, you must first master structure, then if you find that there are deeper issues that need to be resolved before a client can change, be prepared to refer your client on, or to undertake further training yourself.

This book will not make you a structural bodyworker as such, but it may help you embark upon some preliminary, safe experiments in gently reorganizing structure, and help you to alleviate some of your clients' structural or postural issues in the short- to medium-term. Your success in these endeavours will, I hope, encourage you to consider some of the excellent training programs now widely available in various schools of structural bodywork in many countries throughout the world (see Appendix 1 for training institutions).

SECTION

1

BACKGROUND AND HISTORY OF STRUCTURAL BODYWORK

STRUCTURAL BODYWORK: AN OVERVIEW

INTRODUCTION

Human bodies have a structure that can be eased, balanced and, to a certain extent, refashioned. Any effects of structural change will be reflected in all aspects of our being – not only in how we move and function in the world, but also in how we think and feel. *Structural bodywork* is a modern somatic practice that directly modifies our structure, evoking within it greater order, length and alignment. Structural bodywork integrates the human structure. The emerging structural balance brings with it greater freedom and grace in how we function as human beings. By the intelligent application of *bodywork* techniques, both ancient and modern, *structural bodyworkers* can align the human structure, reducing the biomechanical stresses within it, and helping us to find healthier, more balanced and efficient ways of living.

The changes that arise from structural bodywork can prompt a radical shift in our awareness and in the quality of our everyday experience. A body that is structurally balanced will have a freer, lengthened posture, more generous movement possibilities, a greater sense of vitality, and more resilience to meet the inescapable challenges and stresses of life. Structural bodywork is at its very core an *embodiment process* – a process that can awaken the 'self sensing' of the body (Hanna 1980), that can help us become more centred and comfortable in the body, that can even help us take joy in our physicality. Such an awakening can be a vital antidote to the dissociation from the body that is such a disturbing feature of modern life.

The word *structure* has come to have a specialized meaning in the realm of structural bodywork. Its meaning will be clarified throughout this book but, in essence, it refers to the integrated wholeness of the body's connective tissue network and includes the whole spectrum of connective tissue structures, from the fascial web to the skeletal superstructure. Structural bodyworkers, however, have a particular interest in the fasciae of the body since, of all the connective tissues, these are the most amenable to change. Ida Rolf was one of the first of the somatic pioneers to stress the importance of the fascial web, calling it 'the organ of structure' (Rolf 1977), and since her time structural bodyworkers have been refining its meaning. The word *fascia* has taken on a broader meaning than a strictly anatomical definition and is often taken to include other connective tissue structures such as tendons, ligaments, bursae, retinaculae, cartilage, perichondrium, the periosteum, joint capsules, meninges, basal laminae, serous and mucous membranes and organ capsules – all composed mostly of collagen fibres, all different metamorphoses of 'the one fascia'.

STRUCTURAL DYSFUNCTION

If we look around any busy street we will see everywhere what Ida Rolf (1977) liked to call 'random bodies' (see Fig. 1.1). These are bodies exhibiting the outward signs of structural dysfunction, with stooped, swayed or rigidly held backs, collapsed or 'pumped' chests, poke necks, Chaplinesque feet, hyper-extended knees, shoulders that are hunched, 'military squared' or too elevated. In other words, bodies wavering between collapse and overcompensation in their struggle with gravity. And these are just the obvious and visible signs. Less obvious are the hidden structural imbalances that manifest as inelegant and restricted gait, inefficient movement patterns, stressful work habits or an oppressive sense that this body is just not functioning as it should.

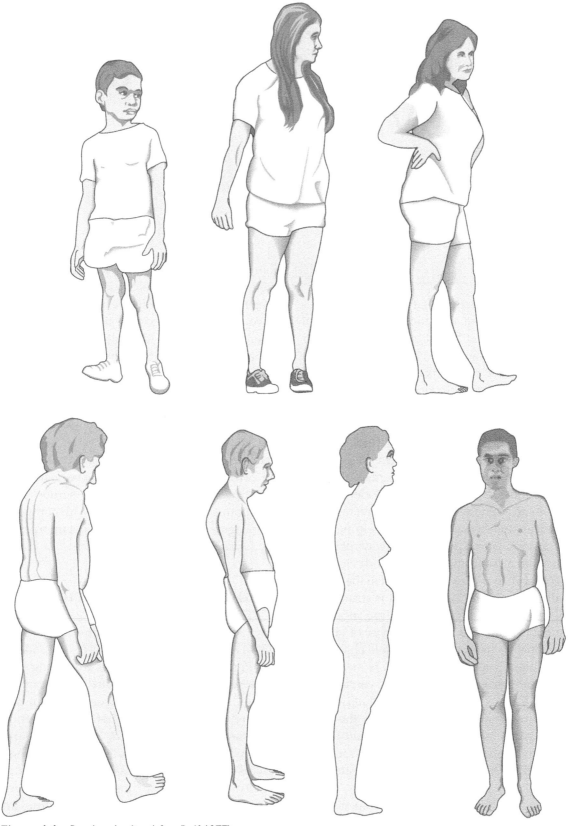

Figure 1.1   Random bodies (after Rolf 1977).

Structural dysfunctions in bodies typically arise from:

- long-term effects of gravity on an unbalanced posture
- poor ergonomic habits, sometimes made inevitable by poorly designed work environments
- asymmetrical patterns of body use – arising either from habit, from handedness and other lateralized preferences, or from the demands of non-symmetrical activities
- postural adaptations to injury – typically subconscious attempts of our *sensory-motor intelligence* to avoid or minimize pain
- postural adaptation induced by diseases and deficiencies
- gradual adaptation of soft tissues to repetitive strain or emotional stress
- congenital and developmental factors such as asymmetries of the skeleton
- the results of emotional or 'character' armouring.

Becoming set in our ways

All of these conditions encourage and perpetuate movement patterns that are inhibited, constrained and inefficient. These restricted movement patterns will, in their turn, impose an uneven pattern of strain upon the soft tissues of the body, with some tissues receiving too much mechanical stress, and some not enough. Soft tissues, from the structural bodywork perspective, refer to the fascial and myofascial networks of the body. These fasciae respond to such stress in characteristic ways: there is a tightening, a stiffening and an increase in fibrosity, and there may also be an adaptive shortening or lengthening of the tissue. In all cases there is a *diminished capacity for the tissue to lengthen*. An insidious 'vicious cycle' is established (see Fig. 1.2) – as this network of soft-tissue restrictions gradually infiltrates the body, it maintains then deepens the neuromuscular habits that brought it about in the first place. We become literally 'set in our ways', in the same sense that a jelly sets: the tissues gel, conforming more and more to our everyday postures and habitual patterns of usage.

This 'setting' process is a kind of short-term wisdom on the part of the body. It is just one aspect of a necessary and conservative group of processes within our overall somatic organization that strives to maintain a homeostasis, to keep us *as we are,* to maintain a kind of balance, whether or not that balance is healthy in the long run. It is as if our sensory-motor intelligence is saying, 'This is how this body wants to behave, so let's help it do just that!' This leads to the strange paradox – that even the most obviously collapsed and habitual

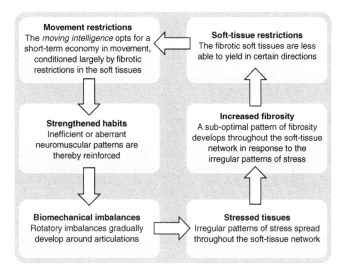

Figure 1.2 A vicious cycle showing the interplay of habit and soft-tissue restriction.

posture is, in the shorter term, the most economical way of being. It would take more energy to 'stand up straight' than to submit to the prevailing structural form. So, despite the fact that dysfunctional postural patterns may give rise to all manner of secondary problems, such as undue stress on joints and soft tissues; compression or entrapment of the nerves, blood vessels and the viscera; restriction in respiration and so on, it is still the most energy-efficient way of existing within the current structural arrangement. This is why it is so easy to slump, almost unconsciously, into the old patterns – and why these patterns reassert themselves when we tire or do not pay attention to our bodies.

The converse of this disturbing scenario is that if our habitual patterns become more efficient and balanced, then these too can become consolidated at the tissue level. It is not just bad posture that can become fixed and habitual. Structural bodywork is based on the fundamental premise that this vicious cycle can be reversed; that the compromised soft tissues can be mobilized, establishing more balance within the soft-tissue network, reducing the overall level of stress upon the soft tissues, encouraging more efficient neuromuscular coordination, and opening the way to more generous movement possibilities. Hence the fundamental approach of structural bodywork is to release the compromised soft tissues and then invite new movement with proprioceptive educational techniques. With a judicious use of both structural and functional interventions at different stages of this work, structural bodywork can promote dramatic improvements in posture and functionality (see Fig. 1.4 at the end of the chapter). And, as Figure 1.3 implies, functional intervention need not merely assist

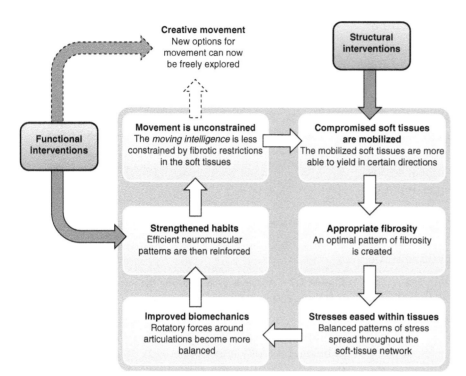

Figure 1.3 The vicious cycle is reversed.

in normalizing movement and posture by restoring the status quo; it can present the extraordinary prospect of evoking a true creativity in movement, of allowing a higher order of functionality to emerge. New and improved functional patterns will then positively feed back into maintaining a more balanced structure.

STRUCTURAL BODYWORK – A COMPLEMENTARY APPROACH

There is growing enthusiasm in the general public for complementary (or alternative) therapies, which encompass a dazzling array of methods, both ancient and modern. More and more they are being accepted as benign and effective alternatives to allopathic medicine: the model of health and treatment that has long been dominant in the West. This growing acceptance and trust is mirrored to a certain extent even within the medical profession itself, which is becoming by degrees much less dismissive of alternative approaches and seeing them as truly complementary to its work. Increasingly, we find multidisciplinary clinics that cross the medical–complementary divide. Surveys in Westernized countries show that a substantial proportion of the population now use alternative practitioners and take unprescribed alternative medicines (MacLennan et al. 1996). People who regularly use such practitioners generally believe

complementary approaches to be more consistent with their overall philosophical orientation to life, particularly involving such concepts as holism and self-responsibility. Health consumers are making informed choices, believing that both medical and complementary approaches can serve different aspects of their health goals and aspirations at different times. There is a kind of 'mix and match' philosophy emerging in which consumers do not deny the validity of either tradition but use the specific insights of each to meet their own requirements. For many, visiting an alternative practitioner is a positive choice rather than a reaction against allopathic medicine (Astin 1998).

Structural bodywork is not as widely known as some other alternative modalities such as homeopathy, naturopathy, osteopathy, or even Swedish massage. However, in the world of somatic therapies, structural bodywork is widely seen as the pre-eminent approach to easing structural dysfunctions, and certainly this reputation has some basis; the pre-requisites for entering structural bodywork training programs are exceptionally high, with entrants often having already successful careers in other somatic fields such as massage or physiotherapy. Students emerge from these trainings grounded in a deep experience and understanding of human structure and with a broad knowledge of biomechanics and scientific kinesiology. On account of this, structural bodyworkers tend to be among the most highly

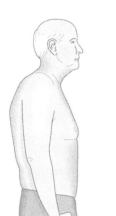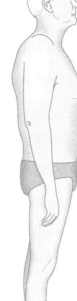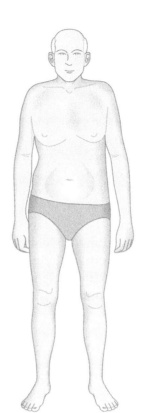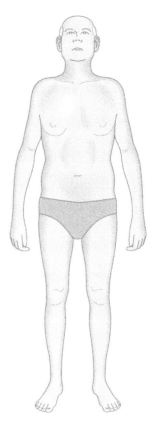

Figure 1.4 Before and after Rolfing.

trained and highly respected of contemporary somatic professionals.

Historically, the various systems of structural bodywork have been administered by official bodies, usually established by their founders to train and certify new students. Like all such institutions they tend to be highly proprietorial and to guard their methodologies most fiercely, often patenting their approach and its brand name. This attitude is understandable; it is due in part to the genuine need to protect valuable systems from abuse and facile imitation. In many cases, however, this vigilance has led these organizations to become exclusive, self-serving and anti-competitive. Happily though, this guild-like mentality appears to be on the decline.

So, at the beginning of the new millennium, it is 'interesting times' in the world of somatic therapies. A highly creative fusion of techniques and approaches is now taking place. And as part of this sea change, structural bodywork is becoming more widely recognized by both the general public and other somatic practitioners. Many massage therapists are moving into structural bodywork as an area of specialization, and many physiotherapists are seeing aspects of this approach as an invaluable adjunct to their work.

BODY-SHAPING TECHNOLOGIES

Historically, most cultures have evolved technologies that attempt to alter our physical appearance or structure. Many of these technologies have a cosmetic intent: ranging in practice from corsetry to ritual scarring, from the neck-lengthening of Nubian women to the foot-binding of young females in pre-Maoist China, and from the lip-stretching of Niu Gini tribesmen to the head-binding among the ancient Mayan aristocracy. Such practices modify the body's structure to satisfy a culture's 'body aesthetic', or to formalize aspects of social status; rarely do they actually improve human functionality. On the other hand, many body-shaping practices have had a truly therapeutic intent. Among the ancient Greeks, Hippocrates and Galen advocated steam and traction as a way of dealing with *kyphosis*, and used primitive traction and compression devices as means of dealing with perceived deformities such as scoliosis or 'hunchback'. These practices survived into medieval times and were practiced throughout the European and Arab worlds (Harris 1993), and indeed modern variations of the same devices are still in use today.

For centuries, yogic practice in the East has taught the need for structural alignment. Hatha yoga is a highly evolved and coherent set of practices for producing a lengthened and opened body. Although there has been nothing comparable to yoga in the West, there exists a long tradition of structural craftsmen and craftswomen – the 'bonesetters' – working successfully outside the prevailing medical establishment (Burch 2002). In the late nineteenth century came the development of osteopathy and chiropractic, as well as the orthopaedic branch of Western medical science led by Dr James Cyriax, Dr James Mennell and others. Then, in the 1960s Rolfing® emerged as the foundational form of structural bodywork. Each of these systems has developed a unique approach to modifying human structure. Thus, from the earliest times through to the present, there seems to have been an almost universal understanding that the human body is, to a certain extent, plastic.

The West has always had its cosmetic traditions and technologies, along with concerns about body shape and body image. In recent times, however, this concern has become almost obsessive. Whole industries – diet, gym and fitness, fashion, cosmetics, and cosmetic surgery – have developed to service this obsession. All of these industries tend to emphasize the most external and visible aspects of our being and urge us to conform to the current body aesthetic. Some approaches, like gym work or strict, formulistic exercise systems, can indeed modify structure, but they often lack a coherent set of guiding principles and are just as likely to reinforce old, unbalanced patterns as to provide any real structural benefits. Although structural bodywork certainly has the potential to evoke dramatic and visible changes in posture and physical appearance, as an approach it is much more concerned with how we move and feel. It has more to do with our sense of ease and comfort in our bodies, and with our sense of embodiment. Nevertheless, if clients are seeking a cosmetic improvement, then structural bodywork can certainly provide it (Fig. 1.4).

REFERENCES

Astin J 1998 Why patients use alternative medicine: results of a national study. Journal of the American Medical Association 279: 1548–1553

Burch J 2002 Roots, flowers and pollen: an historical outline of manual therapies. Structural Integration 30(3): 35–40

Hanna T 1980 The body of life. Healing Arts Press, Vermont, pp vii–xiii

Harris J 1993 History and development of manipulation and mobilization. In: Basmajian J, Nyberg R (eds) Rational manual therapies. Lippincott, Williams and Wilkins, Baltimore, pp 7–19

MacLennan A et al 1996 Prevalence and cost of alternative medicine in Australia. The Lancet 247: 569–573

Rolf I 1977 Rolfing: the integration of human structures. Harper and Rowe, New York

CHAPTER 2
A BRIEF HISTORY OF STRUCTURAL BODYWORK

TRADITIONAL APPROACHES TO STRUCTURE

Prior to Rolfing®, there were only a few systems that had investigated human structure in a systematic and scientific way – chiefly Hatha yoga, osteopathy, and the work of a few isolated therapists such as Françoise Mézières (Mézières 1947). Prior to the twentieth century, yoga was without doubt the most detailed and far-reaching attempt at investigating human structure and of devising a systematic set of strategies for changing and improving it. The whole realm of yogic practice is vast and all-encompassing and, in truth, the structural aspect is only a very minor part of this system. Structural alignment is seen as secondary to the spiritual and meditational practices of yoga, and the opened body that results from Hatha yoga is seen not as an end in itself but as a means of enabling practitioners to have a stable seat in meditation. By using a combination of muscular stabilization and skeletal leverage, assisted by specific breathing practices, Hatha yoga is able to open up fascial planes. As a system, it has been refined over several millennia, and its technology for change is of a very high order.

On reaching the West in the nineteenth century, yoga had to adapt somewhat to Western values. Now, classes tend to be large and to have more general, and therefore less individualized, instruction. As with all group-based teaching approaches, a student's individual and idiosyncratic problems are often overlooked. Many styles of Hatha yoga now exist; some are rigid and formulistic, while others honour the structural individuality of all the students and will modify their practices to suit the individual. So, although yoga as taught in the West has great potential for improving structural balance, in practice it has often become simply a way of maintaining a *lengthened* structure, and this is not necessarily an *integrated* structure.

Osteopathy was the first modern Western approach to see structural integrity as an essential component of health. It tends to view structure primarily through the skeletal system, and in practice works by gently mobilizing the soft tissues then freeing up the capsular restrictions around joints. Rolfing, on the other hand, emphasizes the fascial network of the body. It works through a unique, systematic process of soft-tissue manipulation, usually much more forceful than the techniques of osteopathy, which is designed to lengthen the shortened soft tissues and which, when combined with elements of postural and movement education, helps to re-align and balance the body's structure.

The twentieth century has witnessed a spectacular growth in scientific research and a vast accumulation of information about the human body. Throughout this period, the biomedical model has been the dominant health paradigm. It is a reductionist approach to understanding health that focuses on disease and the relief of symptoms, and although it is usually very successful in doing what it does, the larger view of the *person* is missing from the biomedical world-view. With the growth of this approach came the seeds of an inevitable reaction against its excesses and a questioning of its values. As a result, alternatives both new and ancient are now offered; alternatives that speak of health as a complex web of relationships, rather than as an absence of disease.

Parallel with this extraordinary period of scientific achievement was a less visible trend. Towards the end of the nineteenth century a *natural health* movement was appearing throughout Europe. Echoes of this movement can be found in such diverse places as the communal theories of Tolstoy, the Naturism movement, the sanatorium movement (with its spas and water treatments), and in gymnastic and movement systems such as eurhythmy. From the turn of the twentieth century through to the 1940s, a scattering of somatic innovators, usually working in isolation and unknown to each other, were quietly refining their ideas and practices. These men and women 'devoted their lives to developing strategies for recovering the wisdom and creativity present in breathing, sensing, moving and touching' (Johnson 1995), and included innovators like Elsa Gindler, F.M. Alexander, Moshe Feldenkrais and Ida Rolf. Some of them were trained in science but were not afraid of challenging its orthodoxy. Then, between the 1940s and 1960s, their systems that had been so long in germination suddenly sprang to life with startling synchronicity. Many and diverse somatic systems emerged, and although many of these systems originated in Europe, it was in the United States that this flowering became most visible. The period coincided with the *human potential movement* and the birth of humanistic psychology. Centres like the Esalen Institute in California flourished and there was a widespread openness to the torrent of new ideas flowing parallel with the mainstream. There was a hunger for real alternatives in all aspects of Western life. It was the dawning of the New Age.

Elaborate structural and functional bodywork systems sprang forth during those frenetic times, along with the discovery in the West of a host of alternative systems of internal medicine (though *alternative* only to the Western biomedical model; in their own cultures they were usually mainstream!). There were complex constitutional approaches like homeopathy from Germany, energetic systems from China and Japan, Ayurvedic medicine from India and the three-humours system from Tibet. At that time also, chiropractic and osteopathy became 'respectable' and Rolfing became more widely known and practiced, along with a host of other somatic approaches.

ROLFING

Ida Rolf – somatic pioneer

In this somatic renaissance, an outstanding pioneer of structural bodywork was Dr Ida P. Rolf (1896–1979) (Fig. 2.1). She was a brilliant and original American scientist who began her career as a research biochemist and later turned her formidable intellect to dealing with the structural and physical problems of her family and friends. She originally called her work *Structural Integration*, but some of her clients at Esalen jokingly remarked that they were going to be 'Rolfed' or 'Rolfed

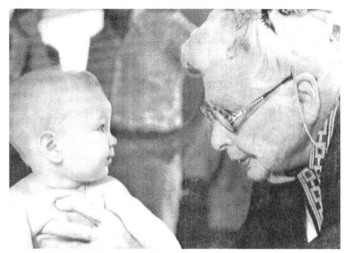

Figure 2.1 Ida Rolf (reproduced with kind permission from Ronald Thompson).

over', so the word 'Rolfing' was coined and is today a registered service mark with The Rolf Institute. However, her words 'structural integration' remain as the best generic description for this kind of bodywork, and this is the name that she preferred.

Dr Rolf had a profound belief in the ideals of yoga and held that a lengthened and aligned body not only fostered physical health, but psychological, emotional and spiritual health as well. Like the followers of yoga, she believed that a body organized around a vertical line was freer to respond to all of life's demands and better able to accommodate the ceaseless influence of gravity. She was also inspired by the wisdom and the holistic vision of Dr Andrew Taylor Still, the founder of osteopathy, and shared his belief that structure and function are absolutely interdependent. Having studied with some of the 'first generation' osteopaths, she learned their approach to soft-tissue manipulation and then, over a period of some thirty years, developed and refined her methods. This culminated in her unique approach to enhancing the body's capabilities – Rolfing Structural Integration.

Her approach is admirably summarized by one of her first students, Jan Sultan:

Dr. Rolf's premises held that gravity bore on the body as a major 'environmental' factor in its well-being. She observed that to the extent the structure was organized around a 'central vertical line,' representing gravity's influence, it would operate relatively free of compression, actually drawing support from the gravity dynamic. Conversely, because of the body's segmental organization, gravity will act on individual segments when they are displaced away from the same central vertical axis.

This adds compressional loading to the structure and sets up an adversary relationship with gravity.

The synthesis of Dr. Rolf's thinking lay in the observation that the connective tissue was the organ of adaptation to the structural struggles in the gravity field. This tissue can change the direction and density of its fibres with changing demands of the body. She saw that this mechanism of adaptation could be used to support a higher level of organization in the body if it were manually freed from its habitual 'set' and the person educated to utilize that freedom; to repattern their structure towards alignment with the central vertical axis of gravity's effect.

(Sultan 1986)

Structural bodywork today owes a great debt to Dr. Rolf's pioneering work, and much of her rich conceptual legacy remains. Some of her key insights were that:

- gravity is the most fundamental (though least acknowledged) environmental influence upon us
- the body is a plastic medium, due primarily to the plasticity of the fascial network
- the fascial network is a seamless whole, and local changes will be reflected throughout its entirety
- structural enhancement evokes functional improvement (the most important enhancements being: the generalized lengthening of tissues, an improved agonist/antagonist balance, an increased bilateral symmetry, and the unwinding of torsional patterns)
- structural improvements will promote a healthier metabolism and improved tissue nourishment
- incremental small structural changes are integrated more successfully than larger ones
- the sequencing of structural interventions is vital, both within a session and over a series of sessions
- change at the structural level of organization will inevitably evoke changes at all other levels – the metabolic, the functional, the emotional, the psychological and perhaps even the spiritual.

The recipe

Ida Rolf taught Rolfing as a structured series of ten sessions, each sixty to ninety minutes in length. Each session had a central theme, a number of structural goals, and a prescribed sequence of structural interventions (Brecklinghaus 2002). This was the so-called 'recipe'. As a teaching tool, this recipe was a highly effective means of empowering inexperienced students at the beginning of their careers as structural bodyworkers. It allowed

---

Box 2.1   Basic themes of the Rolfing 10-session recipe

SLEEVE SESSIONS

1. respiration
2. balance through the legs and feet
3. lateral line – sagittal balance

CORE SESSIONS

4. base of core, midline of the legs
5. abdomen, psoas for pelvic balance
6. sacrum – weight transfer from head to feet
7. relationship of head to rest of body – primarily occiput–atlas (OA) relationship, then to rest of body

INTEGRATING SESSIONS

8. balance between upper and lower girdles
9. balance between upper and lower girdles
10. balance throughout the whole system

---

them to perform often highly potent work without yet having developed the skill of 'seeing' a client's structural deficiencies. Its refined sequencing of structural interventions seems to help most clients. Thousands of students have embarked upon the uncertain seas of structural integration guided by this map (Box 2.1).

The recipe, however, was a standardized protocol and as such could hardly be expected to deal with the huge range of structural variations found among clients; it was bound to fit ill with certain structural or body types. Dr Rolf insisted that her students follow the recipe; however, she herself often paid scant heed to it. There are many anecdotal accounts in which she departs seriously from her own protocol, which tends to support the idea that the recipe was intended as a learning tool that could be modified, or even abandoned, once the underlying principles were understood. Nowadays there are many variants of the recipe, although most remain very close to Rolf's schema.

Gravity as the therapist

Ida Rolf felt that many of the dysfunctional bodily patterns found today are the result of the body's failure to intelligently negotiate its relationship with gravity. She believed that part of the integration process involved the re-establishment of a balanced relationship with gravity, that 'Gravity is the therapist'. In her own words:

One individual may experience his losing fight with gravity as a sharp pain in the back, another as the unflattering contour of his body, another as constant fatigue, and yet another as an unrelenting threatening environment. Those over forty may call it old age; yet all these signals may be pointing to a single problem so prominent in their own structures and the structures of others that it has been ignored: they are off-balance; they are all at war with gravity.

(Rolf 1977)

Part of Rolf's vision of the integrated structure was the idea that, within the field of gravity, a body will work best if organized around a vertical midline and that there is an ideal structural arrangement that will support this.

Somatic Platonism

Don Hanlon Johnson (1980), himself a trained Rolfer, speaks of what he calls the 'Somatic Platonism' of Rolfing and other systems, which is the belief that there exists an underlying ideal form for the human structure and that the job of bodyworkers is to usher their clients towards this ideal form. Rolf herself speaks of this ideal form:

Form and function are a unity, two sides of the same coin. In order to enhance function, appropriate form must exist or be created. A joyous radiance of health is attained only as the body conforms more nearly to its inherent pattern, this form, this Platonic idea, is the blueprint for structure.

(Rolf 1977)

For Ida Rolf, this ideal form was a body with minimal spinal curvature, a reduced lumbosacral angle, a 'horizontal' pelvis, and with minimal segmental displacement from a vertical midline – usually referred to as 'the Line'. This kind of postural 'template', however, was not unique to Ida Rolf; variations of a similar ideal alignment are found in many systems, including modelling and deportment systems, ballet, Pilates, physiotherapy, scientific kinesiology (Kendall et al. 1971, Basmajian and Nyberg 1978), orthopaedic medicine and even in certain monastic traditions. Johnson questioned the practical usefulness of this view of human structure, arguing that it limits our vision of what can be achieved through this work, as well as setting us up for failure when we cannot help our clients to meet this ideal. The question of an idealized human form will be explored in greater detail in Chapter 13, but it should in fairness be said that many of these systems have evolved since their inception and have undergone considerable refinement from their early, often rigid, belief systems around postural 'correctness'.

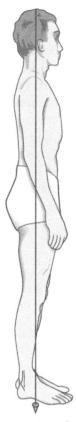

Figure 2.2 Typical representation of an ideal alignment, with the gravity line falling from the mastoid process, through the middle of the shoulder and hip joints and in front of the ankle. (Based on photo in Kendall's classic text (Kendall et al. 1971).)

For instance, the Rolfing approach now has a much fuller appreciation of different kinds of postural predisposition (Sultan 1986), and the postural ideal of the original Pilates approach has shifted away from its early ideal of the 'flat back' towards the more benign 'neutral spine' (Latey 2002) (see Fig. 2.2).

EARLY OFFSHOOTS FROM ROLFING

In somatic as in religious history, schism seems inescapable. A number of Rolf's original students broke away to develop variations and extensions of her work. An underlying factor in all these departures was the gradual realization that structural work, despite its obvious transformative potential, was often not enough. By itself, it did not necessarily address functional shortcomings, nor did it directly address the wider humanity of clients by considering their emotional and psychological wellbeing. At a purely structural level, Rolf's work did not seem to acknowledge readily that there might be different structural types, different degrees of sensory-motor intelligence, different capacities to respond to this work. It is clear that Rolf herself came to realize some of these limitations in her original approach. She responded by encouraging the development of a movement-based approach, *Rolfing Movement Integration*, to supplement her structural work and to help clients make that vital transition from structural change to a higher order of functionality. Although she believed that structural work could be psychologically transformative, in practice she never made an explicit connection between the structural and the psychological ways of working, believing that those inner aspects could be left to look after themselves. It is clear that Rolf herself in no way regarded this as a limitation of her approach. Her approach is primarily about integrating structure, and if secondary side benefits arise from the work then so be it. Her pragmatic viewpoint is summed up in her well-known words, 'All this metaphysics is fine, but be mighty sure you've got physics under the metaphysics' (Feitis 1978).

There are many offshoots that have developed from Rolf's pioneering system. It is a tribute to the power of her original ideas that so many derivative systems have branched from the central trunk of Rolfing. We will look briefly at some of the more important ones.

Hellerwork – Joseph Heller

Joseph Heller (Fig. 2.3) was one of Ida Rolf's earliest students and later became the first president of the Rolf Institute when it was founded in 1976. He came to believe that the process of structural change demanded a simultaneous shift in attitudes and core beliefs. Clients needed to feel not only a postural or structural shift, but also a shift in how they engaged with their lives. He felt that structural work could be made more potent and vital if it included two other parallel strands: an emotional–attitudinal exploration of key life issues, plus some very specific movement explorations that were intimately related to these life issues. So, as a result of his broad interest in structural integration, movement education, humanistic psychology and somatic awareness, he synthesized his new form of bodywork, Hellerwork, and went on to found his own teaching organization in 1978.

His approach took the structural themes of Ida Rolf's 10-series but extended the series to include an eleventh session designed to assist clients to take their self-discoveries out into the world. Each session was structured around a potent theme, charged with many levels of meaning, and with titles such as 'inspiration', 'standing on your own two feet', 'reaching out', 'holding back', 'losing your head' and 'coming out'. Hellerworkers are

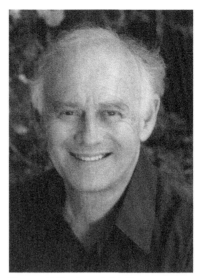

Figure 2.3 Joseph Heller.

taught to perform myofascial interventions that are virtually identical to those specified in the traditional Rolfing 10-series, but they also engage their clients in a dialogue around the sessional theme, and with their movement explorations draw from them new ways of interacting with their world.

Like Rolfing, Hellerwork also has evolved since its inception, although students are still taught an 11-series, which is used as the basic and foundational recipe for all their work. It is significant, however, that Joseph Heller wished above all that clients be well served and he urged his students to apply all their knowledge and training, such as that which came from other bodywork modalities, from yoga or tai chi, from other movement trainings, from a psychological or medical background, or from their own intuitive sense of what the client needed. Hellerworkers therefore have many options for dealing with the specific needs of their clients, the only caveat placed upon them is that they declare to their client which system they are using with them at any time during the process.

Postural Integration – Jack Painter

Like Joseph Heller, Jack Painter (Fig. 2.4) is an eclectic thinker. Influenced deeply by the psychological ideas of Wilhelm Reich and their later recasting as Bioenergetics, he has explored widely in the fields of Gestalt psychotherapy, bodywork and Eastern energetic systems. Although not a student of Ida Rolf he received work from her and her students. He integrated the Rolfing 10-series recipe into a comprehensive framework for fostering personal growth known as Postural Integration. He understood the difficulty that many people have in

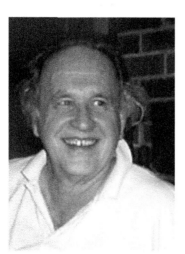

Figure 2.4 Jack Painter.

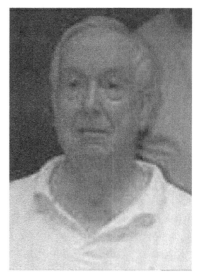

Figure 2.5 Dub Leigh.

making meaningful changes in their lives and felt that this deep behavioural conservatism is intimately related to what Reich had called 'body armouring' or 'character armouring'. He believes that a more complete approach to working with people must include working with their bodies in order to, as it were, remove the layers of armouring (Painter 1987). He does not regard his approach as belonging to the psychotherapeutic tradition, which he believes does not empower the client sufficiently.

> *I consider myself more a coach or guide to self-regulation... the expression of our energy, emotions and attitudes is not something added to or coordinated with work on the fascia – it is literally there in the body or bodymind. In a deep stroke we express in our tissue what we are and what we feel.*
>
> (Painter, personal communication 2002)

So, while clients are receiving bodywork they are given space to express emotional and life issues, facilitated by Gestalt-style dialogue and working 'in the present', while the opening of the body and the emotions is deepened by Reichian breath work.

Zen Bodytherapy – William 'Dub' Leigh

'Dub' Leigh (Fig. 2.5) is one of a small group of individuals who studied Rolfing under Ida Rolf, and the Feldenkrais method under Moshe Feldenkrais (Leigh 1987). Taking the Rolfing 10-series as a basic sessional framework, he incorporated aspects of joint manipulation and trigger-point therapy into his approach. He developed a complex model of body reading and assessment that went beyond a mechanical examination of the clients' postural organization to include their movement qualities, emotional tendencies and habits of muscular tension.

After practising and teaching bodywork for twenty years Leigh moved to a Zen monastery in Hawaii. His Zen teacher was Tanouye Tenshin Roshi, a martial arts master who had also mastered the movement of energy, 'ki', for healing. Tanouye Roshi and Leigh worked together for six years to develop Zen Bodytherapy, incorporating Rolf's emphasis on deep work for structure and Feldenkrais' emphasis on movement exercises for function. Zen Bodytherapy adds the use of focus, breath, and 'ki' to accelerate the change possible with bodywork.

Other derivatives of Rolfing

Other systems that were inspired by Dr Rolf's work are CORE bodywork, developed by George P. Kousaleos, and SOMA Bodywork developed by Bill M. Williams, one of the first students of Ida Rolf. Both systems retain something like a 10-session series and aim at balancing and integrating the human structure in gravity.

THE PRINCIPLES OF STRUCTURAL INTEGRATION

So, while some of Rolf's former pupils sought to extend or augment her work, others have aimed to broaden and deepen it. Since her death in 1979 there has been an ongoing process of enquiry and exploration within the Rolfing community. This intellectual ferment has led to a true evolution of the conceptual framework behind Rolfing.

Some of Rolf's earliest pupils attempted to take her method beyond a sterile, formulistic approach and enquired deeply into the principles that lie behind effective work of this kind (Maitland et al. 1995). This line of enquiry looked to discover and refine the small number of principles needed to provide effective, individualized strategies for structural work. They comprise three principles, the *adaptability* principle, the *palintonic* principle, and the *support* principle, under a governing meta-principle, the *wholism* principle. When understood, these principles can help practitioners decide: 1) What do I do first?; 2) What do I do next?; and 3) When am I finished? (Maitland 1995), without recourse to a fixed sequence of interventions such as the recipe.

It was acknowledged that there was much wisdom inherent in the recipe, and that although it represented a strategic set of interventions based on principles, it was a recipe nonetheless (Maitland 1995). This was quite a radical departure from the Rolfing tradition, and it was this questioning of the recipe as the central pillar of Rolfing that was one of the main factors that led to the creation of the two leading organizations that exist today for training in Structural Integration: *The Rolf Institute* and *The Guild of Structural Integration.*

These same pupils also came to see that although the recipe was an effective approach for dealing with some kinds of postural organization, it proved less effective for other kinds, or even had a disorganizing tendency. So to have a wider relevance, Rolfing needed a practical way of understanding the dynamics of different kinds of postural organization. This practical need led to the development of the *internal–external model,* an original and effective means of assessing clients' postural tendencies and of strategizing effective work to balance their structure (Sultan 1986). This model will be explored more fully in Chapter 13.

New directions – Renaissance persons

More recently within the world of structural bodywork, there has been a movement towards greater interdiscip linary contact and cross-fertilization, sometimes even taking the form of unabashed borrowing – extracting whatever works from whichever tradition. Today's structural bodyworkers are looking beyond the boundaries of their training and are exploring related disciplines to widen their repertoire of skills. Many are incorporating the subtleties of visceral manipulation and cranio-sacral therapy. Others are integrating joint mobilization and indirect spinal manipulation into their soft-tissue work (Maitland 2001). Erik Dalton has developed a unique synthesis of myofascial and skeletal work in his *Myoskeletal Approach* (Dalton 1998). Yet others have found that their experience of structural bodywork, as giver or receiver, has acted as an intellectual catalyst, prompting them to enquire seriously into related areas of human function and experience. This explosion of somatic exploration is yet another of the extraordinary legacies of Ida Rolf's pioneering work.

Judith Aston, one of Ida Rolf's earliest pupils, struck out from the Rolfing community to create her unique approach to exploring movement and posture, Aston Patterning (Aston 1999). James Oschman, cell biologist and teacher, was inspired by his Rolfing experience to explore the science of structure and the energetics of bodywork modalities (Oschman 2000). Other practitioners have explored deeply into the role that the embodiment process can play in the healing of severe physical, emotional and psychological trauma (Levine 1997, Redpath 1995), a path also explored by Pat Ogden, former structural integrator and the developer of Hakomi Integrative Somatics. Rosie Spiegel, like Ida Rolf herself, saw enormous health benefits flowing from the Yoga tradition and in her book (Spiegel 1994) she shares her insights into the parallel traditions of yoga and Rolfing. Will Johnson has developed an embodiment-training program that integrates a Western somatic embodiment approach with Buddhist meditational practice (Johnson 1993, 1999). Others have used their structural insights to move into industrial and corporate settings in order to assist with the burgeoning problems of repetitive strain syndromes (Goodwin 2003, Rossiter 1999). Tom Myers went on to develop his extraordinarily *anatomy trains* metaphor, which is an extremely useful way of visualizing the global myofascial lines of clients (Myers 2001).

And of course the borrowing goes both ways; many of the so called 'deep tissue' techniques that are now being taught at massage schools have actually been abstracted from Rolfing. Although they are undoubtedly useful in treating regional problems, these techniques can easily be misused without the guiding rationale of a holistic approach.

REFERENCES

Aston J 1999 Aston postural assessment workbook: skills for observing and evaluating body patterns. Psychological Corp

Basmajian J, Nyberg R (eds) 1978 Rational manual therapies. Williams & Wilkins, Baltimore, pp 7–19

Brecklinghaus H 2002 Rolfing structural integration: what it achieves, how it works and whom it helps. Lebenshaus, Gundelfingen

Dalton E 1998 Myoskeletal alignment techniques: deep tissue routines for today's manual therapist. Manual and videotape set, http://www.erikdalton.com

Feitis R 1978 Ida Rolf talks about Rolfing and physical reality. The Rolf Institute, Boulder

Goodwin S 2003 Carpal tunnel syndrome and repetitive stress injuries: ways to avoid it and work with it; a Rolfer's perspective. Massage and Bodywork 17(6): 67–78

Johnson D H 1980 Somatic Platonism. Somatics 3(1): 4–7

Johnson D H 1995 Bone breath and gesture: practices of embodiment. North Atlantic Books, Berkeley, pp ix–xviii

Johnson W 1993 Balance of body, balance of mind: a Rolfer's vision of Buddhist practice in the West. Humanics Trade Paperbacks, Atlanta

Johnson W 1999 The Liberation of Sensations. Rolf Lines 27(1): 6–7

Kendall O, Kendall F, Wadsworth G 1971 Muscle testing and function. Williams and Wilkins, Baltimore, p 19

Latey P 2002 Modern Pilates: a step-by-step at home guide to a stronger body. Allen and Unwin

Leigh W S 1987 A Zen approach to Bodytherapy. The Institute of Zen Studies, Honolulu

Levine P 1997 Waking the Tiger: healing trauma. North Atlantic Books, Berkeley

Maitland J 1995 The Ten Series as a set of strategies based on the principles of Rolfing. Class notes in Rolfing training

Maitland J 2001 Spinal manipulation made simple: a manual of soft tissue techniques. North Atlantic Books, Berkeley

Maitland J, Salveson M, Sultan J 1995 The principles of Rolfing. Class notes in Rolfing training

Mézières F 1947 La gymnastique statique. Edition Maloine, Paris

Myers T 2001 Anatomy trains: myofascial meridians for manual and movement therapists. Churchill Livingstone, Edinburgh

Oschman J 2000 Energy medicine: the scientific basis. Churchill Livingstone, Edinburgh, p 66

Painter J 1987 Deep bodywork and personal development. Bodymind Books, Mill Valley

Redpath W 1995 Trauma energetics: a study of held-energy systems. Barberry Press, Lexington

Rolf I 1977 Rolfing: the integration of human structures. Harper and Rowe, New York

Rossiter R, MacDonald S 1999 Overcoming repetitive motion injuries the Rossiter way. New Harbinger Publications, Oakland

Spiegel R 1994 Bodies, health and consciousness: a guide to living successfully in your body through Rolfing and yoga. SRG Publishing, San Carlos

Sultan J 1986 Towards a structural logic. In Flury H (ed) Notes on Structural Integration 1: 12

STRUCTURAL BODYWORK IN THE CONTEXT OF OTHER COMPLEMENTARY THERAPIES

There has been an unprecedented growth in new complementary (or alternative) therapies. The frenzied pace of this growth has been quite bewildering, and the cross-fertilization between old and new stock is producing some strange and exotic hybrids. Each new system is providing a different map, a different view of the human organism; each is focusing on different details, and different *levels* of detail within the whole person. Like the three blind men and their elephant, each system is focusing on different aspects of the whole phenomenon, *often taking these aspects to be the whole*. So how can we begin to find order in this wild profusion, and what is the place of structural bodywork in all this?

THREE CORE COMPLEMENTARY PRACTICES

One perspective for understanding the scope of modern complementary practice is to look at three core practices, which are the three broad spheres of specialization and training – the *somatic*, the *constitutional* and the *psychological–emotional* (see Box 3.1).

Somatic practitioners

work with the living body in all its structural and functional aspects. They use either their hands or their voices to communicate with the somatic intelligence of their clients, attempting to evoke a higher level of functionality.

Constitutional practitioners

deal with the deeper levels of our physical organization: the systemic, biochemical, metabolic or energetic aspects; they attempt to create balance within these less visible systems, often giving their clients something to 'take'.

Psychological–emotional practitioners

deal with the inner life and its outward behavioural aspects, the psychological and emotional aspects of our experience; they listen and talk to their clients in order to resolve and balance internal conflicts, or to broaden self-knowledge.

Box 3.1 includes only those approaches that have an 'alternative' flavour: that are non-mainstream. Hence, conventional Western medical approaches are not included, but neither are the psychological–emotional ones that have developed within academic contexts, such as Freudian psychotherapy, or the cognitive and behaviourist approaches to psychotherapy.

The model is clearly an oversimplification. It could well be argued that certain approaches should be categorized differently. Some of the more comprehensive systems like Chinese medicine or Shiatsu do include both somatic and constitutional elements, while other systems such as Hellerwork or Postural Integration include both somatic and psychological–emotional components. Many practitioners calling themselves 'holistic' would claim that their work encompasses several or all of these core practices; however in fact it is quite rare to find what we might term 'true renaissance persons', that is, practitioners who are equally skilled in more than one of these core practices. By and large this model does resonate with how the public views complementary approaches, and it is reflected in the curricular structure of most complementary health colleges where students tend to emerge as bodyworkers, naturopaths or counsellors.

Box 3.1   Three core complementary practices

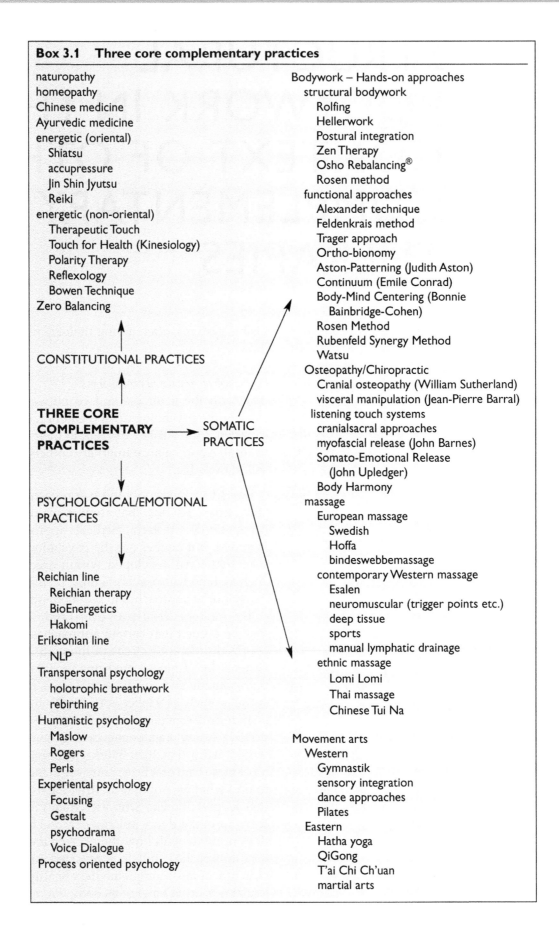

naturopathy
homeopathy
Chinese medicine
Ayurvedic medicine
energetic (oriental)
   Shiatsu
   accupressure
   Jin Shin Jyutsu
   Reiki
energetic (non-oriental)
   Therapeutic Touch
   Touch for Health (Kinesiology)
   Polarity Therapy
   Reflexology
   Bowen Technique
Zero Balancing

CONSTITUTIONAL PRACTICES

THREE CORE COMPLEMENTARY PRACTICES → SOMATIC PRACTICES

PSYCHOLOGICAL/EMOTIONAL PRACTICES

Reichian line
   Reichian therapy
   BioEnergetics
   Hakomi
Eriksonian line
   NLP
Transpersonal psychology
   holotrophic breathwork
   rebirthing
Humanistic psychology
   Maslow
   Rogers
   Perls
Experiental psychology
   Focusing
   Gestalt
   psychodrama
   Voice Dialogue
Process oriented psychology

Bodywork – Hands-on approaches
   structural bodywork
      Rolfing
      Hellerwork
      Postural integration
      Zen Therapy
      Osho Rebalancing®
      Rosen method
   functional approaches
      Alexander technique
      Feldenkrais method
      Trager approach
      Ortho-bionomy
      Aston-Patterning (Judith Aston)
      Continuum (Emile Conrad)
      Body-Mind Centering (Bonnie
         Bainbridge-Cohen)
      Rosen Method
      Rubenfeld Synergy Method
      Watsu
Osteopathy/Chiropractic
      Cranial osteopathy (William Sutherland)
      visceral manipulation (Jean-Pierre Barral)
   listening touch systems
      cranialsacral approaches
      myofascial release (John Barnes)
      Somato-Emotional Release
         (John Upledger)
      Body Harmony
massage
   European massage
      Swedish
      Hoffa
      bindeswebbemassage
   contemporary Western massage
      Esalen
      neuromuscular (trigger points etc.)
      deep tissue
      sports
      manual lymphatic drainage
   ethnic massage
      Lomi Lomi
      Thai massage
      Chinese Tui Na

Movement arts
   Western
      Gymnastik
      sensory integration
      dance approaches
      Pilates
   Eastern
      Hatha yoga
      QiGong
      T'ai Chi Ch'uan
      martial arts

ANOTHER PERSPECTIVE ON COMPLEMENTARY PRACTICE – MAITLAND'S THREE PARADIGMS OF PRACTICE

It has already been suggested that some kinds of practice are inherently broader in scope than others. Chinese medicine, for instance, comprises a vast constitutional system encompassing acupuncture, herbal and moxa treatments and different kinds of massage. It is inherently a bigger, more complete system than say foot reflexology or Swedish massage. Maitland (1992, 1993) offers a perspective that is very useful in clarifying the nature of different complementary practices. He suggests that all complementary approaches can be categorized into three fundamental paradigms of practice: relaxation, corrective or holistic (see Fig. 3.1). Although in his paper he limits the discussion to massage and bodywork practices, he does suggest that a similar analysis could equally be applied to any other kind of complementary practice.

Relaxation approaches are intended to encourage the relaxation response and alleviate pain, and include practices such as relaxation massage and biofeedback. Corrective approaches are centred upon the treatment of the symptoms of structural or functional dysfunctions.

For these practices a more extensive training is required than for relaxation approaches and, therefore, assessment procedures tend to be more detailed and refined. Maitland cites chiropractic, deep-tissue therapies and neuromuscular re-education as examples of these approaches. Holistic or integrative practices, he says, 'are devoted to enhancing the natural tendency of the whole person to seek higher and higher orders of functioning and well-being'. He sees Rolfing, homeopathy and acupuncture as being integrative practices in this sense.

Maitland points to a hierarchical relationship between the approaches; namely that a relaxation approach cannot produce a corrective outcome except perhaps accidentally. Similarly, a corrective approach cannot have an integrative outcome except accidentally, although it can achieve all the benefits of a relaxation approach. A holistic approach can achieve everything that can be achieved through both relaxation and corrective approaches, while at the same time it works to harmonize a whole system. Maitland sees corrective approaches as a by-product of the Cartesian tradition: the reductionist perspective that understands the body as composed of parts, of being a 'soft machine' rather than an integrated, unified whole.

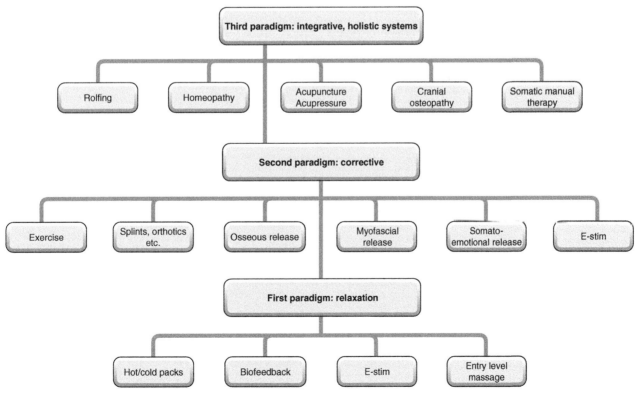

Figure 3.1 Maitland's three paradigms of practice.

In a later paper (Cottingham and Maitland 1997), the authors suggest that these three approaches may be used sequentially (and even concurrently) in the treatment of somatic dysfunctions by alleviating symptoms, restoring balance and alignment, and promoting efficient postural and movement patterns.

This analysis offers a perspective into the scope of complementary practices to see whether their intent is to relax, to correct or to balance, and whether they are complete practices or just collections of techniques without a unifying rationale.

REFERENCES

Cottingham J, Maitland J 1997 A three-paradigm treatment model using soft tissue mobilization and guided movement-awareness techniques for a patient with chronic low back pain: a case study. Journal of Orthopaedic and Sports Physical Therapy 26: 3

Maitland J 1992 Rolfing: A third paradigm approach to body-structure. Rolf Lines 20(2): 47–49

Maitland J 1993 Das Boot. Rolf Lines 21(2): 1–7

CHAPTER 4

WHAT IS STRUCTURAL BODYWORK?

DEFINITION

Structural bodywork

is a 'hands-on' somatic practice that attempts to enhance posture and flexibility, and to encourage more efficient movement patterns by inducing relatively long-lasting changes to the body's structure and educating clients into embodying these changes functionally.

This definition of structural bodywork emphasizes that the main aim of this approach is shared with all other somatic modalities: to improve the quality of our client's functionality. But it also highlights its defining difference: that it works by effecting structural change at a tissue level. The soft-tissue changes of structural bodywork are intrinsically different to those of massage, being fascial rather than tonic, and are longer lasting. This definition also includes those structural bodywork approaches that have a more psychological flavour. The educational aspects that are a necessary component of these approaches can take many forms, including proprioceptive, movement-oriented and work directed at a psychological and emotional level. This definition accepts that some structural changes cannot be accepted by the body without an accompanying emotional or psychological shift.

THE MAIN CHARACTERISTICS OF STRUCTURAL BODYWORK

Structural bodywork:

- is a holistic approach
- balances the structure rather than fixes somatic dysfunctions

- is a strategic, systematic process
- is an individualized approach
- proceeds through the cumulative effects of small changes
- is a lengthening process
- works within the fascial network.

A holistic approach

The *New Oxford Dictionary of English* defines *holism* as a philosophy 'characterized by understanding the parts of something to be intimately interconnected and explicable only by reference to the whole'. Of holistic medicine it states, 'Medicine characterized by the treatment of the whole person, taking into account mental and social factors, rather than just the symptoms of a disease'.

So what does it mean to say that structural bodywork is a holistic approach? It certainly does not mean that it addresses the whole person. All approaches that claim to be holistic are really only relatively so; the *wholeness* of an individual is simply too vast to comprehend. However, if we take a systems view of the whole person, if we accept that a person encompasses many layered and interpenetrating systems (the human being as a 'system of systems'), then we can address and perhaps even begin to understand a *whole system* within the *whole person*. Structural bodywork considers the entire fascial network by looking at the relationships between its parts and how it relates to its 'neighbouring' systems: the skeletal–articular, neuromuscular and central nervous system (with its somatic and autonomic aspects), as well as the emergent emotional and psychological aspects of our being. We can therefore say that structural bodyworkers aspire to be holistic in working with the structural aspects of the client, and that success depends largely on how holistic in scope their work becomes.

Balancing rather than fixing

Unlike corrective or remedial approaches, structural bodywork is not primarily symptom driven and does not necessarily or immediately seek to address *where* clients are hurting; it looks beyond the immediate symptoms to find an underlying pattern that may have given rise to that symptom or cluster of symptoms. It looks for deeper causes. Very often the place that first registers pain is really the 'weakest link' in a complex web of imbalances, or the place that has become overworked because other parts are not participating enough and sharing the functional burden. Ida Rolf often used to say 'Where you think it is, it ain't', suggesting that the cause of somatic distress is often not obvious, and rarely at the point of pain.

Suppose a client is suffering from wryneck. It is quite natural to want to alleviate the discomfort. If the discomfort is the result of recent injury, such as a minor strain or just the recent effect of a bad sleeping position, then symptomatic treatment is entirely appropriate. If the condition is acute then a structural approach is out of the question in the short term since we cannot ask the sensory-motor intelligence to integrate structural changes at the same time as it is organizing the body to avoid pain. If they have the remedial skills, structural bodyworkers will often focus on relieving the discomfort of their client's acute conditions, with the intention of addressing the broader structural issues later on, once the acute problem has settled.

However, this wryneck may equally be the end result of a complex web of interrelated causes, the 'last straw', as it were, so that applying a heat-pack, giving some light massage or performing some joint mobilization is likely to be just a partial solution. It may alleviate the discomfort in the short term and speed the healing of tissues locally, but it will not address the underlying network of causes and a repetition of the problem is likely. Any experienced somatic therapist will at some time have played the game of 'chase the pain' or 'chase the symptoms' – the saga of fixing one locus of pain only to have it appear elsewhere. It is highly likely that the underlying web of causes needs to be investigated in this case.

We have already mentioned the important distinction between corrective–fixing approaches and holistic–integrative approaches. Maitland (1992) takes as an example of the fixing approach the use of an isolated strategy such as joint mobilization. He states that an approach:

whose therapeutic goal is joint mobility and whose theoretical commitment is to conceptualizing the body as a mechanical thing composed of parts, will ultimately fail to recognize the ubiquitous presence of compensatory, adaptive strain patterns throughout the body. Simple joint mobilization without any understanding of how these patterns reinforce structural dysfunctions can only produce temporary change.

Being a holistic approach, structural bodywork holds as a core assumption that balancing the structural system as a whole will reduce the overall level of biomechanical stress within it. The system then becomes more robust and resilient, and there will be less likelihood of painful conditions recurring. Ida Rolf herself saw this process in thermodynamic terms in that we are attempting to increase the order, decrease the 'entropy' in the structural system (Feitis 1978). In fact her description of order within the human body has strong resonances with chaos theory and the emerging science of complexity (Lewin 1993).

The primary aim of structural bodyworkers is to balance the structure of their clients, not to fix their aches and pains. Yet it is usual to find that these aches and pains do spontaneously disappear, sometimes so gradually and non-dramatically as to pass unnoticed by the clients themselves! In fact many clients have to be reminded that their first impulse for seeking treatment was to deal with their pain. If the client's problems are severe or recurrent then it is usual to find that, after the process of structural balancing, painful episodes become less frequent and, when they do occur, the recovery time is speedier.

A strategic, systematic process

Structural bodywork is strategic and systematic. Changes throughout the myofascial network system cannot be made all at once. The work therefore proceeds stepwise by a series of approximations towards a more harmonious condition of structural balance. This implies that a series of sessions are required, with enough time between to allow the organism to assimilate the changes. The process is strategic because the *sequencing* of the structural interventions is critical. Certain structural outcomes can only be achieved if prior ones are achieved and sessions often contain interventions designed to allow for change at a later stage. As an example, it would be pointless trying to address the 'head forward syndrome' by merely working with the neck, because the organization of the chest, spine, and tilt of the pelvis would all need to be addressed, and these in turn are influenced by the connections between the pelvis and

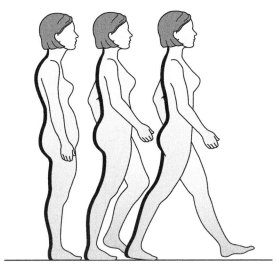

Figure 4.1 Progress in the Rolfing series (drawings based on photos of one of Ida Rolf's clients) (Rolf 1977).

the legs, and so on (see Fig. 4.1). The head forward syndrome is best understood as a whole body pattern in which the forward head is the most obvious feature. Some general guidelines for sequencing structural work will be examined in Chapter 14.

An individualized approach

Each person's structure is unique. Certainly there are some structural patterns and themes that are widespread, and some important generalizations can be made about these common patterns, but effective structural bodywork must be tailored to the client's structural idiosyncrasies. Interventions must be specific and selected with care, and the approach can never be entirely protocol-driven. Non-individualized approaches are common in many gyms, yoga and exercise classes in which everyone gets the same treatment, regardless of their structure or condition. The same tendency exists in formulistic massage approaches in which practitioners apply an unvarying sequence of strokes to their clients. While non-individualized approaches can be entirely appropriate for maintenance purposes, they can only go so far in addressing the individual's idiosyncratic needs. The individualized approach also happens to be much more interesting for the practitioner, with each client presenting a unique challenge.

The cumulative effects of small changes

Bodies are conservative; they take time to change.
Ida Rolf (Feitis 1978)

Any structural change in the body will require a period of relearning, of integration. Definite changes that have occurred in the tissues and the sensory-motor intelligence will need to adapt to a body that feels different, that has new degrees of freedom. New patterns of muscular recruitment will need to be established, or old patterns modified. This must take its time. The dramatic changes so often seen in the before and after photos of Rolfing clients are achieved gradually. The strategic pacing of structural bodywork sessions honours the integration process and accepts that gains are cumulative and assimilated gradually.

Structural bodywork is a systems approach that has much in common with ecology. We can view the body as a vast ecosystem containing various semi-autonomous systems that have definite interrelationships with each other. Ecologists recognize that any large-scale intervention in an ecosystem will invariably have unforeseen consequences, which are often bad. We see this in the catastrophic side effects of large-scale damming, strip mining, deforestation, and irrigation. This has parallels in a complex system such as the human body; here too, large-scale interventions tend to have unforeseen consequences – also often bad. It is recognized that large-scale structural interventions, such as the surgical lengthening or shortening of any part of the musculoskeletal system, are very difficult to assimilate. The results of drastic orthopaedic surgery can require long periods of rehabilitation before functionality returns. Structural bodywork therefore allows time between interventions to allow the whole system to readjust at all levels.

Structural bodywork as a lengthening process

In all Rolfing work, we are involved in a lengthening process. If there were a law against lengthening a body, Rolfing would be out. I'm not kidding, completely. Rolfing involves lengthening. That's the only way you can straighten a body.
Ida Rolf (Feitis 1978)

One of the main strategies used by structural bodyworkers is to free up and lengthen tissue that has either adaptively shortened or lost some of its resilience, that is, lost some of its ability to lengthen effectively. Figure 4.2 is a simplified model of a joint or articulation. It shows tissues spanning each side of the joint – tissues that, broadly, could be called agonist and antagonist (without, at this stage, being too specific as to whether it is muscular, fascial or ligamentous).

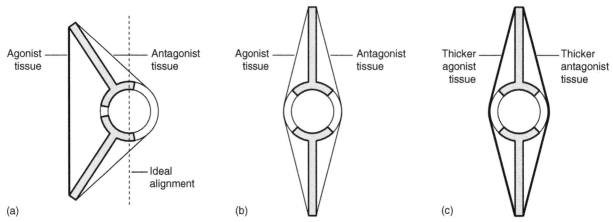

Figure 4.2 (a) Bones are held out of alignment by shortened tissue on one side and lengthened tissue on the other; (b) an ideal, balanced arrangement around a joint. Optimal connective tissue density allows easy lateral movement in both directions; (c) increased fibrosity in all soft tissue around the joint. The bones are aligned but with compromised ease of movement and increased compression on the joint. (Based on original drawings by Dr Hans Flury.)

Figure 4.2a presents the typical short–long imbalance around an articulation in which the agonist tissues have adaptively shortened and the antagonist tissues have adaptively lengthened from their optimal working lengths. This maintains a misaligned relationship between the skeletal elements. It is apparent that in order to create a more efficient alignment of the bones, the antagonist musculature must work harder to overcome the elastic resistance of the shortened agonist tissue.

Figures 4.2b and 4.2c present a balanced relationship between the agonist–antagonist tissues. However this 'balance' may be of different kinds. Figure 4.2b demonstrates an optimal balance that allows maximum ease of movement around the joint, with a healthy resilience in the connective tissues. This is the ideal. Note that there can also be sub-optimal balance, one involving a generalized shortening around the joint. Figure 4.2c represents the case in which the agonist and antagonist tissues alike have become more fibrotic and have lost their optimal resilience. This is usually the end result of a generalized tightening of the musculature around a joint, sometimes referred to as a 'holding pattern' – a habitual, relatively continuous pattern of high tonus in all of the musculature around a joint. All groups respond by becoming too tight and by working harder than necessary, and in the longer term stimulating the investing fascia into becoming more dense and fibrotic. Movement in either direction then becomes limited by the inelasticity of the opposing tissue. This will inevitably result in higher energy expenditure for all rotatory movements around that joint and an increased burden of compression on the joint surfaces.

These scenarios require different lengthening strategies: those of *balancing* and *decompression*. Balancing involves establishing or re-establishing a balanced relationship between the agonist and antagonist tissues, by lengthening only those tissues that have adaptively shortened (see Fig. 4.2a). Decompression works by mobilizing all the compromised tissue – agonist and antagonist alike (see Fig. 4.2c).

An obvious question arises at this point: what can we do about tissue that has adaptively lengthened *and is already too long*? It will be suggested later in the book that lengthened tissue can usually be left to look after itself. As the shortened tissue lengthens there will be less neurological inhibition of its lengthened antagonists, which will naturally strengthen and shorten with the exercise involved in everyday movements.

Working within the fascial network

Ida Rolf was one of the first to emphasize the importance of the *fascial network* as an anatomical system. She called it 'the organ of structure' since its most obvious function is to provide the structural support for the human body. As a system, it had received little attention from the medical profession, even though it has some remarkable properties, and more of its functions are being discovered all the time. It is in fact the most extensive system in the human body, being more extensive than even the nervous or circulatory systems (in fact it forms the supportive superstructure of both these systems). It ranges in scope from coarse macrostructures such as the iliotibial tract to the diaphanous wrapping of individual muscle cells. It is connected and continuous from the grossest to the finest levels. In the words of Ida Rolf (1977):

> *In the myofascial system as whole, each muscle, each visceral organ, is encased in its own fascial wrapping. These wrappings in turn form part of a ubiquitous web that supports as well as enwraps, connects as well as separates, all functional units of the body. Finally, these elastic, sturdy sheets also form a superficial wrapping serving as container and restraining support for the whole body – this is the so-called superficial fascia, lying just under the skin.*

Oschman (2000) has broadened this vision even further by showing that fascial continuity extends even to a sub-cellular level and that the continuum of what he calls 'the living matrix' actually crosses cell boundaries and links up with the cytoskeleton, the micro-filamentous superstructure within individual cells.

Fascia responds to the mechanical stresses borne by the body through a process of adaptive shortening, lengthening, thickening and tightening. It constantly adapts to our habitual postures and to repeated patterns of usage. Structural bodywork attempts to free up this compromised tissue so that a higher level of functionality can emerge.

Fascia is much more than just a containment system of the body; movement scientists are now beginning to recognize the crucial role played by the fascial network in creating efficient movement patterns. Our bodies are able to harness the elastic recoil properties of fascia to create economical, efficient rhythmic movement. Kinetic energy is stored as potential energy in the stretched fascia, which can immediately be released, or 'recycled', in further movement. This inherent rhythmicity in our structure will be explored in Chapter 10.

REFERENCES

Feitis R 1978 Ida Rolf talks about Rolfing and physical reality. The Rolf Institute, Boulder

Lewin R 1993 Complexity: science at the edge of chaos. Phoenix, London

Maitland J 1992 Rolfing: a third paradigm approach to body-structure. Rolf Lines 20(2): 47–49

Oschman J 2000 Energy medicine: the scientific basis. Churchill Livingstone, Edinburgh, p 66

Rolf I 1977 Rolfing: the integration of human structures. Harper and Rowe, New York

STRUCTURAL BODYWORK: SOME FREQUENTLY ASKED QUESTIONS

WHY DO PEOPLE COME FOR STRUCTURAL BODYWORK?

Ida Rolf characterized two broad groups of people who came to her for work: those who were hurting and those who were seeking a way to facilitate change in their lives. In her words:

> There are two types of people who come to a Rolfer. One has what I so elegantly call a bellyache, and wants you to get that bellyache out. The other's ache is an overly absorbing recognition of the fact that he is unhappy. He is unwell, uneasy. He wants to know why, he wants to move on, he wants to know more.
>
> Ida Rolf (Feitis 1978)

And when clients speak to me of their aspirations when beginning this kind work, the most common reasons they give are that they wish:

- to relieve their aches and pains
- to deal with what they perceive as their postural problems
- to overcome movement restrictions and a lack of flexibility
- to work with somatized emotional problems
- more rarely, to achieve some kind of cosmetic result.

Clients often arrive having worked with many different kinds of practitioner and will often speak of their pain 'history' – a sequence of stressful or traumatic episodes that has gradually brought them to their present unbalanced state. Sometimes their main concern is their overall comfort level; they may have aches and pains that they relate to poor posture, and certainly the biomechanical imbalances of poor posture can lead to discomfort. Sometimes it is a functional inefficiency arising from structural imbalances that are often sensed as a lack of energy. Sometimes it is for purely cosmetic considerations; clients wish to look straight, or do not like their shoulders rounding forward.

Cosmetic considerations cannot be dismissed as mere vanity or just the need to conform to the current body-aesthetic. Most humans are acutely attuned to reading the body language of others, which is achieved mostly at a subconscious level by appraising their posture, facial expressions and how they move. Acknowledging that certain postural configurations indicate certain feeling states, such as depression, lack of confidence, anxiety or bravado, they often wish to deal with the deeper causes of the signals that their bodies are sending to the world.

Many clients see structural bodywork as a way of changing their outlook, their *being*. In the mid-twentieth century, psychologists began to notice that psychological disorders were often reflected in a disorganized somatic self (Feldenkrais 1949). Freud's protégé, Wilhelm Reich introduced the concept of 'character armouring', describing how strategies of muscular tension can be used for the suppression of feelings. He suggested that there was now a cogent alternative to the 'talking cure' in dealing with psychological issues, which was to work directly through the agency of the body. Feldenkrais pointed out that, until this point, there was a strict taboo against working with the body in a psychotherapeutic context and that all touch between client and therapist was frowned upon. More recently however, somatic, or 'body-centred', psychotherapeutic systems have begun to suggest that therapists can help clients organize their psychological and emotional life by helping them to organize their physical presence, to live more embodied lives. This has resulted in a clear trend towards a blending of the roles of the somatic therapist and the psychotherapist. There seem to be two historical strands at work here: a Reichian strand, which came from a 'head based' psychological tradition trying to become more somatic in its orientation, and a bodywork approach trying to become more psychological in its orientation, as exemplified in the work of Heller, Painter and others. Whether there is a true middle ground here remains a moot point.

It is interesting to note that many traditions regard postural 'correctness' as having a spiritual dimension. Our language contains many words that have a strange ambiguity in that they express parallel physical and emotional meanings. 'Attitude' can mean one's posture or bearing, or it can mean one's perspective or sentiment. 'Flexibility' can mean suppleness or elasticity, but it can also mean a willingness to compromise or accommodate, that is, a behavioural flexibility. 'Upright' can mean erect, but in the Christian tradition, it means principled and honourable. And in various religious traditions, such as yoga, Zen and Jesuit monasticism, the correction of posture is seen as a necessary part of spiritual development. There seems to be a universal acknowledgment that if you change your posture, you change how you feel, and for many people this is the real reason they seek structural bodywork.

IS THERE ANY RESEARCH INTO THE BENEFITS OF STRUCTURAL BODYWORK?

There has been a considerable amount of research in the fields of massage and osteopathy, but little in other alternative modalities. For Rolfing, however, there has been a small but significant body of research that has established, among other things, that it can decrease pelvic tilt, improve agonist–antagonist coordination, decrease vagal tone (a measure of autonomic activation), and reduce anxiety (Cottingham 1985). It is preliminary research that shows only gross correlations; it does not show which elements of the Rolfing process are most potent, nor does it exclude the possibility that other somatic therapies can produce similar results (we know for instance that almost any form of benign touch can have beneficial effects on the immune system).

However, there has been an immense amount of qualitative or 'action research' in the area of structural bodywork, with much individual enquiry, exploration and daily problem solving conducted by the practitioners themselves. There is a real wisdom that can emerge from the shared, collective clinical experience of thousands of practitioners working with thousands of clients

over many years, and networking with other practitioners. This wisdom is more a body of folklore than a system of validated knowledge and can be likened perhaps to the *Materia Medica* of homeopathy, which is a huge repository of anecdotal evidence that is an extremely useful resource, athough not necessarily organized along scientific lines. This folklore is obviously pre-scientific, often in agreement in its generalities but almost inevitably at odds in its specifics. And as in the history of all practical knowledge, there is a point at which it must move beyond the collection and classification of data into the next stage – of clarifying its theory, testing it, and becoming a true applied science (Flury 1988).

Since the days of Ida Rolf there has also been an immense amount of research into the biochemistry and biomechanics of connective tissues, while in the field of sports medicine there has been some useful research into the techniques and efficacy of stretching. The results of this research will be examined in Chapter 9.

HOW IS STRUCTURAL BODYWORK DIFFERENT FROM MASSAGE?

Massage therapy can provide excellent benefits to clients: a measurable reduction in tonus levels, improved local circulation, reduction of stress, improved immunological response, quicker healing of injury, reduction of oedema, and so on. These results, though highly desirable, are usually relatively short term and require frequent follow-up treatments. The techniques of structural bodywork can give much the same kind of results as massage, but result in longer lasting changes to the overall structural organization of the body that can indeed be lifelong if clients are able to integrate them fully into their movement repertoire.

CAN STRUCTURAL BODYWORK DEAL WITH SKELETAL ASYMMETRIES LIKE SCOLIOSIS?

Structural bodywork is a very effective way of dealing with the structural imbalances of scoliosis. As can be seen in Figure 5.1, a combination of myofascial and osteopathic approaches can produce remarkable changes in the relatively young (Dalton 1998). We know, however, that bony deformations tend to consolidate in time, and that the potential for completely reversing these changes in adults is limited. Wolff's Law tells us that bones do

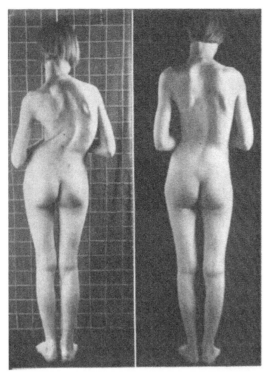

Figure 5.1 Improvement in scoliosis after thirty months of myofascial and osteopathic work. Client of Erik Dalton (Dalton 1998).

adapt to the stresses applied to them and can change shape even in adulthood; bony tuberosities, crests and condyles can enlarge and densify from the effects of stressful exercise. In the opinion of one Advanced Rolfer:

When scoliosis is in an advanced stage, some vertebrae can actually degrade to a cone shape that can no longer be modified. In spite of this, we can work to release compensations and let the body be more at ease.

(Mazzali Fulgenzi 2000)

One can speculate that if the process of structural bodywork does balance the tensions within the myofascial network and remove the major stresses then, in the longer term, perhaps even skeletal form may be remodelled. However bony changes do not occur quickly, so it is unlikely that this question will be answered in the near future. This being said, there is much anecdotal evidence to suggest that the segmental asymmetry of scoliosis can be markedly reduced, even in adults, and the stresses that arise from asymmetrical muscle usage can be greatly eased by balancing the fascial network. 'Even if Rolfing sometimes induces only limited decrease in rotations (mainly in adults), easing the compensations makes the client more comfortable' (Mazzali Fulgenzi 2000).

IS STRUCTURAL BODYWORK REALLY ABOUT IMPROVING POSTURE?

Kisner (1985) defines posture as 'a position or attitude of the body; the relative arrangement of body parts for a specific activity, or a characteristic manner of bearing one's body'. This is the static conception of posture which many of us have, as if there were only one way of standing, one way of sitting, and so on. Such definitions tend to hide the extraordinary and dynamic neuromuscular process of moving and being within the field of gravity, all the unconscious proprioception and response of the anti-gravity musculature. A seemingly static posture is as surely a function as walking, throwing or jumping. For this reason, Feldenkrais disliked the word 'posture', considering its Latin roots suggest a certain fixedness, like a 'post'. He coined the word 'acture', preferring its connection with the roots of the word 'action'. Posture is not a static condition, but rather a state of dynamic equilibrium in which the nervous system coordinates the myofascial and skeletal systems to maintain a continuity of stance or orientation within the field of gravity.

One of the questions most frequently asked of structural bodyworkers is 'Why is keeping a good posture so difficult?' From our earliest days we are being given postural advice, ranging from crude imperatives like 'Sit up straight', 'Chest out, stomach in', 'Stop slouching', 'Tuck your tail under', 'Pull those shoulders back, soldier!' and so on, to quite refined suggestions from the Alexander approach: 'Let my neck be free in order that my head may go forward and up …' Why then is it so difficult to follow these suggestions? Why is it that we can follow them when we remember to, but that as soon as we forget we revert to the more ancient pattern? Ida Rolf suggests that in order to understand this problem we need to draw a vital distinction between the concepts of *posture* and *structure*, and explained it like this:

It's rare to find a person with structural integrity, a body stacked properly with respect to gravity, free to move … Mind, I'm not talking about posture. I'm talking about structure. Posture is holding your structure as well as you can. When the structure is properly balanced, good posture is natural. A man slouches not because he has a bad habit but because his structure doesn't make it easy for him not to slouch. Structure implies the relationship of parts and it implies gravity. In school they never make you feel you are living in a gravitational field. We know about gravity in architecture. We know that buildings show strain to the degree that they deviate from an optimal relation to gravitational pulls. In buildings we recognize the origins of these strains but in bodies we don't.

(Gustaitis 1975)

In this context, 'structure' refers to the integrated cooperation of the major structural elements of our physical reality, the skeletal and the fascial systems – our personal architecture. Our posture then is a functional pattern in which our neuromuscular system is constantly at work balancing our structure against the effects of gravity and other external forces. So it is correct to say that one important aim of structural bodywork is to help clients achieve better posture, and the approach is through freeing up the structural restrictions that make it difficult to maintain efficient alignment. However, posture is just one function that structural bodywork addresses; a whole spectrum of functional patterns can be effectively enhanced by this approach.

REFERENCES

Cottingham J T 1985 Healing through touch: a history and a review of the physiological evidence. Rolf Institute, Boulder

Dalton E 1998 Myoskeletal alignment techniques: deep tissue routines for today's manual therapist. Manual and videotape set, http://www.erikdalton.com

Feitis R 1978 Ida Rolf talks about Rolfing and physical reality. The Rolf Institute, Boulder

Feldenkrais M 1949 Body and mature behaviour: a study of anxiety, sex, gravitation and learning. International Universities Press, New York

Flury H 1988 The third finger. In Flury H (ed) Notes on Structural Integration 1: 2–5

Gustaitis R 1975 Rolfing after Rolf. New Realities

Kisner C 1985 Therapeutic exercise: foundations and techniques. F A Davis, Philadelphia, p 418

Mazzali Fulgenzi M 2000 Scoliosis: what to do? Rolf Lines 28(4): 5–13

SECTION 2

OUR SOMATIC ORGANIZATION

CHAPTER 6

HUMAN MAPS

Maps are essential gear for pilgrimages. It is not easy to use them without being led astray.

Don Hanlon Johnson (1994)

Maps are beguiling, empowering, practical, convenient, and profoundly incomplete. They guide us through domains of great complexity without the need for local knowledge. They summarize certain facets of reality without distracting the mind with incidental details. They are also a tacit admission that we rely heavily on conceptual props to help us deal with reality in all its glorious intricacy. Intrinsic to maps are assumptions about which aspects of reality we wish to deal with and which aspects we wish, in a sense, to disregard. This is true of all types of maps, including standard territorial maps, maps used in all conceptualized systems, maps used within all complementary health approaches, and maps used in structural bodywork. In this section we will look at maps generally in the world of somatic therapies and identify those maps that are specific to the conduct of structural bodywork.

We have already seen in Chapter 3 how each complementary modality offers a different view of the human being, focusing on different details and different levels of detail within the whole. Every modality has its own unique selection of maps, models, views and schemas of the human territory. And they are always merely a selection from that vastness that is the human being. So at the heart of all modalities, whether ancient or modern, medical or complementary, is a systematic process of elimination (though not necessarily a conscious one), in which we decide which aspects of the whole human it is important to look at and investigate, and which to ignore. This makes all therapists specialists.

So, as the quotation from Johnson implies, maps have their dangers; and not just the common error of 'mistaking the map for the territory', but the graver error of mistaking the territory for the whole known universe. On the road to understanding in any field, if there is a tendency, calculated or otherwise, to exclude anything from our enquiry, then it automatically limits or stalls any progress in thinking. Therefore, it is vital that, as complementary health practitioners, we know our maps and the assumptions underlying them, which so often remain unacknowledged. We need to realize that the view of the human being taken within our discipline is limited; *it is necessarily incomplete.* Failure to understand this may (and so often does) lead us to believe that our system can do more than it can. But if we take the time to reflect upon and understand our maps, we become less fixated on our own systems and more accepting of the potential validity of others. It gives the freedom to explore and respect other systems, and to realize that complementary therapies are, as the name ought to imply, *complementary,* not only to conventional medicine, but to other complementary therapies as well. This understanding leads to the realization that, as individual practitioners, we cannot do everything and that it is vital that we develop a sound referral network in our practices, and are willing to pass on clients who we feel would achieve more within another modality.

A SCIENTIFIC MAP OF HUMANS

Figure 6.1 is a structural map of a human that summarizes much of the domain of biological science, encompassing the vast territory of anatomy, physiology and biochemistry (Tortora and Grabowski 1993). It shows an elegant and hierarchical layering of systems within systems, with the emergence of different orders of function at each level. This view is the culmination of the analytical and reductionist approach to understanding humankind that started with Descartes and developed throughout

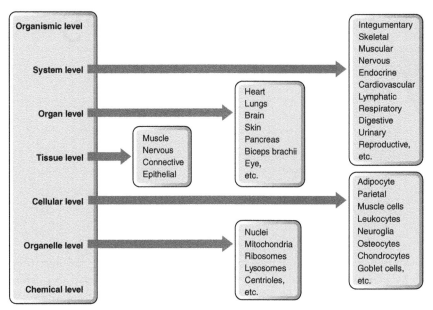

Figure 6.1 A scientific map of a human showing different levels of structural organization (after Tortora and Grabowski 1993).

the scientific revolution. It sees an organism as the integrated collaboration of organ systems, such as the skeletal, digestive, circulatory and respiratory systems. Each organ system is seen as consisting of two or more organs that work together towards some systemic end. Each organ is seen as composed of a combination of the four basic types of tissue – muscular, nervous, connective or epithelial. Each tissue is characterized by specific kinds of cells supported with specific kinds of extracellular matrix. Each cell is seen as including a complex arrangement of organelles, and each organelle is seen as an orderly arrangement of biochemicals.

The above figure is an extremely useful map for summarizing the domain of Western biological science as each of its levels represents vast amounts of specialized knowledge and enquiry. However, this map also covers much of the ground of Western complementary approaches, which have staked their claim on the same territory. Later on we will examine which particular aspects of the scientific map have been considered relevant to the structural bodywork worldview. This map does not try to be all-inclusive; it consists of those aspects of man that biological science has chosen to examine according to its own methodologies. But just what does it omit? It does not extend below the chemical level, down to the subatomic level of organization of matter (it would probably be argued that subatomic phenomena are not relevant at the organismic level of organization). Nor does it extend upwards into the emergent properties of the whole organism by representing its behavioural, psychological, emotional, social and species characteristics. This map does not relate in any obvious way to

other constitutional maps that are in much currency in the world of complementary therapies, such as the Chinese and Japanese meridian systems, or the Ayurvedic dosha system.

This map also has nothing to say about how the organism experiences the world, nothing to say about emergent properties like *self-sensing* and *awareness.* Yet these are the very functions that stand at the heart of true somatic approaches. So, as useful as this map is for structural bodyworkers, it must be supplemented with other dimensions: emergent functions like proprioceptive awareness and feeling, and all of the behavioural, psychological, emotional and energetic aspects of our being. For a more complete map of the domain of structural bodywork, another point of view is required – the somatic viewpoint.

THE SOMATIC VIEWPOINT

The adjective *somatic* has come to have a rich meaning in the world of complementary therapies, and is used for defining broad categories of practice, as in somatic therapies, somatic approaches, and somatic psychotherapy. Indeed it is now used to identify the whole field of somatic exploration and enquiry, which is known as Somatics. The word 'somatic' is derived from the ancient Greek word for body, soma, and has come to have two distinct though related meanings. There is the long-established usage within biological science referring to the physical or corporeal body; the *New Oxford Dictionary,* for instance, says: 'somatic, adj., of or relating to the body, especially as distinct from the mind'.

In this sense it is used in such phrases as: psychosomatic disease, somatic cells (as distinct from germ cells), the somatic nervous system, and so on. It is this broad meaning that has been adopted in naming one of the three core complementary practices (see Box 3.1, p. 22); all of these somatic practices deal with the palpable human body in this general sense.

More recently however, the term somatic has acquired a more specific meaning within the world of complementary therapies. Thomas Hanna (1980), one of the founding thinkers in the new field of Somatics, has sought to differentiate the terms *body* and *soma*. He defines soma as 'the living body in its wholeness' or 'the body as experienced from within', whilst the body is the externally referenced perception of the same phenomena. We see the body of others but sense the soma of ourselves. Other thinkers have emphasized this categorical distinction. Nicoll (1952) states:

We can all see another person's body directly. We see the lips moving, the eyes opening and shutting, the lines of the mouth and face changing, and the body expressing itself as a whole in action. The person himself is invisible.

He goes on to say that the internal and external perspectives are irreducible to each other, categorically different. In discussing this distinction and its relationship with the emerging field of Somatics, Hanna writes:

Somatics is the field which studies the soma: *namely the body as perceived from within by first-person perception. When a human being is observed from the outside – i.e., from a third-person viewpoint – the phenomenon of a human* body *is perceived. But, when this same body is observed from the first-person viewpoint of his own proprioceptive senses, a categorically different phenomenon is perceived: the human soma.*

(Hanna 1995)

The third-person perspective is the basis of the scientific observation of all phenomena, including the human body. It is the body perceived and studied as an external object – as it is so elegantly summarized in Figure 6.1. This perspective does not take into account the subjective experience of the particular body being looked at. However, the *somatic perspective*, the first-person perspective, takes the subject's inner experience as being paramount; that is, how that body experiences itself through proprioceptive self-sensing and feeling. Practitioners using somatic approaches have, as a primary aim, the enrichment of the subjective experience of their clients. They attempt to engage the attention of their clients in an exploration of the quality of their own inner sensorium and feeling experience. They challenge them to track the changes taking place and to sense the differences that emerge from the work. So, if we look back once again at the three core complementary practices (Box 3.1, p. 22) we find that many of the modalities defined there as somatic are so in the biological sense, but not in the sense described by Hanna. Some modalities, like Feldenkrais, Continuum and Rolfing are firmly grounded within the somatic viewpoint, while others, such as routine, mechanical massage approaches (except in a more minor way), are not. Similarly, psychological–emotional approaches like Hakomi are grounded within the somatic perspective and others, like the behaviourist or cognitive approaches, are not.

This is not to say, however, that the somatic point of view is intrinsic to complementary systems alone. All therapeutic approaches depend upon both perspectives; it is a question of degree. Even within an extreme biomedical approach, in which objective tests and the careful examination of signs and symptoms are the chief path to diagnosis, practitioners still need the information that comes from a simple question like: 'How do you feel?' Conversely, somatic approaches cannot avoid a third person perspective; after all, as somatic practitioners we can never have our clients' experience for them. We can only infer the nature of their experience by observation, by reading the external signs, and then extrapolating from our own experience. Again, it is stressed that somatic approaches differ from other approaches merely in the importance they place upon aligning their clients with their inner experience, by helping them to experience their experience. Structural bodywork is just one of many somatic practices that make this attempt.

So why is the somatic perspective so significant to the domain of structural bodywork? Structural bodyworkers have long noticed that their work is simply more effective when they engage the client's attention in sensing the changes that are taking place in them, opening them to the richness of their own sensorial life. And they notice that their work is less effective when they treat their clients as passive receivers of their work, as clay to be moulded into shape, almost without the client's participation. Our sensory-motor intelligence is such that if a new pattern is deeply sensed as more efficient or pleasurable, it is much more likely to be accepted and integrated into our movement repertoire. Clients' sensitivity in listening to their body and sensing changes is to a certain extent predictive of how successful a structural bodywork approach will be with them.

A UNIQUE STARTING POINT

When people come to a somatic practitioner for the first time it is a pivotal moment. They are at a unique starting point – the first day in the rest of their somatic life. They bring with them a unique constitution, a unique history, their unique sensitivities and sensibilities. There is a vast spectrum in the levels of their preparedness for somatic work, many different levels of sensory-motor intelligence, and a huge variance in the use and abuse their bodies have received in their life so far. Thus, it is highly unlikely that a single proprietary approach will suit them exactly.

Some people have spent their lives with an extreme outward orientation of their perception; they have never really taken the time to listen in to their body and have never allowed their attention to 'come home', to rest and settle inside. This may include people who may have played a lot of sport, danced, or who are quite athletic and seem to revel in their physicality. Many who have taken these paths are externally driven, believing in gain through pain, and although extremely fit and healthy may actually have bodies that are quite insensitive. The subtlety of yoga or Alexander Technique may be beyond them, but the inherent directness of a structural manipulative approach, however, may be a more suitable way to put them more in touch with their bodies.

We live in a culture that encourages the outward flow of our attention; it is the culture of 'the ten second sound bite'. Only a few practices such as meditation, tai chi, chi kung, yoga and true somatic therapies attempt to reverse the flow in order to encourage an internally directed attention. Hanna observes that often our attention is so externally diverted that it is only pain that can awaken us to our somatic dysfunction, and that sometimes even the early mild signals of pain may not reach the threshold of our awareness and so may pass unnoticed. He has even given this tendency the status of a syndrome, calling it *sensory motor amnesia* (Hanna 1988). This means that while we can expect some clients to have a deep sensitivity to their process, others have only a fairly gross level of self-sensing. It is important to keep this fact in mind. As somatic practitioners we can observe the immediate and short-term changes occurring in our clients and can imagine that this is relatively permanent. We may observe the visible signs: their walking is more fluid or there is a healthy resilience to the tissue, but it so often happens that some clients find it difficult to sense these changes, even when you point it out to them.

Part of the skill of the structural bodyworker, then, is to find ways to awaken clients to a fuller experience of themselves through a greater perception of the quality of their movement, their alignment and the sensations of their own tissues. It may not be possible to sense the reorganization occurring at the level of their connective tissues, but they can experience the results of it in the overt signs, such as easier gait, reduced bodily stress and an extended range of movement, and in having a sense of the aesthetic in their movement – that it is well executed, inherently graceful, organic or efficient. And we, as structural bodyworkers, can also help the client learn to delve into and differentiate, through sensation, the different states of their tissues: whether densely stuck or healthily resilient, vaguely sensed or full of vitality, tense or relaxed, turgid or soft. Hence it is vital that the somatic viewpoint be integrated into the maps of structural bodywork. It is also vital that we, as somatic therapists, should ourselves have at least started the journey along the road of somatic awakening. How else can we talk about it?

THE MAPS FOR STRUCTURAL BODYWORK

The maps for structural bodywork have been inherited partly from the biomedical model, partly from yoga and osteopathy, and partly from dance and movement science. And, encouragingly, maps from other cultures are entering the mix – particularly Eastern energetic concepts. Some forms of structural bodywork have incorporated certain psychotherapeutic models into their map collection, while most have taken on board the overriding somatic perspective. Structural bodywork accepts the scientific map as outlined in Figure 6.1, but brings a more unifying perspective to bear upon it. For instance, it sees the connective tissue network less as a tissue type, more as an overriding organizer of the human form. Labelling connective tissue merely as one of several tissue types does not give a sense of the intelligent wholeness and the essential unity of the network.

LEVELS WITHIN OUR SOMATIC ORGANIZATION

All multicellular organisms that move must possess at least:

- a system of executive control
- a locomotory system
- a morphology or architecture.

From the vastness of the human being, these are the systems we directly contact and seek to change through the structural bodywork process, with the intention of influencing the emergent processes of complex behaviour and the somatic awareness that arises from the integrated life processes of the whole organism. The terminology of biology acknowledges the tight integration of these systems with each other: with the term *neuromuscular* relating the systems of executive control and locomotory, and the terms *musculoskeletal* and *myofascial* reflecting the inseparable connection of the locomotory system with the architecture of the body.

These closely integrated systems are, however, quite hierarchical in their internal structural organization as they consist of layered and nested systems, with each layer having its own functions, intelligence, sphere of influence and semi-autonomy. The higher elements control the lower elements, whilst the lower elements have a constraining influence upon the higher levels of the hierarchy, providing real-time limits in what they are able to realize.

At the lowest (or structural) level is the morphology or architecture of the body (and from here on in we will stay with the word 'architecture', in keeping with Dr Rolf's predilection for architectural analogies). The

architecture refers to the properties and the disposition of the structural materials from which a body is composed: bone, cartilage, ligaments, tendons, bursae, synovial sheaths, retinaculae, interosseous membranes, fascial sheaths and fascial hydrostatic bags, plus all the 'semi-liquid material' that is enclosed within these bags. This is the unanimated body; a body with its somatic nervous system turned off. This architecture is animated by the contractile properties of muscle fibres under nervous system control, which together comprise the neuromuscular system.

At the highest (or functional) level is the executive control that emanates from the central nervous system. This system is itself hierarchical in its organization, with whole-body functions initiated at the higher centres of coordination and control within the sensorimotor cortex, cerebellum and basal ganglia; other functions coordinated from further down the spinal cord, at the level of the brain stem, and the lowest level (reflex activity) mediated purely at the spinal cord.

Let us look now at these three systems and show how they relate to those aspects of the scientific map that are most important for structural bodywork. Figure 6.2 shows the emergent behaviours that are of central interest to structural bodyworkers and also other conceptual

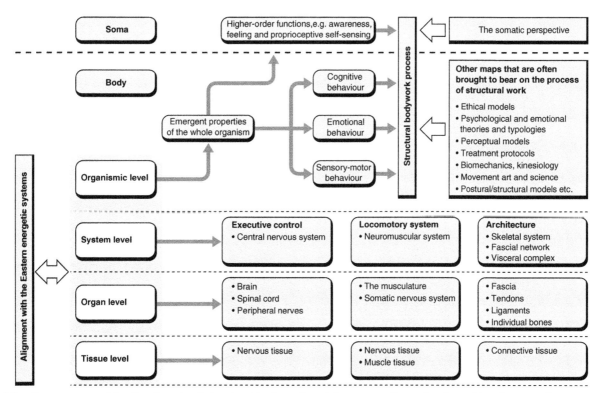

Figure 6.2   A map summarizing the domain of structural bodywork and the perspectives often brought to bear on the process.

maps that are often brought to bear on the process of structural bodywork, such as psychological theories, ethical constructs, prescriptions around the therapeutic relationship, aspects of movement science, structural models and so on.

REFERENCES

Hanna T 1988 Somatics – reawakening the mind's control of movement, flexibility, and health. Addison-Wesley, Reading, Massachusetts

Hanna T 1995 What is somatics. In: Johnson D (ed) Bone, breath and gesture: practices in embodiment. North Atlantic Books, Berkeley, p 341

Johnson D 1994 Body, spirit and democracy. North Atlantic Books, Berkeley, p 200

Nicoll M 1952 Living time. Eureka Editions, The Netherlands, p 3

Tortora G, Grabowski S 1993 Principles of anatomy and physiology. HarperCollins College Publishers, New York

CHAPTER 7

THE TECHNIQUES OF STRUCTURAL BODYWORK

Ultimately, all somatic approaches aim at giving our clients greater somatic awareness, more freedom of movement, more options for movement, greater efficiency of movement, more pleasure in movement, less discomfort and less mechanical wear and tear. If we look at the broad gamut of somatic approaches in Box 3.1 (p. 22), we note that the approaches vary considerably in how they attempt to reach these ends. Each system has its own characteristic goals, assessment strategies, procedures, protocols and maps, plus a 'toolbox' of techniques that are specific to it. Alexander teachers would no more consider using soft-tissue mobilization techniques than chiropractors would consider using subtle manual suggestion to draw out the improved functionality that may arise from their manipulations.

All techniques used by therapists are quite specific as to which level of our somatic organization they address. For instance, the techniques of myofascial and osseous release directly address the architecture, while the subtly informative hands of an Alexander teacher directly address our sensory-motor intelligence, the functional level of our organization. Sometimes, even entire approaches are dedicated to addressing only one level of their clients' organization, for example the Alexander technique and connective tissue massage (Bindegwebbsmassage). This may be entirely appropriate if that is exactly the work that a client requires; however, working at one level is likely to be somewhat limiting, arbitrary and artificial, since important aspects of the client's needs are likely to be overlooked. Inevitably, a singular technique can address only a narrow aspect of the somatic organization. Approaches that employ a combination of techniques can address more. However it is approaches that can address the wider spectrum of our somatic organization that will

have the widest applicability, particularly if they have an overriding holistic orientation.

Some of the better-known approaches work purely at the highest level of somatic organization, that is, the level of whole-body neuromuscular organization. They work both locally and globally to influence global neuromuscular patterns, and include approaches like:

- the Alexander technique
- the Trager® approach
- the original complete Proprioceptive Neuromuscular Facilitation (PNF) system (the contract–relax stretching protocol that is often called PNF is actually only a fraction of the system)
- the Feldenkrais method
- the Continuum® approach
- Hatha yoga
- the martial arts
- Rolfing Movement Integration.

These aim to enhance our somatic awareness, improve the efficiency of functions, give more movement options, induce less stress on the body and promote greater coordination – in short, to promote an integrated functionality. The techniques these systems employ are largely educational and use either verbal or manual cuing, or direct imitation ('Do it like this'), in order to communicate new movement possibilities to their clients. These systems often have an unacknowledged 'trickle down' rationale, which is the assumption that if you can change the outward behaviour then the benefits will eventually be felt at the lower levels, particularly in the gradual adaptation of the soft tissues to the new patterns of movement.

Another class of techniques operates at an intermediate level of neuromuscular coordination, even at the level of spinal reflexes. For the techniques in this class, the intention is to influence relatively local tonus patterns, usually around a specific joint or articulation, with less emphasis on whole body functioning. This work may be intended to allow greater lengthening of muscles or stimulate them to fire more consistently through a range. They include such neuromuscular techniques as:

- the muscle energy technique
- the PNF contract–relax techniques and eccentric resistance techniques
- the CRAC (contract–relax–antagonist–contract) approach
- trigger point therapy
- the strain–counterstrain approach
- the positional release approach.

These techniques work locally to affect the proprioceptive regulation of local muscular tonus. Used alone, these techniques belong to Maitland's corrective or fixing paradigm and their results are not necessarily integrated into stable whole-body movement patterns.

Other techniques focus on effecting mechanical changes at the tissue level of our somatic organization, our architecture. They work locally to release local soft-tissue restrictions. These techniques include:

- deep tissue massage
- passive stretching
- myofascial release
- soft-tissue mobilization (Bindegwebbsmassage)
- joint mobilization
- osseous release (including both indirect techniques and high velocity low amplitude thrusts).

(It should be noted in passing that traditional massage techniques are not included here, since their main intention is to produce a short-term relaxation response and not a structural change).

The intention of these techniques is to increase the range and quality of movement around articulations by releasing mechanical restrictions, for instance, by easing restrictions in the periarticular tissues around facet joints, by giving more resilience to the fascial sheaths or by gently challenging ligamentous limitations. There is a growing body of evidence to suggest, however, that many techniques that aim at changes at the tissue level are in fact facilitated neurologically by a resetting of local proprioceptive output from the surrounding connective tissues, which results in releases that were once thought to be purely mechanical. This has been demonstrated, for instance, with the high velocity release of

facet joints. Where once the effects of such manipulations (such as a reduction of spasm) were thought to be due to the mechanical freeing or stretching of the facet joint capsule, it is now thought to be due to the resetting of the tonus levels in the immediate muscular environment, a decrease in 'gamma bias'. Schleip (2003) suggests that the measurable increase in fascial resilience following direct technique myofascial release is due in part to a local resetting of tonus levels, via a number of local feedback loops in the surrounding tissues. In fact, more advanced dissection techniques are showing that the fascia, tendons, ligaments and joint capsules are very densely innervated, having perhaps the highest number of proprioceptors of any organ or system. This class of techniques often work on the unacknowledged assumption of the 'filter up' effect; that if you release restricted tissues then the intelligent body will automatically respond to these changes and begin to move more efficiently. The degree of this 'filter up' effect, however, seems to depend largely upon the sensory-motor intelligence of the client.

These soft-tissue techniques are mirrored to a certain extent in the releasing techniques of physiotherapy and the more direct approach of orthopaedic medicine. These mainstream disciplines achieve similar outcomes using techniques such as:

- traction
- cross-friction massage
- taping
- the surgical shortening, lengthening or repositioning of muscles, ligaments or bones
- various kinds of fasciectomy for addressing compression, tunnel or compartment syndromes (for instance releasing the carpal tunnel or the anterolateral compartment of the lower leg)
- the use of mechanical aids that force or redirect structural adaptation (shoe orthotics, Harrington rods, splinting, body casts, leg braces, corrective shoes and so on)
- the strengthening of ligaments by inducing fibrosis (by prolotherapy or cross-friction massage)
- the shrinking of connective tissue using microwaves.

Figure 7.1 illustrates in an approximate way the correspondence between the somatic levels of our organization and the techniques and approaches typically used to address them. What is not illustrated by this diagram, however, is the fact that although structural bodywork approaches focus on effecting structural changes at the level of our architecture, they also attempt to evoke

Somatic level	Body systems	Typical functions	Typical techniques	Typical approaches
Executive control Sensory-motor intelligence	• Cortex • Cerebellum • Basal ganglia • Alpha motor system • Brain stem • Gamma motor system • Spinal cord	• Orchestration of whole body response • Initiation of novel movement • Immediate solutions to movement problems • Integration of kinaesthetic information • Startle reflex • Tonic neck reflexes • Postural reflexes such as the Landau response **Simpler reflexes such as:** • stretch reflexes • reciprocal inhibition • post isometric response	• Spoken guidance • Tactile guidance • Demonstration and imitation **Neuromuscular techniques such as:** • Muscle energy technique • Contract/relax stretching	Feldenkrais Alexander Aston-Patterning Continuum etc. Movement arts (see Box 3.1) PNF
Locomotory system	• The musculature • Motor units	• Coordinated firing of motor units • Sarcomere contractility	Neuromuscular techniques	PNF
The architecture	• Myofascial system • Skeletal system • The viscera	• Visco-elastic and visco-plastic properties • Compressive resistance • Semi-liquid hydraulic properties	• Cross frictions • Traction • Soft-tissue techniques • Myofascial release • Osseous release • Visceral manipulation	• Structural bodywork • Rolfing • Hellerwork • Postural integration etc. • Ostoepathy • Chiropractic

Functional domain

Structural domain

Figure 7.1 The correspondence of techniques and the levels within our somatic organization.

fresh functional patterns, employing many of the techniques used by the more educational approaches such as Alexander and Feldenkrais. This will be clearer as we explore the nature of structure and function in the next chapter.

THE IMPORTANCE OF ADDRESSING ALL LEVELS OF OUR SOMATIC ORGANIZATION

So if we consider these two facts: that clients' starting places will be extraordinarily varied, and somatic techniques invariably focus on only one level of our somatic hierarchy, then it is clear that many approaches, by themselves, cannot offer a full solution to our clients' needs. There may, by happenstance, be a close correlation between what a client needs and what a practitioner can offer, but the more complete somatic therapist will be able to work at a number of different levels within the client's somatic organization. Ultimately, the minimal requirement of a structural bodyworker is to have a range of skills that include some in each of the three groups of techniques: soft-tissue releases, neuromuscular releases and integrative techniques, and knowing when to use them. Without this range of skills, bodyworkers will need to select their clients carefully, appraising who will respond to their work and who needs referring on to another kind of practitioner.

THE NEED FOR AN INTEGRATED APPROACH

Many somatic practitioners have emphasized the need for an integrated approach using several levels of technique, believing that structural and functional approaches are appropriate at different phases of treatment. For instance, Cantu and Grodin (1992) state:

the sequencing of treatment includes beginning superficially with a manual approach, and working gradually into deeper tissues. Once the deeper tissues are accessed and affected, elongation of the structures becomes facilitated. When optimal length and mobility are established, neuromuscular re-education is emphasized to prevent recurrence, as well as postural integration. The progression from a light manual approach (mechanical), and then to an emphasis on movement and posture (movement approach) is the key to complete treatment.

Cottingham and Maitland (1997) recommend a treatment model for use within a physiotherapeutic context, based on Maitland's three-paradigm schema (see Chapter 3 and Fig. 3.1, p. 23). Here the authors suggest a treatment protocol that works at three levels: within the relaxation paradigm – essentially pain modulation procedures; within the corrective paradigm – manual techniques and exercises to correct faulty biomechanical alignment, and within the integrative paradigm – guided movement to improve postural and movement patterns. They emphasize that although this work can be performed sequentially, in actual fact there can be a huge overlap in the application of these different levels of approach, and work within the three levels often proceeds concurrently.

A THREE-LEVEL MODEL – FROM RELEASE TO INTEGRATION

In the practical section of this book it will be recommended that therapists who wish to explore the structural bodywork approach can begin their exploration by employing a simplified three-level protocol (see Fig. 7.2) that closely parallels the Cantu–Grodin and Cottingham–Maitland protocols mentioned above.

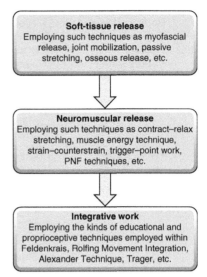

Figure 7.2 A simplified three-level protocol for structural bodywork.

As was stated in the introduction, this protocol will not make you a structural bodyworker as it lacks the overriding holistic rationale that is necessary for real structural integration. However, it will allow you to make some initial explorations in gently reorganizing structure, and can give results which, although not a complete structural rebalancing, can alleviate some of your clients' structural problems in the short to medium term.

The complete structural bodyworker requires skills in at least three levels in order to produce real and lasting structural change, and best results can be achieved by progressing through the three levels of somatic organization. First, at the tissue level, there is generally a lengthening or softening process that brings more length and resilience to shortened tissue. This is rarely sufficient for lasting change. Sometimes clients with a high degree of sensory-motor intelligence can integrate this kind of work directly into their overall somatic organization, but for most clients at least some integrating work is essential. Neuromuscular techniques can then be used to assist the released muscles in 'knowing' that they can lengthen. This class of techniques is aimed at modifying responses at a relatively low level of neurological organization and not a whole body response – essentially changing the mapping on the sensory-motor cortex. Finally, this local pattern needs to be integrated into the whole body functions of standing, sitting, walking, reaching and all complex movement patterns. This requires proprioceptive education, somatic awareness, integration and coordination.

This protocol assumes that for most clients both structural and functional work will be necessary, the relative amount of each depending greatly on individual needs. It also suggests that if structural work is required, it should either precede functional work or run in parallel with it. So in the next section we will look more closely at the concepts of structure and function, which stand at the heart of the structural bodywork approach.

REFERENCES

Cantu R, Grodin A 1992 Myofascial manipulation: theory and clinical application. Aspen Publishers, Gaithersburg, pp 20, 25–57

Cottingham J, Maitland J 1997 A three-paradigm treatment model using soft-tissue mobilization and guided movement – awareness techniques for a patient with chronic low back pain: a case study. Journal of Orthopaedic and Sports Physical Therapy 26: 3

Schleip R 2003 Fascial plasticity: a new neurobiological explanation. Journal of Bodywork and Movement Therapies 7(1): 1

STRUCTURE AND FUNCTION

There is no real difference between structure and function; they are two sides of the same coin. If structure does not tell us something about function, it means we have not looked correctly.

Dr A. T. Still (the founder of Osteopathy)(1899)

There are many apocryphal tales surrounding the great somatic pioneers, Ida Rolf and Moshe Feldenkrais. One is that in the early days of their association in England they agreed to divide the somatic world into two empires (rather like politicians who had just carved up Europe after World War II); Ida Rolf developing the process of *structural integration,* and Moshe Feldenkrais the process of *functional integration.* Time passed and they each separately fashioned their own unique systems; however, they managed to preserve a running dispute that lasted the rest of their lives, each asserting that their process was the superior.

Many years passed, and on the occasion of Ida Rolf's eightieth birthday, a huge party was organized to which all the luminaries of the Rolfing world were invited. Included, of course, was Rolf's old friend and sparring partner, Moshe Feldenkrais. When all the formalities were over, these two old antagonists got together and, ignoring everyone else, spent the rest of the evening continuing their favourite dispute about the role of structure and function, with the course of their argument going something like this: 'Function determines structure!' (Feldenkrais), 'No, no, you old fool, structure determines function!' (Rolf) and so on for the rest of the evening.

We know that both were inclined to exaggerate a point to provoke critical thinking in those about them (and perhaps also out of sheer cussedness!), and that neither seriously held the extremes of these viewpoints. Rolf's respect for the genius of Feldenkrais is evident in her writings in which she acknowledges his insights into the neuromuscular patterns of anxiety. And from the earliest years of her exploration, Dr Rolf employed various movement techniques to support the structural aspect of Rolfing – 'tracking', 'Rolf yoga' and re-patterning exercises. Later on she promoted Judith Aston's movement work, and then *Rolfing Movement Integration.* She knew that soft-tissue manipulation by itself was not enough to guarantee an improvement in functionality.

And neither did Feldenkrais hold to an extreme functional view. He was Rolfed by Ida herself. And in a touching (but still guarded!) testimonial for her book, *Rolfing* (Rolf 1977), he wrote, 'when Ida Rolf integrates structure, as nobody else can, she improves functioning. Rolfing was a revealing and unforgettable experience for me.' We also know that some of her students worked very hard on the steely psoas that Feldenkrais had developed from his years of Judo, and that he was even known to use these structural release techniques on his own clients (for, like all the great somatic innovators, he was a skilled borrower).

STRUCTURAL AND FUNCTIONAL APPROACHES – A PRACTICAL POLARITY?

Structure refers to our physical form or, in biological terms, our morphology; function refers to the behavioural patterns effected by structures. The Macquarie Dictionary (1989) for instance defines function as 'the kind of action or activity proper to a person, thing, or institution', and structure as 'Biol[ogical] mode of organisation; construction and arrangement of tissues, parts, or organs'.

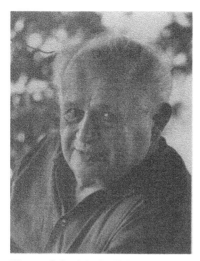

Figure 8.1 Moshe Feldenkrais.

Feldenkrais (Fig. 8.1) believed that our structure is moulded by the interaction of our genetic inheritance with the sum result of all the movements that the body has enacted throughout its life. The central rationale of his approach is that, as human beings, we are largely unaware of our movement patterns (our functions). The ways that we have found to solve the movement problems presented by life are not necessarily the most sound or efficient. His method involves, first, guiding our attention to our movement patterns so that we discover *how* we move, then offering new movement options that may be more efficient or more pleasurable, and then helping us integrate these new options into our larger movement repertoire. To him, change in function is about learning: he believed that the profound functional changes that arise from this work ultimately modify our structure.

Rolf, on the other hand, believed that structural changes are the key to functional improvement. She believed that structural reorganization of the body would allow it to intelligently renegotiate its relationship with gravity, so that new ways of standing, moving and being would spontaneously emerge:

You can change human beings. You can change their structure, and in changing their structure you are able to change their function. Structure determines function to a very great degree and to a degree which we can utilize. The basic law of Rolfing is that you add structure to the body. In so doing you are demanding a change in function. This is the basic reason why Rolfing works as it does.

Ida Rolf (Feitis 1978)

Rolf's works offer many examples of how structural change brings forth functional change: sometimes the dramatic and visible shift in postural organization evident in the before and after photos of Rolfing (see Fig. 1.4, p. 11); and sometimes more subtle and less visible changes such as the shift in muscle usage from *sleeve* to *core* (in her terminology), which can be experienced as a feeling of effortlessness in movement and a sense of lift in posture.

When we look at the historical development of the field of Somatics, it certainly appears that the newly emerging modalities naturally aligned themselves towards the opposite ends of the structural–functional spectrum. At the functional end we have approaches such as the Alexander Technique and the Feldenkrais method, in which the stated intention of the approach is *to evoke functional change through learning*; and at the structural end we have Rolfing, osteopathy and chiropractic in which the intention is *to evoke functional change through structural change*. It is important here to restate the major contention of this book: that all modalities can and do assist clients, but the most successful strategies will appropriately address every level of their somatic organization, and this usually means both structural and functional work in different degrees, depending on the individual.

THE BIRTH OF STRUCTURE AND FUNCTION

Since structural bodyworkers are working primarily in the structural realm, it would be useful to clarify the meaning of 'structure' and 'function' from an anatomical and developmental perspective.

In human embryogenetic development, shortly after conception, the fertilized egg develops into a blastosphere: a hollow sphere of cells. These cells are undifferentiated and seemingly identical in every respect; they do not yet exhibit the huge range of different cell structures and functions that are found in the mature organism. After about a week the process of differentiation begins (see Fig. 8.2). The cells swirl, migrate and begin to differentiate. They organize themselves into two primitive germ layers, which are the ectoderm and endoderm. Then, in between these layers emerges a third layer, the mesoderm. There follows an amazing developmental cascade in which each of these three layers undergoes an extraordinary sequence of growth, folding and invagination, which ultimately develops into a major cluster of related organ systems within the body (see Box 8.1). The ectoderm will transform into the skin

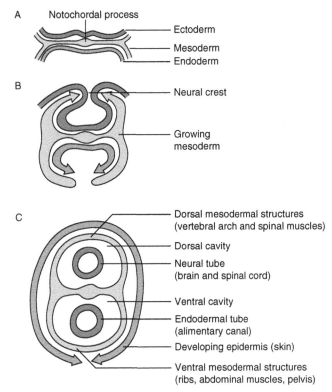

Figure 8.2 The growth of the mesoderm.

Box 8.1

ECTODERM

tissues of the central nervous system
epidermis of skin
hair
eyes, ears and other senses

MESODERM

skeletal and cardiac muscle
most smooth muscle
cartilage, bone
other connective tissues
blood vessels and blood cells
dermis of skin

ENDODERM

the respiratory tract
the digestive tract
the digestive organs

---

and nervous system, the mesoderm into the connective tissues and muscles, and the endoderm into the internal organs or viscera. Schultz and Feitis (1996) give a more detailed account of this extraordinary process.

As structural bodyworkers our main focus will be on those systems that arise from the middle layer, the mesoderm. These systems are:

1. the connective tissue network (particularly the skeletal and fascial systems), and
2. the muscular system (particularly the skeletal muscles).

These are the tissues that we will actively engage and seek to change. The ectodermic systems, too, will be important because we work through the skin (with its vast collection of nerve endings) and will necessarily engage the central nervous system, but these systems are perhaps more the central concern of somatic therapists with a functional emphasis (like Feldenkrais and Alexander Technique practitioners) who work more with sensory-motor coordination and integration.

From a structural perspective it could be argued that the endodermic system (the visceral complex) is of lesser importance to the structural bodyworker. It may be an extraordinarily complex and intelligent system, but from the point of view of gravity it is just bags of jelly (in the same way that a computer, despite its complex functionality, could equally be used as a doorstop or an anchor!). The visceral complex can be considered as a 'semi-liquid' aspect of our material reality and we move as if our core space were a large balloon packed with smaller, jelly-filled balloons. Some animals need to tighten their abdomen during running to prevent this semi-liquid mass from 'sloshing around' too much. However, the visceral complex has its own soft connective tissue network, with suspensory ligaments and the fascial wrappings of organs, and in the opinion of many osteopaths and structural bodyworkers the condition of the viscera can have both a mechanical and a reflexive influence on our posture and movements. When grosser myofascial interventions fail to produce the expected result then visceral work is often the next step.

THE BODY'S ARCHITECTURE

Ponder this question for a moment: 'If it were possible to remove all the cells from the human body, what would be left?' Our anatomical training might lead us to answer something like: 'Not very much' or 'Just a pool of liquid – gastric fluids, lymph, synovial fluid and the like'. But in fact a great deal would be left, for instance, most of the skeletal material, bone and cartilage; most of the connective tissue network, ligaments, joint capsules, bursae, fasciae and tendons, as well as a lot of fluid – in fact all the extra-cellular materials in the body. When we come upon animals that have died in the wild, what we find are the skin, tendons, ligaments and the bones. And although eventually all will be returned to dust, it is the watery, cellular materials that disintegrate first, leaving behind the more durable, structural parts.

It is sobering to realize that a large part of our material reality is non-cellular. Our structure is composed of real structural materials in the same way that bridges and buildings are composed of steel, glass, concrete, plastics and carbon fibres. And like these familiar structural materials from our engineering world, our bodily structural materials have physical properties such as tensile and compressive strength, elasticity, plasticity, electrical conductivity, and so on. The behaviour of our bodily structural materials can best be understood within that branch of physics called *mechanics* – and be seen as responding to Newtonian forces. So in a sense, structural bodyworkers are the engineers of the human body (though of course not only engineers) in that we roll up our sleeves and tinker with its structure to help it work more efficiently.

However, our bodily building materials differ from architectural building materials in one major (and extraordinary) respect, which is that they are self-adapting. They can transform themselves in response to the forces applied to them. Interpenetrated by living cells, these materials have a unique relationship with the rich tapestry of life processes that surround them. They live at a slower pace and have a less vigorous metabolic life than their resident cells, but are actively serviced by them. There is a specialized group of cells whose job is to support and maintain these structural materials by debriding damaged or redundant tissue and manufacturing new materials according to the greater needs of the organism as a whole. Would that our own architects and engineers could devise buildings that could intelligently and unobtrusively modify their internal structure to meet the demands we place on them!

Our somatic bricks and mortar

What are the building materials of our bodies? What are our somatic bricks and mortar? The most pervasive structural material is collagen fibre, comprising as much as 40% of the body's protein. Later we will look at this remarkable substance in more detail, but suffice to say that in different forms and configurations, collagen unifies our whole structure; it is literally the glue that holds us together. In fact old-fashioned wood glue was

prepared from the boiled down collagen of the skin, ligaments and bones of animals. In our bones, collagen fibres combine with bone salts to forge the most rigid of our connective tissues. In connective tissue proper, collagen fibres and ground substance (the all-pervasive extracellular lubricating gel) combine with other kinds of fibre (elastin and reticulin) to create a vast array of connective tissues, each suited precisely to their local conditions.

These structural materials have some extraordinary properties; collagen fibres have a tensile strength greater than steel, yet form tissues of great elasticity and pliability. They give the iliotibial tract the resilience of tyre rubber, and yet shape the delicate reticular tracery of the spleen. Think of the strength and durability of leather (the preserved dermis of the cow) or the density of bone, which can resist compressive forces in the order of 2 000 pounds per square inch (approaching 14 000 kPa). Our somatic bricks and mortar are real structural materials with some remarkable properties. As a unified whole they are the *yin* (or passive aspect) of the mesodermic system. The contractility of muscle cells is the *yang*.

The yin and yang of our structural reality

The body's structural materials and their resident servant cells are one major outflux of the mesoderm; the muscle cells are the other. These two subsystems have very different properties: the connective tissues are essentially non-cellular and metabolically passive, whilst the muscle cells are cellular, metabolically active, and actively contractile. These form the passive and active elements of our structure and so can be described as the yin and yang of our structural reality, being our structural connective tissue materials and the actively contractile elements that provide the motive power to move them. But what we normally call 'muscle' is more properly seen as an inseparable fusion of muscle cells and their fascial environment: contractile units suspended in an ocean of fascia, which is the most abundant connective tissue in the body. In fact, muscle tissue is 50–60 per cent fascia.

A MAP FOR STRUCTURAL BODYWORK

We can now summarize the components of the three embryogenetic organ systems from a structural bodywork perspective. Figure 8.3 relates to the earlier one (Fig. 7.1, p. 45) and shows a layering of processes with increasing complexity, intelligence (or information processing capability) and other emergent properties. Like

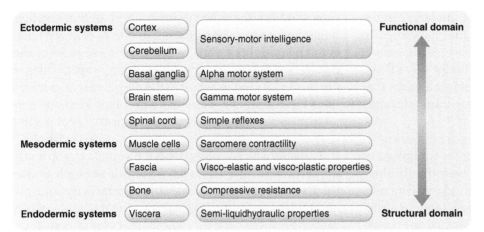

Figure 8.3 Elements of the embryogenetic systems that relate to structural bodywork.

all maps it does not describe the whole territory, but it does present, in a hierarchical form, all the elements essential to structural work.

Some models for understanding human structure

The mesodermic subsystems work together along with other systems to form a completely functional, organic whole. What forces are at play? What are the structural dynamics of a system such as the human body? Many structural and functional models have been offered, some from biological science, some from the somatic pioneers and, interestingly, some remarkable insights have emerged from architectural science.

A robotic model

The mechanistic model, found in older kinesiological texts, portrays the human being as a system of skeletal levers impelled by muscular pulleys, making it a 'soft machine' (Maitland 1992). It paints a robotic picture that leaves huge areas of our functionality unexplained. This is not to say that the bones do not act as levers, but simply that this is an extremely limited and partial description, ignoring for instance the oscillatory behaviour of the all-encompassing fascial network (Fig. 8.4).

A building block model

As mentioned earlier, Ida Rolf was very fond of using architectural analogies in her discussion of human structure and used various models to highlight different aspects of our structural dynamics. One was a building block model that saw structural segments, such as the thorax, pelvis and limbs, stacked in vertical alignment somewhat architecturally. This thinking is very evident in her 'Little Boy Logo' (see Fig. 8.5). This model is useful in visualizing the kinds of segmental displacements that can occur in an unbalanced structure (what she called a 'random body'). However, such an analogy

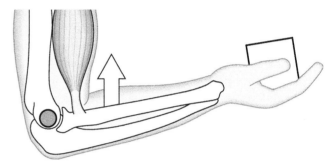

Figure 8.4 A robotic model – the body as a collection of skeletal levers like this.

cannot be taken too far. Like buildings we do need to be balanced within the field of gravity, and compressional forces from gravity do indeed act longitudinally through our upright skeleton. But in truth a human being does not stand in the same way that a gothic cathedral stands: there are no level surfaces within the body to build up from, and our bones do not, in fact, even touch one another (Flury 1989).

The 'blocks in a sack' model

Rolf also offered a 'blocks in a sack' model that portrayed the body as an organization of blocks enclosed within an elastic envelope (see Fig. 8.6). This model emphasizes the structural importance of the superficial and deep fascial network, and seems to anticipate the tensegrity model from the world of modern architecture. The tensegrity model has proved extremely useful in the description of living structures from the cellular level to a macroscopic level.

Tensegrity systems – 'Continuous tension and local compression'

Buckminster Fuller, the architect and inventor of the geodesic dome, coined the term *tensegrity* (from 'tensional

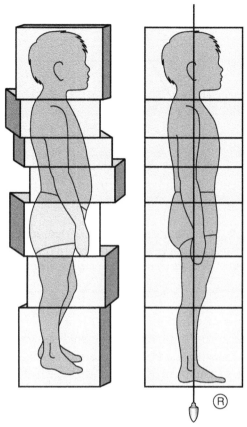

Figure 8.5 'Little Boy Logo' – the body as a stack of blocks or segments (Rolf 1977).

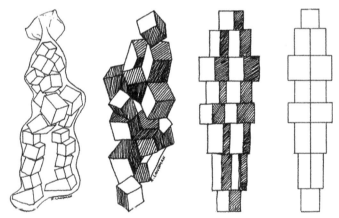

Figure 8.6 'Blocks in a sack' model (reproduced with the kind permission of Alan Demmerle).

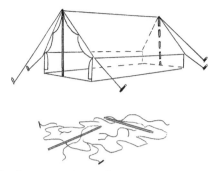

Figure 8.7 A tent as a tensegrity structure

etc.) as they employ a clever combination of two kinds of material element – those that are strong when compressed, and those that are strong when stretched. All materials in fact have both compressive and tensile properties. However some traditional building elements such as posts, poles, struts and columns are employed to capitalize on their compressive strength, which means that they can effectively resist crushing forces that are applied to them. Other elements, such as cables or sheets, are utilized for their tensile strength and can effectively resist forces that would stretch or lengthen them. Tensegrity structures combine these two kinds of structural element and mutually balance their tensile and compressive qualities in such a way that the compressive elements do not actually touch one another. Some aspects of the human structure can perhaps be best understood as tensegrity systems.

One remarkable property of a tensegrity system is that if an external force disturbs its internal equilibrium, it will yield but will do so in a way that distributes the stresses and loads evenly throughout the whole system, with all the elements sharing the workload. What a design advantage this would be for an organism: to have a system that inherently avoids loading some parts too much.

The tent tensegrity structure
A tent is a tensegrity structure, as shown in Figure 8.7. Here the poles are the compressional elements and the fabric the tensional element. If we look at the disassembled tent we have poles with many degrees of freedom, and the tent fabric that by itself lies in a random, chaotic heap. But when they are arranged together, with tension strategically placed through the fabric, and compression through the poles, they form a whole with a real structural integrity. The tension in the fabric acts to space and position the poles appropriately. The poles preserve an appropriate span and tension in the fabric.

integrity') to describe a principle for designing lightweight integrated structures that deliver great stability with minimal material. Tensegrity structures are different in principle from the traditional columnar structures that employ a 'ground up' stacking of compressive elements (bricks, stone, concrete, steel posts and struts,

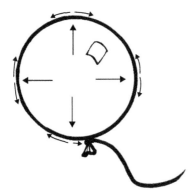

Figure 8.8 A balloon (or hydrostatic bag) as a tensegrity structure.

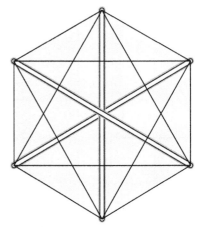

Figure 8.9 A simple tensegrity structure. This octahedral tensegrity structure can be constructed from three sticks and three elastic bands. The sticks do not rely on the contact in the centre.

Fluid mechanics

A balloon is also a tensegrity structure, although at first glance it might not seem so. Not only solids have compressive qualities; the whole field of hydraulics is based on the principle that fluids and gases can resist compressive forces. So there is another class of structure that conforms to the tensegrity principle, that is, the balloon or hydrostatic bag (see Fig. 8.8).

A balloon is compressed air surrounded by rubber. The tensioned skin of the balloon is compressing the air inside and, conversely, the skin is being placed under tension by the expansive tendency of the pressurized gas within. This tension is communicated evenly throughout its whole surface area so that the balloon is a balanced combination of compressive and tensional elements – a tensegrity structure. Having such a structure, a balloon is self-balancing. Externally applied forces will deform the structure redistributing the force evenly throughout. Once the force is removed, however, the balloon will return to its former shape. We will see later that tensegrity structures of both the tent and balloon design can be found within the human structure.

A tensegrity model

You can get a practical understanding of the tensegrity principle by constructing the model in Figure 8.9 from elastic bands and dowels or tongue depressors. You will find that the whole has a real structural integrity and is resilient enough to regain its shape after you gently deform it. In fact, it regains its shape with a bouncy rhythmicity. This is the oscillatory dance of potential and kinetic energies that is inherent in the tensegrity design.

The behaviour of the human body is beginning to be more fully explored within scientific kinesiology. It is increasingly apparent that the elasticity of connective tissue within a tensegrity arrangement goes a long way towards explaining the rhythmic, elastic, undulatory behaviour of our bodies. Later, it will be shown that economical rhythmic movement such as walking must harmonize with the body's inherent undulatory properties at a structural level and that part of our job as bodyworkers is to assist our clients to discover the rhythmic harmony inherent in their own structure. This rhythmic aspect of our biological inherency will be examined in more detail in Chapter 10.

The human body as a tensegrity structure

Our human structure can be understood as conforming to the tensegrity design. Our bones (like the tent poles) are the compressional elements; the fascial sheaths, tendons and ligaments (like the tent fabric) are the tensional elements. The fascia serves to maintain the appropriate spatial relationships between the skeletal elements. If we could turn off the tonus of the muscle fibres entirely we would be left with a true tensegrity structure, that is, bones organized into a skeleton by the spanning fascia.

Imagine that by some miraculous intervention we could dissolve away all materials from the human body except the fascia; what would remain would be a perfect representation of the human form, with spaces to represent all the muscles, bones, organs and cavities of the body. However, this fascial spectre could not last a moment because the relentless force of gravity would instantly act, and like a tent without pole it would slump to the floor in a random heap. (Here we are using the word fascia in its broadest sense, to mean all of the binding connective tissues: myofascia, aponeuroses and tendons, ligaments, synovial capsules, and even the periosteum of bones.)

If we could repeat the experiment, but this time dissolving away everything except the bones, then what would momentarily remain would be a skeleton, followed by the clattering of a disarticulated and jumbled heap of bones because there was nothing to bind them together or maintain their normal spatial configuration.

But if, in a third experiment, we could dissolve away all the materials except the fascia *and* the bones, then what would remain would still retain a recognizably human form as it would still remain an integrated and coherent whole, despite the fact that it would be collapsed and unresponsive. Like the fabric of the tent, it is the fascia, ligaments and other connective tissues that maintain the appropriate relationship between the bones by maintaining an appropriate spacing and span. *It is fascia that creates the unified skeleton.* It takes the integrated properties of the fascial and skeletal systems to create a true tensegrity structure, but like all such structures it would be relatively inert, relatively static. It would be internally stable but would respond only to externally applied forces, particularly gravity, and would be unable to initiate movement from within itself. With its neuromuscular system turned off, it would be a body with structural integrity but which could not move of its own accord.

Hans Flury (1997) has been one of the foremost thinkers in helping to clarify the meaning of structure in the field of structural bodywork. Of structure he says:

> *Structure is the spatial arrangement of all the parts of the body, determined primarily by the fascial net, as it manifests in the absence of any muscle activity in the body and with no outside forces acting on the body. This spatial arrangement can be called the 'structural body.' It is evident that we can never see the structural body directly because there always exists muscle activity in the body, and outside forces are always acting on the body.*

Even with this definition of structure, we could see the structural body directly by removing all muscular tension and removing all outside forces, including the influence of gravity, although that would be under the rather extreme set of conditions of someone floating in outer space under general anaesthetic! (see Fig. 8.10). This is not in fact a fanciful suggestion: a human body under such conditions would necessarily 'give in' to all its internal structural tensions and would assume a form that accurately represents that body's true structure. Would the body tend to flex as a whole, or extend as a whole? This would surely show which internal forces within the structure would need to be balanced by muscular tension when in gravity and in full function.

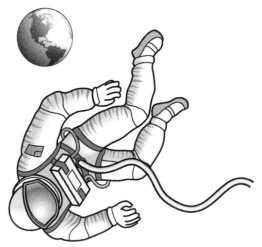

Figure 8.10   An anaesthetized spaceman, showing his real structure.

In order for the structural body to perform even the most rudimentary act of standing upright, another element needs to be added as a means of intelligently varying the pattern of tension throughout the fascial network. This is performed by the coordinated contraction of muscle cells, organized into motor units, and under the control of the central nervous system. The neuromuscular system supplies the orchestrated pattern of tensions to the fascia, which then communicates them through tendons and aponeuroses to the bones and hydraulic bags, thus allowing the whole structural body to balance harmoniously within gravity. The muscle cells supply the motive power, and the central nervous system supplies the control.

It is important to note that not all the contractile force of the musculature is conducted directly through to the skeleton; some is utilized to tighten fascia (the iliotibial tract for instance) and some is used to maintain the form of key hydrostatic bags (the other type of tensegrity structure in the body). Our tissues are about 75% water, which is most evident in a relaxed state. Think of a relaxed cat (in full parasympathetic mode!), for instance, which can almost be poured from your hands. Our bodies contain many balloons, or fascial bags, filled with semi-liquid contents: our muscles within their myofascial sheaths, the viscera within their peritoneal 'bag', the heart in its fibrous pericardium, and the lungs within their pleural containment. Indeed, our entire organism as a whole is contained within the embrace of the superficial and deep fasciae.

The structural integrity of a hydrostatic bag comes from the interaction between the compressive tendency of the surrounding sheath and the tendency for the fluid contents to resist compression. If we take for instance the abdominal cavity; the viscera are contained within a fascial bag, the peritoneum. The muscles surrounding this bag are the breathing diaphragm, the pelvic floor and the abdominal muscles. A coordinated contraction of these muscles (i.e. the valsalva manoeuvre) will both reshape and firm up the peritoneal bag in a way that can actually give structural support to the thorax above, and stiffen the spine. So we can look at the human body as an integrated combination of two kinds of tensegrity design: the tent and the hydraulic bag or balloon.

THE UNITY OF THE STRUCTURAL AND FUNCTIONAL BODIES

So far we have explored the internal dynamics of the body, but we know that bodies also exist within a larger environmental context. On earth, the most significant environmental influence is gravity. Other external forces may impinge on the body from time to time, but gravity is the ever-present force to which the functional body must constantly adapt.

The *structural body* responds to two sets of forces: those generated from within itself and those received from without. Muscular forces act from within the structure, constantly harmonizing it with the pull of gravity and other external mechanical forces that may impinge upon it, for instance impacts from other bodies or forces of acceleration.

Our structural body can be understood largely in terms of the two kinds of tensegrity structure: the skeletal–fascial complex and fascial hydraulic bags – fascial balloons with either hard or soft fillings (Flury 1991). Our *functional body* can be understood as our structural body animated by neuromuscular dynamics. So, when we look at a human being in motion, are we seeing a structure or function? In fact we are seeing both. Any action, even the simple act of standing upright, will require:

- the structural body, being a tensegrity system that consists of the coordinated interaction of the structural properties of the materials from which we are built – the compressive strength of bone; the tensile strength of the fascial web; and the hydraulic behaviour of the semi-liquid contents of the fascial bags
- the functional body, which consists of a structural body that is animated by a coordinated pattern of neuromuscular activity, including the maintenance of pressure in the visceral hydraulic bags through muscular tonus

- an environmental context dominated by the constant pull of gravity.

The above can be stated as a simple formula:

Functional body = Structural body + neuromuscular coordination (within the context of gravity and other forces)

So what does this formula mean for the structural bodyworker? This way of looking at bodies can clarify and define the central concerns of our work. It tells us where we work and why. Since the intention of structural bodyworkers is to evoke functional change through structural change, the practical focus of the work is to evoke change in the structural body. The structural body consists of a skeletal–fascial complex. Since in the short term we cannot change the shape of bones, it is the fascial net that we work with. This means that the fascial net becomes the main focus of our work. In the words of Ida Rolf 'A bone is where it is by way of how it is carried by the soft-tissue. So a Rolfer's job is with the soft-tissue. The bones are the landmarks, but our job is with the soft-tissue' (Feitis 1978).

Working to influence the fascial net is the defining characteristic of the structural bodyworker; working to influence tonus patterns (the coordinated firing patterns of the musculature) is the defining characteristic of the functional bodyworker.

A change of shape caused by a change of the fascial net is a structural change. It is plastic in nature. A change of the tonus pattern also changes the shape of the body, but this is elastic in nature.

(Flury 1997)

SUMMARY

This chapter began with the structure versus function debate of Rolf and Feldenkrais and clarified the meaning of these terms to help define more clearly the respective domains of the structural and functional somatic therapist.

Function is ultimately initiated and ruled by the central nervous system but, as was stressed in Chapter 7, there are many levels to our somatic organization. And although the higher organizing functions of cortical processes are at the top, the movement patterns they initiate are necessarily conditioned by what the structure will allow in real time. Our sensory-motor intelligence is constantly making choices about what is economical in our movement, what is pleasurable (or at least what does not cause pain), and will usually (although not always) take the path of least resistance. And the path of least resistance is largely defined by our structure. Our structure has a major influence on what is economical in movement and will therefore condition and temper greatly how we move. Our structure will be a constant, underlying, unconscious determinant of our movement patterns, thereby making certain patterns statistically more likely to occur and others less likely.

Nevertheless, the body will not always take the path of least resistance, and the body will not always respond to the input of the structural bodyworker; sometimes the body has its own deep reasons for remaining unbalanced and inefficient. Godard (2000) uses the poignant term *libidinal efficiency* to point to the fact that sometimes a body will choose discomfort or postural inefficiency as a means of supplying a deep emotional need that overrules the need for physical comfort. Even with the best structural bodywork available, a body will not allow itself to shift from its old patterns or become more aligned unless it really wants to. For this reason it was mentioned earlier that, if a client is not responding to seemingly sensible structural changes, then it may be necessary to refer on that client to another kind of practitioner.

Later we will look in more detail at the reciprocal pattern of influence between what we call our structure and our functions. We will look at the processes at work that will consolidate our movement patterns into long-lasting structural changes at a tissue level, and how these structural changes then serve to predispose us towards the movement patterns that gave rise to them in the first place. We will also look at the place of the structural bodyworker in interrupting this cycle (see Figs 1.2 and 1.3, pp. 8 and 9).

Ultimately, the structural and functional viewpoints can be reconciled if we realize that structure and function can both be viewed as processes within different time frames. In the words of the great biologist and systems theorist, Ludwig von Bertalanffy (1952):

> The antithesis between structure and function, morphology and physiology, is based upon a static conception of the organism. In a machine there is a fixed arrangement that can be set in motion but can also be at rest. In a similar way the pre-established structure of, say, the heart is distinguished from its function, namely rhythmical contraction. Actually, this separation between pre-established structure, and processes occurring in that structure, does not apply to living organisms. For the organism is the expression of an everlasting orderly process, though, on the other hand, this process is sustained by underlying structures and organized forms. What is described in morphology as organic forms and structures is in reality a momentary cross-section through a spatio-temporal pattern. What are called structures are slow patterns of long duration, functions are quick processes of short duration. If we say that a function such as the contraction of a muscle is performed by a structure, it means that a quick and short wave process is superimposed on a long-lasting and slowly running wave.

The work of structural bodyworkers is defined, but not limited, by working with restrictions within the fascial net: an aspect of our reality that von Bertalanffy would have called a 'slow pattern of long duration'. We will see later how we can assess practically where we need to work within this net, and will look at specific approaches to creating real and lasting change within it.

Now we have defined the territory of the structural bodyworker, we can look in greater detail at the make up of the structural body – the myofascial network and the composition and the properties of fascia.

REFERENCES

Feitis R (ed) 1978 Ida Rolf talks: about Rolfing and physical reality. The Rolf Institute, Boulder

Flury H 1989 Theoretical aspects and implications of the internal/external system. Notes on Structural Integration 1: 15–35

Flury H (ed) 1991 Normal function. Notes on Structural Integration 1: 6–21

Flury H 1997 Grounding structural concepts in physical reality. Unpublished paper

Gallaudet B B 1931 A description of the planes of fascia of the human body. Columbia University Press, New York, p 1

Godard H 2000 Notes from Bodywisdom Conference, Coromandel, New Zealand

Maitland J 1992 Rolfing: a third paradigm approach to body-structure. Rolf Lines 20(2): 47–49

Rolf I 1977 Rolfing: the integration of human structures. Harper and Rowe, New York

Schultz R, Feitis R 1996 The endless web: fascial anatomy and physical reality. North Atlantic Books, Berkeley

Still A 1899 Philosophy of osteopathy. Kirksville, Missouri

von Bertalanffy L 1952 Problems of life. Harper and Row, New York

THE CONNECTIVE TISSUE NETWORK

THE LAYERING OF TISSUES

If we consider the layering of the body's tissues, moving from superficial to deep, we find: the skin, the superficial fascia, the deep fascia and, beneath these layers, the myofascial network, proliferating inwards throughout the musculature towards the core (Fig. 9.1).

The skin

Our outermost layer, the skin, consists of two sub-layers: a thinner outer layer, the epidermis, and the thicker and more fibrous inner layer, the dermis. The epidermis is a complex layer in itself, consisting mostly of epithelial cells with a high content of keratin, which is a protein that toughens and helps waterproof the skin. These cells are produced continuously from an underlying basal layer and gradually migrate to the surface, displaced by new cells from beneath. They gradually dry out and die as they approach the surface, becoming the tough protective outer layer of skin, eventually to be sloughed off at the surface through everyday wear and tear. The dermis is composed mostly of connective tissue but accommodates many nerve endings, blood vessels and other specialized structures such as hair follicles and sweat glands.

The superficial fascia

Beneath the skin is the superficial fascia, which is also known as the subcutaneous layer. It is a continuous

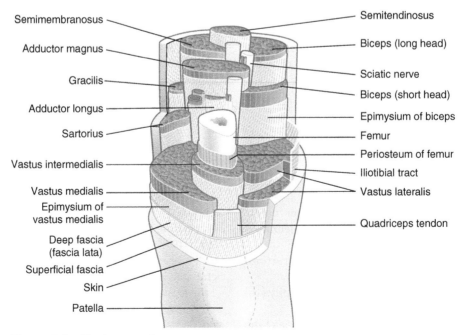

Semimembranosus
Adductor magnus
Gracilis
Adductor longus
Sartorius
Vastus intermedialis
Vastus medialis
Epimysium of vastus medialis
Deep fascia (fascia lata)
Superficial fascia
Skin
Patella

Semitendinosus
Biceps (long head)
Sciatic nerve
Biceps (short head)
Epimysium of biceps
Femur
Periosteum of femur
Iliotibial tract
Vastus lateralis
Quadriceps tendon

Figure 9.1 The layering of tissues.

layer of loose connective tissue that lies between the skin and the deep fascia, and which follows the surface contours of the body. It is webbed by a fine network of the most superficial nerves, blood vessels and lymph ducts, and is the place where layers of subcutaneous fat of varying thickness tend to collect. Although it is the next and deeper layers, the deep fascia and the myofascia, that are of most concern to structural bodyworkers, the superficial fascia does have structural significance. In certain places, particularly over the trunk, it is more durable than the deep fascia, and although it is not as densely fibrous as the deep fascia it does have enough collagen mass to provide resistance to movement. There are considerable differences between individuals in the density of this layer, and such differences may be congenital. These are not just differences in the amount of fat, but also in fibrosity – seemingly in the amount of collagen fibre within the matrix itself. For some, this layer is very thick and tough, somewhat like a thick, tight wetsuit and this will tend to limit all movement. Traditionally, Rolfing addresses this layer quite early in the 10-series as a first approximation in freeing up the structure, before turning attention to the layers of the deep fascia and myofascia underneath. Rolf (1973) states: 'Actual manipulative work with fascia calls to mind the lowly onion. Layer lies within layer. Deeper layers can be affected only as the more superficial ones lose the rigidity that is the signature of imbalance.' Elsewhere, Ida Rolf, in her homely language, calls the work of freeing up the outermost layers 'Taking out the pins'.

The superficial fascia varies considerably throughout the body and takes on specialized roles in different areas. In some places, like the palm of the hand, it is very thin, with a total absence of fat beneath the creases. Here, the close association of the skin with the deep fascia allows little movement or slippage between the layers and makes the palm an excellent surface for gripping objects. In some areas, such as the breasts, the scalp and the soles of the feet, fat is packaged into small connective-tissue compartments. In the soles of the feet this creates a shock-absorbing pad. This same packaging of fat is evident in the dimpling of hips and thighs commonly known as cellulite. It is also this layer that tends to sag in old age as it becomes loosened from the underlying layer.

This layer is easily palpable and, to a greater or lesser degree depending on its fibrosity, may be slid over the underlying layer, the deep fascia. The superficial fascia adheres to the deep fascia but will allow a limited kind of sliding over it, probably only until the fibrous trabeculae connecting the layers become taut. This fact allows us, as structural bodyworkers, to palpate deeper structures by compressing the superficial fascia and sliding it over them.

The deep fascia

Beneath the superficial fascia runs the deep fascia, which is a continuous membrane of dense, irregular connective tissue that flows over the surface of muscles, over superficial bony surfaces (such as the sternum, the anterior surface of the tibia, the iliac crests, the clavicles and so on), and over superficial tendons (such as those of the ankle and wrist). It also branches from the surface occasionally and runs deep to form the sturdier intermuscular septa that separate major functional muscle groups from each other. In the thigh, for instance, it separates the hamstring group from the adductor and quadriceps groups. In a dissected body the deep fascia appears almost as a slick, white second skin or bodystocking, covering the entire surface – bones, muscles and tendons alike – and punctured occasionally by openings or hiatuses through which blood vessels, lymph ducts and nerves enter and leave the superficial fascia. In a freshly dissected body the deep fascia is often transparent but tends to whiten as it dries out; this is the glistening, silvery and extremely tough membrane that you find in some cuts of meat. Sometimes it is delicate, thin and almost invisible; sometimes it is especially thickened in areas that require tensile strength, for example in specialized bands such as the iliotibial tract, the band of Richter or the retinaculae of the ankles and wrists. Occasionally, superficial muscles insert into the deep fascia and influence movement by tightening whole fascial planes. Such muscles include the tensor fasciae latae, the most superficial fibres of the gluteus maximus, the palmaris longus and the platysma.

In his classic treatise on fascial dissection, Gallaudet (1931) describes this layer as:

a sheet of connective tissue varying in thickness and density according to locality. This covers and invests all the so-called higher structures; i.e., muscles and tendons, bursae, vessels, lymph nodes, nerves, viscera, ligaments, joints, and even cartilage and bones, these last by close adhesion to perichondrium and periosteum between the attachment of muscles.

He describes the deep fascia's close adherence to the superficial fascia above, and to the myofascia beneath, by tiny connecting fibrous trabeculae. The trabeculae prevent the complete slippage between and separation of the layers, so that nowhere in the human body can you lift the skin and superficial fascia away from the underlying tissue, as you can, for instance, with a young puppy. Gallaudet also notes that the deep fascia tends to split into separate laminae when it meets a 'higher' structure such as a muscle, reuniting on the other side. This is clearly illustrated in some of the better anatomical atlases: for instance in the beautiful sternocleidomastoid dissection in the Sobotta atlas (Ferner and Staubesand 1982). Gallaudet makes the interesting point that after the deep fascia has been completely reflected (i.e. peeled) from a cadaver, the *epimysium* (the outermost myofascial layer of individual muscles, to be described later) remains intact. Therefore the deep fascia is distinct from (though adhering closely to) the underlying myofascial network, which will now be described.

The myofascial network

Biological entities at all levels tend to have specialized boundaries, or interfaces, that both connect them with and separate them from their surrounding environment, and these are usually membranes of some sort. For muscles, this membrane is the myofascia, which both separates muscles from and connects them to their surrounding musculature. The myofascia packages individual muscles but also forms the internal subdivisions within them. All of the muscles of the body are individually packaged within their myofascial bags, and all of these bags are connected together as one piece; then, as a whole group, they are enclosed entirely within the embrace of the deep fascia. Hence the myofascia meets the deep fascia only at their common, most superficial surfaces. To borrow an analogy from Ida Rolf, if the skin of an orange represents our skin, the superficial and the deep fascia, then the muscles are the individual orange segments and the myofascia is the fibrous membrane that wraps individual orange segments – separating them from each other but also from the skin of the orange (Fig. 9.2).

In Chapter 8 we played with one of the common thought experiments, often used to help visualize the fascial network, in which we imagine a body in which all has been dissolved except the fascia. In this scenario the deep fascia would reveal the overall human shape: the head, the limbs, the trunk and even smaller surface details like the facial details, toes and external genitalia, but also the septa that enclose the major intermuscular compartments. The myofascia, on the other hand, would

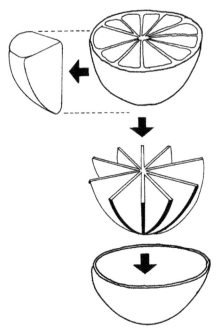

Figure 9.2 Orange analogy from Ida Rolf (Rolf 1977) (reproduced with the kind permission of Alan Demmerle).

reveal the surface outline of each individual muscle as well as its internal fascial structure.

So, while the myofascia wraps and separates the major functional groups of muscles, related forms of fascia form the structural layer of all serous membranes that line the major cavities of the trunk, wrapping and suspending the viscera. Ida Rolf described fascia as 'the organ of support and structure' (1977), and now seems more justified than ever in elevating this network to the level of an organ. Even Gallaudet (1931) suggests that it is more accurately designated as a system.

Since Rolf's early investigations, the fascia has been found to have many functions other than the purely mechanical one of giving form, tensile strength and elasticity to tissue. It also assists in the transport of metabolites, playing host to a variety of cells, and has immunological and other protective functions. It has also been found to have a major biomechanical function in dampening mechanical shocks to the system and in generating rhythmic movement. These properties will be examined in more depth in Chapter 10.

The inner structure of the musculature

Muscles have an extraordinarily complex internal structure that follows a design principle quite widespread in nature and known as fractal patterning. This is the recursive self-duplication of a basic pattern at finer and finer levels of organization. It is found not only in the organization of muscles and nerve trunks, but also in networks that periodically branch or cluster into smaller units of the same intrinsic structure, such as blood vessels, peripheral nerves and bronchioles. In the myofascia this design manifests as 'bags inside bags inside bags'. Alter (1996) illustrates clearly how this recursive patterning continues further down through the contractile and fascial elements, which are the two major sub-components of muscle tissue. The contractile elements start from the myofibril (the basic muscle cell) and fractally divide inwardly through the successively finer elements of the sarcomeres and the myofilaments, and then down to the individual, filamentous macromolecules of the contractile proteins. The fascial elements similarly reduce down from the mature collagen fibre, through the fibril, subfibril, microfibril and the basic tropocollagen molecule.

There are three main levels of muscle organization (see Fig. 9.3). Each muscle is fully enclosed in a tough outer sheath called the *epimysium*. This layer covers the entire belly of the muscle and extends to enclose the outer layers of the muscle tendons, or aponeuroses. Internally, each muscle is composed of long, cylindrical or gently fusiform subcomponents called *fascicles*, each of which is individually wrapped in its own fascial bag called the *perimysium*. Each of these fascicles is a package containing 100–150 muscle fibres, and each muscle fibre is wrapped in its own sheath, the *endomysium*. At each of these three levels within the musculature, the body's 'plumbing' can be found, with nerves and blood vessels traversing these fascial routes (which is a consistent pattern throughout the body). Large vessels are found at the epimysial level and capillaries at the endomysial level. Areolar tissue and intramuscular fat may also be deposited along these routes.

But this subdivision continues further. Muscle fibres are composed of muscle cells, the ultimate contractile unit, and each is individually wrapped in a cell membrane, the sarcolemma, and organized in series along the length of the fibre.

It has been estimated that fascia forms 50–60 per cent of the mass of muscle tissue.

It is important to pause and ponder this fact: that fascia is the abundant, unifying and all-encompassing environment of all muscle cells. This fact alone makes the inherent elasticity of muscles comprehensible and it is important for bodyworkers to realize this. 'Working with fascia' has become a fashionable catchphrase in bodywork circles, and sometimes practitioners talk as if they are working on something other than the musculature; however, they are inseparable aspects of the same system.

Figure 9.4 is a cross-section of the mid-thigh. It illustrates the recursive packaging arrangement of fascial

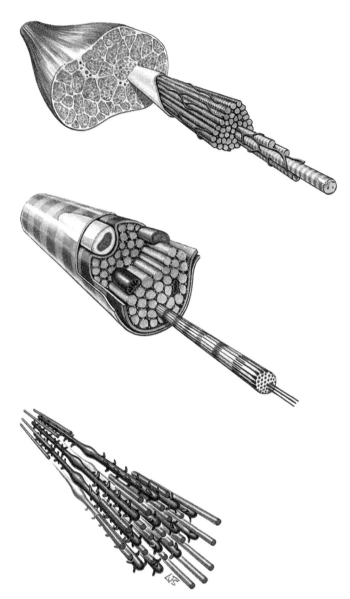

Figure 9.3 The three myofascial levels within the musculature.

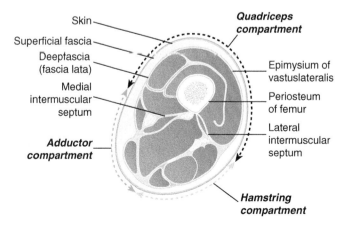

Figure 9.4 Cross section of mid-thigh.

bags. Beneath the skin and superficial fascia is the deep fascia, which in this locality is called the *fascia lata* (or milky fascia in reference to its white colour). It envelops the thigh like a second skin and contains within it the four major myofascial compartments of the thigh: the quadriceps, the hamstrings, the adductor group and the periosteum of the femur itself (which is also a fascial bag enclosing the entire bone). There are also some lesser bags that enclose the sartorius and various neurovascular 'plumbing' routes (every good architect knows that you try to keep all the plumbing together). Within the quadriceps group, the vasti and the rectus femoris are all individually ensheathed within their own epimysial sleeve. Similarly, within the hamstring compartment the hamstrings semimembranosus, semitendinosus and the two heads of the biceps femoris area are each individually wrapped in their own epimysium.

This is a little different from the picture of the musculature that is often portrayed in most anatomical atlases. These texts generally portray muscles as being independent, distinct and individual entities. In fact, the musculature is entirely embedded within a fascial context, and most of the so-called 'individual muscles' are seen as separate only through meticulous dissection and teasing away of the epimysium. As bodyworkers we tend to visualize the 'insides' as they are represented in anatomical texts and atlases. Since most bodyworkers have never performed a dissection, we rely on the representations of anatomical artists who tend to simplify their diagrams to highlight the traditionally accepted or named muscles, and this means stripping away the deep fascia and the superficial epimysium to show the 'important stuff' beneath. It was mentioned at the start of Chapter 6 that our 'maps' are always a simplification, and anatomical illustrations are a prime example; although, of course, this kind of simplification can easily be reasonably justified on educational grounds. Nevertheless, simplification can lead to error. We have inherited and internalized images of the musculature as if all the muscles in the body were separate entities that could glide freely over each other and do their work independently while not affecting their neighbouring muscles. It is much more difficult to visualize and understand the complex dynamics of a system in which *all the muscles are bound together in shared bags*, such that if one muscle shortens it will inevitably drag upon and deform its neighbours.

The traditional structural bodywork representation of the musculature – a potent 'as if'
Ida Rolf freely admitted that many of her explanations as to how her techniques actually work were rationalizations

after the fact (Feitis 1978). Structural bodyworkers from Ida Rolf's time until now have been working with a particular vision of how muscles operate. This idealized conception of the musculature is:

> that in a perfectly functioning body, all muscles are separate entities, each individually wrapped in their own fascial bag, free to glide over neighbouring muscles like silk stockings.

Against this idealized picture of perfect function is juxtaposed a picture of dysfunction in which these independent muscles became 'glued' to each other through injury or abuse, similar to the adhesions known to surgery. According to Rolf:

> following inflammatory illnesses or traumatic injury, layers adhere one to another – they seem to be 'glued' together. They no longer slide but cause adjacent structures to tug on each other, thus contributing to general weariness and tension.

Later, she adds:

> *'Gluing' is an interesting phenomenon. In practically all bodies, on one muscle or another, small lumps or thickened non-resilient bands can be felt deep in the tissue… They apparently form when the fascial envelope of one of the muscles attaches itself to a neighboring fascial surface*

> (Rolf 1977)

This representation of the musculature has entered the consciousness of most bodyworkers; it is powerfully suggested by simplified anatomical drawings and is perpetuated in the teaching of many schools of structural bodywork. This representation of the musculature seems also to have formed the basis for the practical hands-on aspects of structural bodywork in that we use the elbow to break down the adhering layers between muscles and restore the ideal arrangement. A great deal of effective structural bodywork has been performed *as if* this is how muscles work and how they become dysfunctional – a potent 'as if' among many in this field. Yet there is surprisingly little evidence to support this view; it has not been confirmed by cadaveric studies, and for obvious ethical reasons cannot be easily explored in live humans (although it can and has been explored with animals).

'Put it where it belongs and ask for movement'
Ida Rolf gave an enormously powerful practical rule for structural interventions: 'Put it where it belongs and

ask for movement' is one of the so-called 'Rolf laws'. Was she suggesting here that soft tissue can actually be moved around, relocated with respect to adjacent tissues? It is certainly a compelling suggestion, and in a real pragmatic sense it is an extraordinarily useful rule of thumb – another potent 'as if'. If you follow this rule you normally obtain a predictable improvement in functionality, and it is a very practical rule that has been used creatively to augment many different kinds of movement. However, it seems to be based on a picture of muscle tissue that sees each muscle as separated from other surrounding muscles and free to glide over them. This rationale is difficult to maintain if the muscles are bound together in fascial compartments. So what is a more realistic picture of the musculature? If fascial adhesions can develop, just where do they occur? Obviously not in places where there is a natural fascial fusion already. Where are the potential spaces of the myofascial network?

Potential spaces, ectopic bursae and adhesions

What is a potential space in the body? It is a space defined by two surfaces that are in intimate contact yet not bonded, a space that can be opened, like the space between the pages of a closed book. Physics tells us that potential spaces can be very difficult to open as the surfaces are firmly held together by surrounding pressures, and nature abhors a vacuum. This is easily illustrated by trying to separate two sheets of moistened glass. Until the seal is broken the two surfaces cannot be separated, although they can slide over each other. Within the human body, potential spaces tend to be separated by a fine layer of an extracellular fluid such as ground substance, synovial fluid or a specialized surfactant, as in the lung.

An obvious potential space is the scapulo-thoracic articulation, which is the space between the deep surface of the subscapularis and the superficial surface of the serratus anterior. This is a space that allows the necessary sliding of the concave scapula over the convexity of the rib-cage in shoulder-girdle movements such as pushing, punching or reaching (see Fig. 9.5) and, as a potential space, it could conceivably be injected with fluid or with air. There are potential spaces between the visceral organs within the peritoneal bag, again kept separate by a film of fluid. The pleural cavity is another example where there is potential space between the visceral pleura of the lung and the parietal pleura that lines the inside of the thoracic cavity. This potential space likewise has a small amount of fluid separating

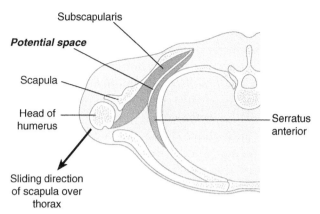

Figure 9.5 Potential space beneath the scapulae.

the lung from the inner wall of the thorax and allows some gliding movement of the surfaces during respiration, but it does not allow them to separate. Occasionally, this potential space can fill with air or bodily fluids, disastrously, as in the case of pneumothorax or collapsed lung.

When there is such a close approximation of internal surfaces, there is the potential for them to become stuck to each other, which is a phenomenon known as adhesion. In medical parlance, *adhesion* has been defined as 'the union of two surfaces that are normally separate, also any fibrous bands that connect them' (O'Toole 1997). This is a well-understood result of abdominal surgery. But adhesions can also occur whenever there is a traumatic interference with any organ boundary, whether through surgery, disease, excessive friction or impact injury. The normal inflammatory processes of granulation and fibrous infiltration can fuse together surfaces that should be separated by a potential space. So where are the true potential spaces within the musculoskeletal system? What are the layers that, ideally, should glide over each other? Can the deep tissue techniques employed by structural bodyworkers actually free up such adhesions? Or are the measurable improvements achieved through soft-tissue mobilization more likely the result of bringing increased resilience to the fascia, rather than a breaking down of hypothesized adhesions?

Surprisingly little has been written about potential spaces within the myofascial system (Prof C dos Remedios, personal communication 2002). We know of large bursal areas, between the scapulae and thorax for instance, as well as ectopic (or floating) bursae, such as those over the greater trochanters. If we take the quadriceps compartment in the thigh as an example, the four 'named' muscles are entirely enclosed within the fascial bag defined by four fascial boundaries: the fascia lata, the two intermuscular septa and the periosteum of the femur (see Fig. 9.4). Therefore, if the quadriceps shorten they will inevitably drag upon other structures that are bound to the common septa. If there is any suggestion of independent or sliding movement between muscles, in this instance it must be between muscles within this bag: that is, between the individual quadriceps. Cadaveric studies have shown that areolar and adipose tissue can be deposited between the fascicles. We can speculate that this will allow some sliding movement between adjacent fascicles in the same way that we can slide the areolar tissue of the superficial fascia over the deep fascia in a limited way. Some authors have suggested that there may be a fluid separation of the fascicles (St George 2001). Dissection of freshly killed animals does tend to suggest that there is a lot of fluid between muscles and they can be easily separated (C Rossi, personal communication 2002).

Anatomist and Rolfer, Gil Hedley, through many dissections of cadavers (which were mostly elderly specimens), has made some interesting remarks about the daily turnover of collagen threads and the build-up of connective tissue. From his dissections he notes that, by and large, over time, structures will tend to adhere to each other, and although some can be teased apart with gentle finger pressure, some require a scalpel. 'There are certain tissue textures that yield readily to your hand or finger. Cotton candy, gossamer threads that are very thin like spider webs. If you touch them they disappear', but in other areas 'You end up having this big solid muck that has cemented the one to the other' (Hedley 1999). He suggests that with lengthy periods of immobilization these fibres will accumulate, become dense and complex, and attract fat deposits. He notes, however, that even in cadavers movement will dissolve the threads.

So a picture is emerging in which there is a continuous turnover of collagen threads – threads that will disperse with movement, or solidify with immobility. Movement is the key.

THE CONNECTIVE TISSUES

The fascial network belongs to the family of tissues in the body called the connective tissues, of which there is an extraordinarily diverse range of forms throughout the body. As a class, these tissues form the most pervasive network within the human body: wrapping, separating, interpenetrating, connecting, supporting all anatomical structures, and forming about 60% of the weight of the body (Heller 1990). This network is even more extensive than the already prodigiously branching vascular and nerve networks. Various imaging techniques have demonstrated the extraordinary density and fineness of the branching networks of our vascular and nervous systems, which seem to proliferate exponentially towards their extremities (see Fig. 9.6). Connective tissues, however, penetrate even further into more 'nooks and crannies' of the body than either of these two systems and, in fact, form the supportive superstructures of both of them: nerve trunks and blood vessels have their own supporting connective tissues. Connective tissues are the matrix in which all else is embedded.

The biomedical view of connective tissue

Connective tissues are usually classified as one of four fundamental tissue types. The Tortora and Grabowski map (Fig. 6.1, p. 38) represents the view in which the four types of tissue are characterized by the unique functions of their cells:

- connective tissue has cells that secrete the structural materials of the body
- muscle tissue has cells that are contractile
- nervous tissue has cells that are irritable
- epithelial tissue has cells that line and secrete vital biochemicals.

However, there is something more elementary about connective tissue; it is the environment in which all the other tissues are created and maintained and, unlike the other three types, connective tissues are substantially non-cellular, consisting mostly of secreted extracellular materials. None of the other three tissue types could exist apart from this matrix. Muscle tissue, for instance, is a composite of contractile cells and their enveloping myofascial meshwork. It is impossible for these contractile cells to generate movement without the unifying presence of their myofascial environment: the epimysial, perimysial and endomysial layers. This fascial framework harnesses the contractile force of all the active muscle cells and gives direction to their combined force, transmitting it to the tendons and beyond. Nervous tissue similarly does not exist independently of its supporting connective tissues. Nerves are enwreathed and supported by connective tissue membranes: for example, the meninges of the brain and spinal cord and the fascia of peripheral nerves, which have a three-level fascial structure that closely resembles that of muscle and consists of the *epineurium, perineurium*

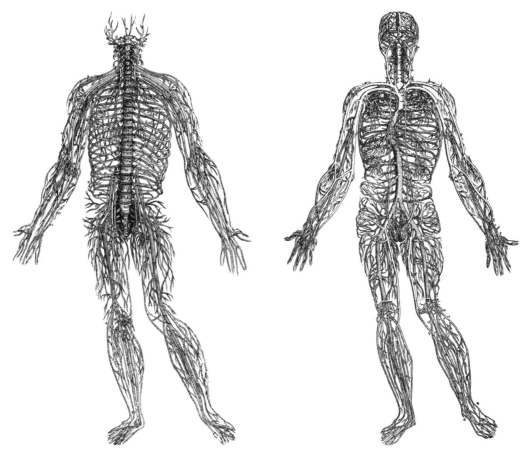

Figure 9.6 The nerve and vascular networks.

and *endoneurium* (see Fig. 9.7). Epithelial tissues, such as the mucous membranes, similarly could not maintain their integrity without the adhesive support of the basement membrane (basal lamina). This is the underlying layer of connective tissue that binds them into continuous sheets or into the globular form of glands. This layer also provides nutrients to epithelial membranes, which are avascular and can only receive nutrients that diffuse through the basement membrane. So there is a sense in which connective tissues are the most fundamental tissue type.

Nearly all connective tissues arise from mesoderm, the middle germ layer that forms between the ectoderm and endoderm in the developing embryo (see Fig. 8.1, p. 49). Developmentally, all structures are guided in growth by connective tissue templates. Bones grow either within a cartilage template or within a fascial matrix; connective tissues form the scaffolding on which muscle fibres form (Schultz and Feitis 1996). The reason that nerves and blood vessels are so often found following along fascial planes is that their growth was originally guided along the plane of a primitive fascial template.

Connective tissues display an extraordinary continuity between all the various structural levels of the body. At the grossest level they maintain the form of the entire organism, containing all within the superficial and deep fascial layers; they provide the structural support for all individual organs, in many cases individually subpartitioning the organs into finer and finer functional divisions; they form the superstructure for the other three tissue types; they are the basic cellular glue at the cellular level of our organization, and, as Oschman (2000) has shown, they can even connect into the microfilamentous superstructure of individual cells.

Connective tissues as composite materials

As outlined in Chapter 8, all connective tissues consist primarily of an extracellular matrix, permeated with a scattering of isolated cells that rarely contact one another. The extracellular matrix itself is a highly variable composite material that nevertheless always contains at least

- some fibrous elements
- a form of the amorphous 'ground substance'.

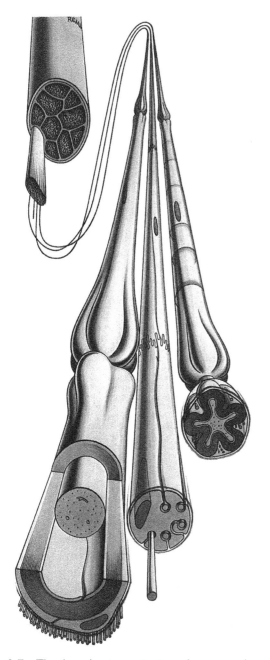

Figure 9.7 The three-level organization of nerve trunks.

Reinforced concrete, for instance, combines the tensile strength of steel with the compressive strength of the surrounding concrete to produce a composite that has the combined properties of the original materials, being strong both in compression and tension. Fibreglass consists of glass fibre embedded within a resinous filler. These materials are almost a case of technology imitating life, since bodies have been making these experiments from time immemorial and have succeeded in creating some remarkable and unique composite materials. Connective tissues have close parallels with some of the composite materials used in industry (S Evanko, personal communication 2002).

The fibrous elements in connective tissue are of three basic kinds: collagen fibres, elastin fibres and reticulin.

1. Collagen will be looked at in greater detail later but, briefly, it is the most abundant fibre within the connective tissue network, forming more than a third of the total protein in the body. It has great tensile strength and is very flexible, even though individual collagen fibres have little inherent elasticity.
2. Elastin, as its name implies, is an elastic fibre, able to lengthen up to one-and-a-half times its unstressed length. It is present in tissues that must resume their shape after stretching.
3. Reticulin is a chemically modified form of collagen that has strands of a much smaller diameter and length than collagen fibres. It is a lighter material that forms the delicate reticular superstructure of the visceral organs.

Ground substance is the ubiquitous, transparent, gooey lubricant of the body that pervades the fibrous elements in the connective tissue matrix and keeps it hydrated. Juhan (1987) distinguishes ground substance from other intercellular fluids that are derived from blood plasma. Ground substance is derived from fibroblastic cells and becomes 'the retort in which all extracellular activities occur'. It is a gel or colloidal substance that contains various water-soluble carbohydrate–protein complexes and can have a wide range of viscosities. It consists of about 75 per cent water and the rest is made up of macromolecules – mostly glycosaminoglycans (GAGs), proteoglycans and glycoproteins. This class of substance tends to be electrostatically attracted to collagen and to have an immense capacity to attract and bind water. The GAG content of connective tissues tends to decrease with age, which is the reason that the tissues of the elderly can become dehydrated and lose their extensibility.

Although these are the basic ingredients, there may be additional elements. Bone, for instance, contains other extracellular materials such as crystalline deposits of bone salts, tricalcium phosphate and calcium carbonate in particular.

We are familiar with composite materials in industry. Our technologists are continually combining materials of diverse properties in order to create new materials that have at least the amalgamated properties of their elements, and perhaps other ones besides. Examples are reinforced concrete, fibrous cement and fibreglass.

GAGs are essentially complex carbohydrate polymers, usually with an attached protein group. They may be unsulphated (hyaluronic acid being the main example) or sulphated (chondroitin, dermatan, heparan, heparin, and keratan sulphates). Hyaluronic acid is a slippery cellular glue that has a lubricating role, particularly in the synovial fluid of joints. The sulphated GAGs are jelly-like substances that have the remarkable property of actively attracting water molecules and binding them in specific arrays around themselves; they are hydrophilic. They help maintain fluid balance within connective tissues, keeping them 'juicy' and providing a lubricating role in the potential spaces of the body, thereby minimizing friction by allowing the free gliding of layers.

Proteoglycans are complex macromolecules consisting of GAGs linked to a core protein. Like GAGs they are intensely hydrophilic. They exert an enormous swelling pressure, which in a fully hydrated form as a component of cartilage tissue can resist massive compressive forces. Glycoproteins are also carbohydrate–protein complexes that have diverse functions, including a role as a basic cellular glue, examples being laminin and fibronectin.

In the connective tissue composites, ground substance acts as the spacer (like the plastic resin of fibreglass) by holding the fibres apart and preventing them from 'matting down', compacting and becoming glued together. It thus maintains a 'critical interfibre distance' between collagen fibres, preventing microadhesions and thereby maintaining the resilience of the tissue. Ground substances also have a key role in the nutrition of cells in transporting dissolved nutrients and metabolic by-products while providing a barrier to microorganisms. It is also no longer believed to be an inert mechanical barrier, but to have an active role in assisting the passage of certain compounds while resisting the movement of pathogens, similar to the way in which water filtration systems allow the free passage of certain sized particles but not others.

Types of connective tissue

Histologists have classified the connective tissues in various ways. This fact is hardly surprising when one considers the huge range of functions these tissues perform and the great diversity of local variation in the specific needs that they fulfil. Figure 9.8 shows the place of connective tissues in the map of Tortora and Grabowski (1993). These authors sub-classify connective tissues as follows:

I.   Embryonic connective tissue
   A.   Mesenchyme
   B.   Mucous connective tissue
II. Mature connective tissue
   A.   Loose connective tissue
      1.   Areolar connective tissue

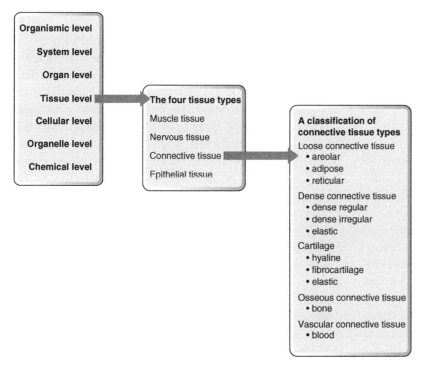

Figure 9.8 The place of connective tissues within the Grabowski–Tortora map.

2. Adipose tissue
3. Reticular connective tissue
B. Dense connective tissue
   1. Dense regular connective tissue
   2. Dense irregular connective tissue
   3. Elastic connective tissue
C. Cartilage
   1. Hyaline cartilage
   2. Fibrocartilage
   3. Elastic cartilage
D. Bone (osseous) tissue
E. Blood (vascular tissue)

As structural bodyworkers it is the loose and dense forms of mature connective tissue that are of most interest to us; they are most relevant to our work, being most accessible to change through mechanical intervention.

Loose connective tissue
Under the microscope, loose connective tissues are distinguished by having a sparser distribution of fibres and a larger proportion of cells than the others types. The fibres form a loosely woven and randomly oriented three-dimensional network that is maintained in suspension by the jelly-like ground substance.

Areolar connective tissue
This contains all three kinds of connective tissue fibre: collagen, elastin and reticulin. It is widespread in the body, forming the superficial fascial layer beneath the skin, and mucous and serous membranes elsewhere. It plays a key role in the function of our musculature, where, in combination with the fascia, it lines muscle walls, allowing some independent movement between adjacent muscles.

Adipose tissue
This is widespread throughout the body and forms an important part of the superficial fascia. Adipose cells store globules of fat that can pad and insulate the skin and also serve as a site for food storage. It is also a kind of general-purpose packaging material for internal organs and similar in function to the polystyrene 'macaroni' in which we package loose articles for postage to stop them rattling around. There is for instance a 'fat pack' that surrounds and supports the kidneys and glues them to the back of the abdominal cavity. There are also fat pads behind the eyes, hence the 'sunken eyes' of people who lose weight quickly. Fat also fills in

spaces around joints and in, and between, muscles (think of the marbled cuts at the butcher shop).

Reticular connective tissue
Composed chiefly of reticulin fibres, this forms the superstructure (or stroma) of organs such as the liver, pancreas and lymph nodes.

It was mentioned earlier that loose forms of connective tissue can be of significance to the structural bodyworker, particularly if there is an increase in density in the superficial fascia; however, it is probably through affecting the dense connective tissues that we can achieve most effect.

Dense connective tissue
Dense connective tissue is marked by a greater density of fibres within the matrix and fewer cells than the loose forms. The fibres themselves are thicker and in closer contact with adjacent fibres. Geometrically they form either parallel or latticed arrays, and may exist in laminated layers with an oblique arrangement of fibres at each layer.

Dense regular connective tissue
This forms key structures such as tendons, aponeuroses and ligaments. The collagen fibres are aligned in ordered arrays, either parallel or close to parallel. This allows the tissue to resist tensile pulls through the long axis of the fibres. Sometimes there is a wave-like crimp to the array that allows a small degree of lengthening.

Dense irregular connective tissue
This forms most of the tensile sheets within the body: the fasciae, joint capsules, the periosteum of bones, the perichondrium of cartilage, heart valves and the heart's investing pericardium, as well as organ capsules such as those of the kidneys. The fibres are mostly collagen and tend to be randomly oriented to resist tensile pulls from various directions. Such latticed arrays contain cross-linkages, or fibres that criss-cross other fibres, fusing at their intersections (possibly through covalent bonding) and knitting them together to form a meshed or latticework structure (Fig. 9.9).

Elastic connective tissue
This forms the key structures of the body in which an elastic recoil is of prime importance: the ligamentum flavum of the spine, the nuchal ligament, the elastic walls of arteries, vocal chords and the bronchioles. The tissue is composed mostly of branching elastin fibres that give these tissues their characteristic yellow colour.

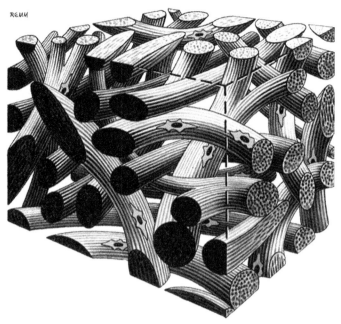

REMM

Figure 9.9 Dense connective tissue (Grays Anatomy 1973).

Having true elasticity, these fibres allow the tissue to regain its original form after being deformed.

Functions of connective tissue

So far we have spoken mostly about the structural importance of connective tissues. They have been found, however, to have a vast range of functions other than simply providing structural support to the body. It was noted earlier that connective tissues are evident at every level of our structural organization, in fact at all of the structural levels outlined in Fig. 6.1 (p. 38), so it can be expected that they should have different emergent functions at each level, from the microscopic to the macroscopic. At a cellular level they have metabolic, immunological, reconstructive and nutritional functions; at the organ level they supply the structural framework that gives stable yet pliant form to organs, and may both package and insulate them. At the organismic level they have important gross biomechanical functions and also provide vital proprioceptive information to the central nervous system.

Connective tissues:

- provide pathways for fluid nutrients and waste metabolites to pass to and from the blood stream, and are thus the main supply route to the more avascular regions of the body
- serve to quarantine infected tissue by providing a semi-permeable barrier to pathogens, thereby delaying the spread of infection

- provide storage sites for metabolic food in the form of fat
- have a protective and immunological function, by harbouring protective cells such as phagocytes, leukocytes, mast cells and fibroblasts
- have a key function in tissue repair after injury or inflammation
- provide vital information to the central nervous system about the forces acting through them (all connective tissues excepting cartilage are richly supplied with nerve endings)
- form the gross wrapping and containment environment at all levels
- assist in cushioning compressive forces within the structure and in resisting tensile forces
- provide a means of recycling the kinetic energy present in the moving structural body by generating oscillatory movement patterns.

Structures composed of connective tissue

All anatomical entities contain connective tissue; however, there are some structures that are composed almost exclusively of it. Their mechanical properties are determined entirely by different combinations of the basic elements, particularly the proportions and types of fibres and ground substance. The structures that consist almost entirely of connective tissue are:

- bones, including cartilage and its fibrous coating, the periosteum
- ligaments, which approximate bone to bone
- tendons and aponeuroses which link muscle to bone or, in a few cases, muscle to fascia
- fascia, the universal wrapping substance of the body
- interosseous membranes which couple contiguous bones
- bursal sacs: flattened, fluid-filled fascial bags that serve to reduce friction in key positions in the body
- synovial capsules that encapsulate and hermetically seal synovial joints
- retinaculae, which reinforce key areas that overlay tendons.

Although this list suggests that these structural elements exist as separate entities, dissection often does not reveal such sharp distinctions. They are all interconnected. As Hedley (1999) notes, there is a certain arbitrariness in the naming of any key connective tissue structures. If we take ligaments, for instance, there are so many specialized thickenings in the connective tissue that we could easily justify having more 'named'

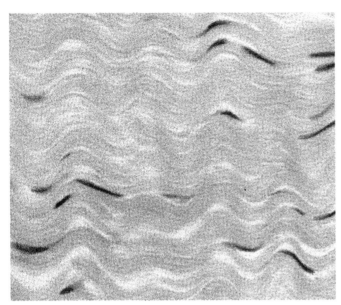

Figure 9.10 Tendon.

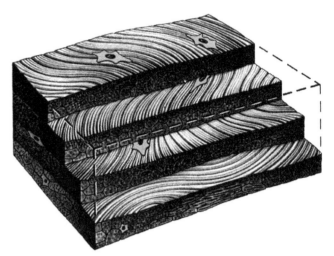

Figure 9.11 Ligament (Grays Anatomy 1973).

ligaments than we have already. We need to keep this in mind when discussing the following structures, since they are sometimes a matter of definition.

Tendons

Tendons are the convergence of all the myofascial structures within the body of a muscle; a gathering together of all the fascial strands of the epimysium, perimysium and endomysium towards the ends of the muscle. They are extraordinarily tough and pliable cords but have little inherent elasticity so as to more efficiently conduct the force of contraction through to the adjoining bone. Too much elasticity would make the timing and coordination of movements very difficult, and yet they are pliable enough to go around corners almost at right angles – beneath the ankle retinaculae for instance. They have a parallel alignment of collagen fibres with a crimped pattern that, magnified, resembles bundles of undulating ribbons. This crimp allows a minor degree of elasticity under tension since the fibres are able to straighten to a limited extent (see Fig. 9.10).

Some tendons, such as the wrist flexors, are enclosed within synovial sheaths that serve to minimize friction as the tendon slides within; others such as the calcaneal tendon are continuous with surrounding areolar tissue, and this has a similar action of minimizing friction.

Ligaments

Ligaments provide stability to joints and oblige them to work through a limited range of motion and to resist forces from many directions. They consist of layered or laminated straps of mostly collagen fibres organized in a slightly less than parallel arrangement. They are less regular in their fibrous configuration than tendons. Their fibres may spiral or layer themselves into oblique arrangements as in Fig. 9.11.

Fascia

The word fascia is derived from the Latin word *fascis* meaning 'bundle'. This name is descriptive of the bundled appearance of the collagen fibre bundles under magnification. Structural bodyworkers think of influencing two kinds of fascia: the deep fascia or bodystocking, and the myofascial network, particularly the more easily reached and worked aspects of the epimysium. In the epimysium the collagen fibres tend to encircle the belly of the muscle but become more parallel with the axis as they reach the tendinous ends. This concentric arrangement around the muscle belly demonstrates just one aspect of the body's ability to recycle the elastic energy of fascia. As a muscle contracts the diameter of the belly increases, thereby tensing the concentric fascial grain. On the muscle's relaxation this stretched fascia squeezes the belly back into shape and assists the muscle to return to its resting length. It may be surmized that this 'pumping' action also promotes circulation throughout the muscle tissue (Fig. 9.12).

The collagen fibres of the major fascial sheaths, however, tend to be oriented in various directions, reflecting the need to resist tensional vectors from many directions. Despite the fact that collagen fibre itself is relatively inextensible, the composite, fascia, has a high degree of flexibility and extensibility; the reasons for this will be discussed later.

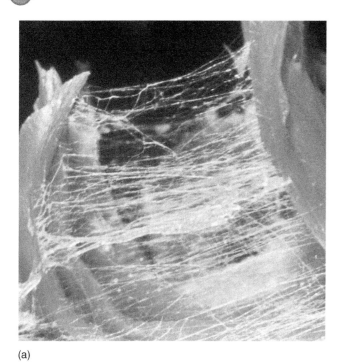

(a)

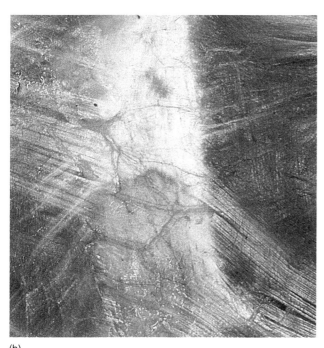

(b)

Figure 9.12   Fascia (Ron Thomson).

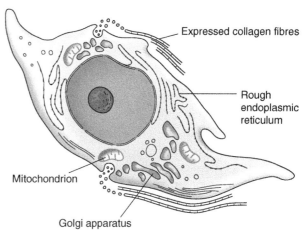

Figure 9.13   Fibroblast.

Expressed collagen fibres

Rough endoplasmic reticulum

Mitochondrion

Golgi apparatus

The histology of connective tissue

Although we have stressed the relative scarcity of cells within the connective tissue matrix, the cells that do reside within the extracellular matrix are vital for its continued functioning. A variety of cells are hosted: some that are stationary and glued to fibres, and some that have a wandering brief.

The main types of cells found within connective tissue are:

- factory cells – fibroblasts, osteoblasts and chondroblasts
- adipocytes or fat cells
- macrophages
- mast cells, which secrete hormones such as histamine, seratonin and heparin
- plasma cells, which are part of the immune system and secrete antibodies
- leukocytes, which are also known as white blood cells.

Fibroblast cells

Fibroblasts (Fig. 9.13) are the most common cell within connective tissue. They are spindle-shaped and manufacture and express all the complex substances used in building connective tissues, that is, the macromolecules that make up both the fibrous and ground substance elements. Related cells, osteoblasts, are specific to the building and maintenance of bone, while chondroblasts build the fibrous component of cartilage. Juhan (1987) comments on the exceptional functionality of fibroblasts, noting that they are unique in being the only cells in the body 'which retain throughout our lives the unique property of being able to migrate to any point in the body, adjust their internal chemistry in response to local conditions, and begin manufacturing specific forms of structural tissue that are appropriate to that area'.

Fat cells

Fat cells are the next most common cell in connective tissue. They are specialized in storing triglycerides, a major energy reserve of the body. They are globular in shape and contain a sac that may be more or less filled with liquid fat. The nucleus and other organelles tend to be squeezed around the cells' periphery.

Macrophages

Macrophages (or 'big eaters') are the reserve foot soldiers of the body, awaiting a call to action. They are generally embedded within the matrix, attached to fibres, but may become mobilized in response to injury, infection or inflammation. Their job is to clear the system of damaged tissue, such as frayed, fragmented or redundant collagen fibres, but they also scavenge for organic foreign elements such as bacteria, splinters and other foreign objects that end up in the body. They thus play a major part in the regeneration of damaged tissue. They attack these materials by engulfing and digesting them in a process known as phagocytosis.

Mast cells

Mast cells comprise about one tenth of the cell population of connective tissue and are found mostly in loose connective tissue. These cells secrete important hormones such as histamine, serotonin and heparin, which are all released during local inflammation. Histamine is of particular interest to manual therapists since it is released in response to localized pressure into tissue and has the function of dilating the local capillaries, increasing the throughput of blood in the area and flushing metabolites away. This vasodilation process gives rise to the characteristic skin redness that follows deep tissue work. It is important in promoting the healing of damaged tissue and in easing localized ischaemic conditions.

About collagen

Collagen fibres are found in nearly all connective tissues but are particularly abundant in cartilage, ligaments, tendons, fasciae and bone. As of 1988, eleven different collagens have been discovered, each genetically distinct (Miller 1988). According to Juhan (1987):

> *Collagen is the longest molecule that has ever been isolated; if one were as thick as a pencil, it would be a yard long. If ever a molecule was designed to make netting and cable, this is it.*

Collagen is manufactured within fibroblasts. Here, collagen precursor molecules, procollagen, are synthesized within the endoplasmic reticulum of fibroblastic cells from available amino acids. These intertwine into a triple helix configuration, forming tropocollagen, a three-ply rope of great strength. These molecules are then expressed into the intercellular space where they polymerize with other tropocollagen molecules to form collagen fibrils, which then aggregate to form individual collagen fibres – a whole of great tensile strength. Vitamin C is essential in this process, and the collagen formation will be depressed if there is a significant deficiency. Vitamin C deficiency diseases such as scurvy are marked by disorders of connective tissue metabolism and can result in weak bones, loosened teeth, fragile capillaries and the compromised healing of wounds.

Collagen has some remarkable properties. It has a tensile strength greater than steel; this means that its individual fibres are very inelastic. They are however remarkably flexible and will bend easily, even though they do not stretch. So how can we then explain the great elasticity found in collagen-based structures, such as fascia, and the lesser elasticity found in ligaments and tendons? This is due more to the particular geometric arrangement of the fibres in the fabric of the tissue. In tendons the fibres are arranged in parallel arrays with a built in crimp (see Fig. 9.10). This allows some lengthening through a straightening out of the crimp. In fascia however it is the latticed arrangement of the fibres that allows extensibility.

Consider the timber lattice in Figure 9.14. Such lattices are popular building items and are commonly used for privacy screening. The diagram demonstrates how a

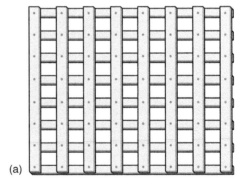

(a)

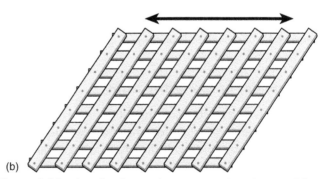

(b)

Figure 9.14 A timber lattice demonstrates how inextensible elements can combine to form a structure that can be deformed.

structural arrangement composed totally of *inextensible* elements can be deformed, in this case by the coupled action of lengthening and narrowing. In this instance, the original shape is not elastically recoverable; it will not return to its original shape unless pushed. But if we take the plastic version of the same latticework structure, often used in gardens for supporting vines, we see how the fused joints give elasticity to the whole arrangement, and it will return to its original shape after being deformed (Fig. 9.15). Figure 9.16 is an electron micrograph of collagen fibres. Note its similarity in structure with the lattices and how the micro-adhesions (known technically as cross-links) fuse the criss-crossed fibres into a latticed arrangement. One can also visualize the spaces between the fibres filled with the gelatinous ground substance and can see that as the tissue is deformed it will tend to squeeze the ground substance around, turning it into a hydraulic 'dampener', and thereby delaying the immediacy of a stretch. Yet another useful analogy is the silk stocking. Silk is a polymerized, macromolecular protein like collagen, and like collagen has a tensile strength greater than steel; yet consider the spring and 'give' of a silk stocking. Its elasticity is due to the woven arrangement of the silk fibres rather than to any inherent elasticity in individual silk fibres. This same principle is expressed in the well-known 'snagged cardigan' diagram (Fig. 9.17) from Ida Rolf's book (Rolf 1973).

Connective tissues and aging

Changes within the connective tissue network typically occur with the aging process, most commonly as an overall loss of fluidity and extensibility. Muscles become less extensible as muscle fibres begin to be replaced with fat and collagen. As the collagen content of muscles increases the collagen itself becomes more crystalline and less flexible; there is an increased 'matting down' of fibres and more cross-linkages are formed. There is a gradual loss of the GAGs within the ground substance, which impairs the tissue's ability to retain water and leads to a dehydration of the tissues. This occurs throughout the connective tissue network, with fascial sheaths, spinal ligaments and arterial walls all tending to become less extensible with age.

With aging, there is also an increase in mineralization of the tissues. Metal salts, particularly of calcium, tend to be deposited between the collagen fibres of ligaments, tendons and fascial sheaths, in a manner similar to that in which bone is formed. This process is usually

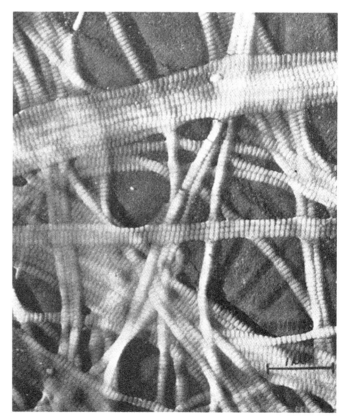

Figure 9.16 An electron micrograph of collagen (from W M Copernhaver, R P Bunge, M B Bunge 1995, *Bailey's textbook of histology*, Lippincott, Williams & Wilkins, Baltimore).

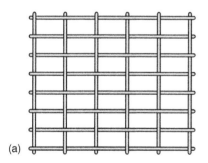

(a)

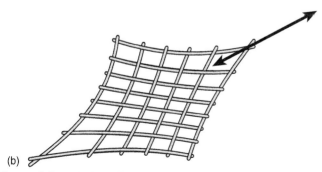

(b)

Figure 9.15 A plastic lattice that does recover its shape after deformation.

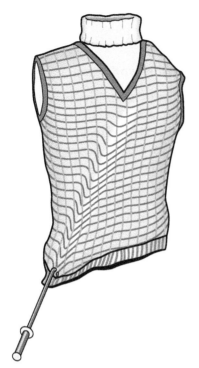

Figure 9.17 The snagged cardigan analogy demonstrating how strain patterns communicate throughout the whole system (Rolf 1977).

attributed to the decreased movement and inadequate circulation common in older age groups, leading to a low-level ischaemic condition in the tissues, which gives rise to areas of reduced biological energy. This reduced circulation contributes to an increasingly acidic metabolic environment; metabolites like lactic and carbonic acids in particular remain too long in the tissues, encouraging both fibrosis and the precipitation of minerals. Tendons and ligaments stiffen and try to become bone; bone spurs form. Elastin also tends to thicken, fray and attract calcium deposits. The calcification of spinal ligaments accounts in part for the increased spinal rigidity found among many seniors; such restriction along our vital axis can be devastating, limiting both movement and respiration.

Many authors have suggested that such degeneration is not inevitable, or at least not so early in life (Hanna 1988). It all points to the need to keep moving. Certainly the descent into rigidity is accelerated when people stop moving, believing this to be an inevitable part of aging. The old adage of 'Use it or lose it' certainly applies.

At the end of Chapter 8 it was concluded that the distinguishing feature of structural bodyworkers is that they attempt to influence the overall structural organization of the body by inducing changes within the fascial network. We will now examine the microstructure of fascia and look at some of its mechanical characteristics to see why it is so plastic.

FOCUSSING ON FASCIA – THE DOMAIN OF THE STRUCTURAL BODYWORKER

Fascia is a specialized tissue in the whole family of connective tissues. Fascial sheaths are continuous and interweave all structures from the dermis to the periosteum. They not only invest and interpenetrate all muscle tissue, but also blend seamlessly with tendons, ligaments and the periosteum of bones. Fascia is the universal wrapping substance of the body. Fascial sheaths are completely continuous and one can reach any part of the body by tracing a path through it. Juhan (1987) calls fascia the *metamembrane* of the body: the 'binding, containing, and shape-giving connective tissue of the body'; he compares it to the function of cellulose in the plant world, which in that realm is the all-pervasive substance of form. However, of all the connective tissues, fascia is the most plastic and open to mechanical change, and is therefore of great interest to structural bodyworkers.

Like all connective tissues, fascia consists of cells (relatively few), ground substance and fibres. It forms membranes of varying densities. Its fabric is composed of interlinking collagen, reticulin and elastin fibres, separated from each other by ground substance. Depending on the structural requirements of the fascia in any area of the body, the fibres can be arranged in parallel to achieve great tensile strength in one direction or organized more into a latticed arrangement to resist stresses from several directions.

We have known for some time that the joint capsules are densely innervated and contain specialized mechanoreceptors that respond to deforming forces within the joint. Recent microscopy has shown that fascia too is highly innervated; it contains myelinated and non-myelinated axons, autonomic nerve fibres, sensory nerve endings and even isolated smooth muscle cells (Schleip 2003). In fact, fascia is one of the most highly innervated systems within the body and it provides a vital source of the kinaesthetic feedback required by the CNS in regulating bodily movement.

Fascia has some unique mechanical characteristics, particularly in its short and medium term response to deforming stresses, and in its extraordinary ability to intelligently modify its own structure in the longer-term to accommodate more efficiently the forces that pass through it. It is self-adapting and self-organizing.

Fascia responds to stress – an extension of Wolff's Law

Fascia shares many features, functional as well as histological, with its connective tissue sister, bone. Neither are inert, and in both there is a continuous turnover of their basic materials. Both respond very intelligently to the stresses that act through them and can actually modify their own structural properties to more efficiently deal with these stresses. Discussing this intelligent plasticity of fascia, Oschman (1989) notes that:

> These changes are of two sorts. First, an overloaded structure may have been gradually reinforced by the laying down of extra collagen fibers… Alternately, some structures may not have been used at their normal capacity; and their fabric becomes, therefore, slowly reduced by the removal of some collagen fibers.

Within the fascial matrix, macrophages are constantly debriding damaged or redundant collagen fibres while fibroblasts are laying down new collagen fibrils where extra support or tensile strength is needed. As new collagen fibrils mature they tend to align themselves along the lines of mechanical stress that pass through the tissue stresses which arise chiefly from the action of the muscles themselves. They may perhaps be guided by the piezoelectric induced fields that surround collagen under stress. Some authors have extended the parameters of Wolff's law to include fascia (Cantu and Grodin 1992). Wolff's law is an early observation about the response of bone to mechanical stress, and states:

> The form of the bone being given, the bone elements (collagen) place or displace themselves in the direction of the functional pressure and increase or decrease their mass to reflect the amount of functional pressure.
>
> (Wolff 1892)

The structure of the entire connective tissue network is in constant flux, so that fascia, like the 'shrink-wrap' plastic sheeting used in the packaging industry, is constantly remoulding itself to conform to our average shape and our everyday patterns of usage.

The metabolic flux of fascia

The opposing forces of synthesis and dissolution, anabolism and catabolism, are an unceasing aspect of our internal chemistry while we live. Drawing upon isotopic evidence, Chopra (1991) notes that, 'Every year, fully 98 percent of the total number of atoms in your body are replaced.' Imagine a house in which a bricklayer is permanently employed in switching bricks: removing them from one part of the house, lodging them elsewhere, discarding some bricks and introducing some new ones. This seems uneconomical to the extreme, so why does the body need to keep its materials in constant flux? What is the biological advantage? Ida Rolf (1977) suggested:

> Connective tissues, particularly the fasciae, are in a never-ending state of reorganization. The continuous metabolic interchange made possible through the intimate relation of fascia with water metabolism allows structural reorganization.

Oschman (1989) proposed:

> Each part of the body, from the smallest to the largest has an average life span ranging from minutes to years; but all structures are always being recreated. This endless cycle of renewal provides a biochemical basis for plasticity; it enables the body to change its shape in response to the ways it is being used.

and he later added the suggestion that metabolic regeneration permitted the rapid adaptation of an organism's structure in response to changes in movement patterns. (Oschman 2000).

Some views on the plasticity of fascia

Ida Rolf was quite explicit about what she believed to be the physiological basis of the great plasticity of the fascial network:

> While fascia is characteristically a tissue of collagen fibers, these fibers must be visualized as embedded in ground substance. For the most part, the latter is an amorphous semifluid gel. The collagen fibers are demonstrably slow to change and are a definite chemical entity. Therefore, the speed so clearly apparent in fascial change must be a property of its complex ground substance… The observable speed of the changes that are induced supports this hypothesis in the light of what we know about the action of colloids and the physical laws governing them. The application of pressure is, in fact, the addition of energy to the tissue colloid. (It is well known in physics that the addition of energy can turn colloid gel into sol).
>
> (Rolf 1977)

This is the so-called 'sol–gel hypothesis' of fascial plasticity.

Authors since Rolf have used the term *thixotropy* to describe the tendency of gels to undergo a phase transition, from gel to sol or sol to gel, by the addition or subtraction of energy, particularly heat energy (Juhan 1987).

This is the same kind of phenomenon as the thinning of oil paint through the mechanical action of stirring. The techniques of structural bodywork usually involve the application of deep slow pressure into the tissues and, according to the sol–gel hypothesis, the mechanical energy derived from pressure is converted to heat energy within the tissues, which induces the phase shift. Oschman (2000) discusses more recent evidence that suggests that sol–gel transitions can result in increased hydration of tissues, leaving a ground substance that is 'more porous, a better medium for the diffusion of nutrients, oxygen, waste products of metabolism, and the enzymes and building-blocks involved in the "metabolic regeneration" process'. He suggests that in the sol–gel phase transition, fibres that may have become shortened or kinked can be freed to their original length, thereby increasing the extensibility of the tissue. He further notes how this same process can release toxins that may have been trapped in tissues for years, which is a proposition that has long been advanced by bodyworkers (and often leads to the parting advice after a particularly deep session: 'Keep the fluids up'). That there is a dramatic change to tissues from this approach is beyond dispute; the actual physical laws and mechanisms at work, however, are disputed.

There has been considerable research into the biomechanics of connective tissue (Alexander 1975, 1988; Cantu and Grodin 1992; Alter 1996). Connective tissues display viscoelastic properties; that is, they have the dual properties of *viscosity* and *elasticity.* Viscosity refers to the degree of stickiness in a semi-fluid substance; its ability to flow. Chewing gum, for instance, can be lengthened and will remain lengthened. Elasticity, on the other hand, refers to the degree to which a substance can resume its original length after deformation or stretching, like a rubber band. But how can a substance have both properties? It is all about timing. For fasciae, a quick stretch and release means that there will be a true elastic response and the tissue will return to its original length. If, however, the tissue is lengthened and held long, then it will return to a different resting length, the degree of which depends on the length of time it was held in the lengthened position. This is a phenomenon known as 'creep'. Research into sports stretching has come to similar conclusions (Alter 1996) suggesting that, for a stretch to effectively modify the tissue, it must be held in a lengthened position for a while. Whether viscoelasticity can account for the immediate response of soft tissues to deep work remains a moot point.

Some authors have suggested that the viscoelastic behaviour may be due to the gradual failure of inter- and intra-molecular bonds between collagen molecule fibres and cross-linking fibres when stressed (Cantu and Grodin 1992). Other investigators have emphasized the behaviour of *composite* materials:

Viscoelastic materials, connective tissues, exhibit time dependent material properties and 'creep' behaviour. … The slower the force is applied, i.e. when enough time is allowed for the liquid component to flow, the more the whole tissue behaves like a liquid. The faster the force is applied, and the less time allowed for viscous damping, the more the load is taken up more directly by the inextensible collagen fibers and the more the tissue behaves like an inextensible steel cable.

(Evanko 2000)

Schleip suggests that the sol–gel hypothesis is insufficient to explain the immediate response of tissues to manually applied pressure (Schleip 1996, 2003). He suggests that the available research shows that the kind of mechanical force applied during structural bodywork is not sufficient to induce the tissue changes that so obviously occur: 'stronger forces or longer duration would be required for a permanent viscoelastic deformation of fascia'. He does, however, see factors such as thixotropy as contributing to longer-term adaptations in the connective tissues. His experiments in Rolfing patients under anaesthesia convinced him that the nervous system must be active during the process if changes are to occur. Schleip suggests that other factors may be at work in allowing such an immediate response in the tissue. Factors such as autonomic response, fluid mechanics and hormonal responses have been mooted. His review of the research demonstrates convincingly that connective tissue is quite densely innervated and has large numbers of mechanoreceptors. He suggests that the short-term plasticity of fascia in deep-tissue work stems from the deep stimulation of the fascial mechanoreceptors, which then operates through two major pathways in the central and the autonomic nervous systems. He suggests that autonomic responses can influence fascial smooth muscle cells and the local fluid dynamics, and by influencing the hypothalamic tuning, which all lead to a 'softening' response in the soft tissues.

Explanations are so often a rationalization after the fact, and despite the different possible explanations, all who have used the more direct form of myofascial release recognize that the 'melting pressure' – a slow, continuously applied load – is extremely effective in producing a softening response in the tissue.

Connective tissue – a perspective of structural bodywork

Many anatomists within the structural bodywork tradition, starting with Ida Rolf herself, have framed a perspective on connective tissue that is rather different to the biomedical viewpoint. Fascia is rarely shown in standard anatomy books. Often it is carefully dissected away to show the muscles beneath as if somehow it gets in the way. There is not the acknowledgement that the totality of the connective tissue network can be viewed as a unitary structure, that is, more at the level of an organ or a system within our overall structural organization. Older surgical techniques tended to ignore its complexity and integrity and would crudely sew all the layers together instead of reconnecting them individually, though this is now changing.

A number of authors within the somatic tradition have visualized the connective tissue network as one continuous and interconnected fabric with a huge diversity of forms. All of these forms are seen as different configurations of the same basic elements that have adapted specifically to local conditions within the body (Rolf 1977, Juhan 1987, Heller and Henkin 1991, Bajelis 1994). Thus tendons, ligaments, aponeuroses, interosseous membranes, synovial capsules, bursae, fasciae, and even bones, are all variations of the one substance, with collagen being the all-pervasive unifying element. Drucker refers to the entire connective tissue network as 'the one fascia'. As an example of this view, one can visualize ligaments and fascia both as metamorphoses of the same kinds of material, with both structures tethering bone to bone, but with different spans and a different density and organization of collagen fibres, and with fascia having muscle cells embedded within its matrix.

Implications for bodywork

The tensile structure of the myofascial network is very dependent upon usage. In this structural view, fascia is always slowly and imperceptibly adapting to the mechanical, metabolic and environmental stresses that act on it. It is always shaping itself according to our habitual postures and average movement patterns. If our postures and movements become limited and fixed, our fascial network will stabilize to that average form, and help maintain the habitual pattern. Like

bone, the fascial web responds to stress by thickening or becoming denser, by laying down new collagen fibres in a direction determined by the stresses that pass through it. (We noted earlier that cells are constantly at work recycling the materials of the connective tissue network.) Paradoxically the fascial network can also thicken in places where there is *insufficient* movement, but in such cases the collagen fibres tend to 'mat down', to fix themselves in a chaotic or 'haystacked' fashion and attract fat deposits because there is not the movement required to align the fibres intelligently. It is as if the structural intelligence of the body is saying 'OK, you obviously don't wish to move this area, so let's make it easier for you not to move it!' This is the kind of 'fibro-fatty intrusion' or contracture that is often seen by physiotherapists when their clients have suffered prolonged periods of joint immobility. This is why modern orthopaedic medicine now tries to avoid total immobilisation after injury or surgery. The newer protocol seems to be something like 'Whatever you *can* do without pain, you *must* do'. So appropriate movement, rather than complete rest, is usually the preferred protocol. Where once a patient undergoing a knee reconstruction would awaken after surgery with a leg in plaster, they now awaken with their leg already in a flexion machine, undergoing gentle flexion and extension movements, which allows the repair of the connective tissues to be 'informed' by the actual movements that the limb will need to undergo later.

An appreciation of the synergistic relationship between form and movement, structure and function, is crucial to the structural bodywork perspective. Movement is seen as necessary for physical health at all levels: for healthy circulation and metabolic efficiency, the maintenance of adequate hydration in connective tissue, the maintenance of joint health and the appropriate span of connective tissues. This is why structural bodyworkers need to see how their clients move and how they stand, and then take special note of areas of the body where there is little movement or more potential for movement. Then, through a skilful use of both structural and functional work they aim to elicit easier, fuller, more coordinated movement patterns.

Congenital differences in tissue density

Busy manual therapists soon realize that there is a wide variability in the qualities and textures of the soft tissues of their clients. At one extreme there are those clients, often of a meso- or ectomorphic body type, whose tissue seems too hard and who, despite the fact that their muscles are hypertoned, may actually be quite weak. It is as if the very density of the tissue is inhibiting free movement. At the other extreme we have those with a soft quality to their soft tissues, as if their 'glue' is too weak. Such clients often have lax ligaments and a tendency to hyperextend at their joints. They may also have hypermobile segments in their spine, which makes it easy for them to fall into slumped postures. They tend to have ecto- or endomorphic body characteristics. And of course there is a spectrum of tissue densities in between these two extremes.

This soft-bodied tendency has long been recognized within the world of structural bodywork and yoga (Rolf 1977, Flury 1989) where it is often seen as dysfunctional. For instance, there are congenital problems with collagen metabolism that can leave people open to dislocations and general collapse. Alter (1996) cites evidence to suggest that there are measurable differences in ligamentous laxity between racial groups, but the anecdotal evidence of many structural bodyworkers is that the difference between individuals is greater than between racial groups.

Tissue density is most definitely a factor that will influence how we work with our clients. The conventional wisdom in structural bodywork circles is that it is more difficult to achieve changes with hard-tissued types, but that once achieved the changes tend to be fairly stable. Soft-tissued types on the other hand are easier to balance but tend to revert to old patterns more easily, and perhaps are more in need of an educational approach.

Is the tissue dense or just tense?

Hard-tissued clients (those with a constitutional tendency towards dense connective tissue) need to be distinguished from those for whom there is a general exaggeration in muscular tonus, the habitually tense, or those we might call 'highly strung' or overwrought. It is as if their tonus 'thermostat' is tuned too high. There seems to be a regulation problem within the autonomic nervous system such that it has become more attuned to sympathetic activation than to parasympathetic. Of course, in time this continual low-level tonus must translate into an increase in the fibrosity of the soft tissues and will lead to their having a denser feel. This can make it difficult at times to distinguish these two armoured types, which is complicated again by the possibility of *both* tendencies being present in the same individual. However, it is important to know the source of the hard-tissue tendency as they each require a different emphasis in their work. For those with a constitutional tendency to dense connective tissue, a systemic approach might be called for (some genetic conditions, mineral deficiency states and connective tissue diseases can predispose to this condition). For the habitually tense, some sort of relaxation education is often indicated, although often they do not respond well to the conventional relaxation education approaches such as yoga Nidra, and progressive relaxation. A movement approach such as Trager work can be an excellent way of working with such clients as it trains them to move in a softer and easier fashion so as to use less energy in rhythmic movement.

REFERENCES

Alexander R M 1975 Biomechanics. Chapman and Hall, London

Alexander R M 1988 Elastic mechanisms in animal movement. Cambridge University Press, Cambridge

Alter M J 1996 Science of flexibility. Human Kinetics, Champaign, Illinois, p 40

Bajelis D 1994 Hellerwork: the ultimate in myofascial release. International Journal of Alternative and Complementary Medicine 12(1): 33–38

Cantu R, Grodin A 1992 Myofascial manipulation: theory and clinical application. Aspen, Gaithersburg, pp 20, 25–57

Chopra D 1991 Perfect health: the complete mind body guide. Three Rivers Press, New York

Drucker D (n.d.) Fascial anatomy. Workbook for Hellerwork students. (not published)

Feitis R (ed) 1978 Ida Rolf talks: about Rolfing and physical reality. The Rolf Institute, Boulder, pp 34, 198, 206

Ferner H, Staubesand J (eds) 1982 Sobotta Atlas of Human Anatomy. Urban & Schwarzenberg, Munich, I, p 265

Flury H 1989 Theoretical aspects and implications of the internal/external system. Notes on Structural Integration 1: 15–35

Gallaudet B B 1931 A description of the planes of fascia of the human body. Columbia University Press, New York, p 1

Hanna T 1988 Somatics: reawakening the mind's control of movement, flexibility, and health. Addison-Wesley, Reading, Massachusetts

Hedley G 1999 Integral anatomy, Part II. Rolf Lines 27(1): 8–12

Heller J 1990 Fascia. Transcript of lecture. In Drucker D (ed.) Fascial anatomy. Workbook for student Hellerworkers. (not published)

Heller J, Henkin W 1991 Bodywise. Wingbow Press, Berkeley

Juhan D 1987 Job's body: a handbook for bodywork. Station Hill Press, New York, pp 64, 66, 70

Miller E 1988 Collagen types: structure, distribution and functions. In: Collagen (ed) Nimni. CRC Press. Vol I Biochemistry

Oschman J 1989 How does the body maintain its shape? Rolf Lines 18(1): 8–12

Oschman J 2000 Energy medicine: the scientific basis. Churchill Livingstone, Edinburgh, p 159

O'Toole M (ed) 1997 Miller–Keane encyclopedia and dictionary of medicine, nursing, and allied health. 6th edn, W B Saunders

Rolf I 1973 Structural integration: a contribution to the understanding of stress. Confinia Psychiatrica 16: 76

Rolf I 1977 Rolfing: the integration of human structures. Harper and Rowe, New York, pp 39, 41, 129

St George F 2001 Myofascial technique. Australian Physiotherapy Association News. March, 15–17

Schleip R 1996 Adventures in the jungle of the neurofascial net. Rolf Lines 24(2): 38–42

Schleip R 2003 Fascial plasticity: a new neurobiological explanation. Journal of Bodywork and Movement Therapies 7(1): 1

Schultz R, Feitis R 1996 The endless web: fascial anatomy and physical reality. North Atlantic Books, Berkeley

Tortora G, Grabowski S 1993 Principles of anatomy and physiology. HarperCollins College Publishers, New York

Wolff J 1892 Das Gesetz der Transformation der Knocken. A Hirschwald, Berlin

THE OSCILLATORY PROPERTIES OF THE FASCIAL NETWORK

When we look in awe at the grace of a gazelle in flight, the poise of a hovering eagle, the stupendous leap of a cat, or the accomplished performance of an athlete or dancer, we are witnessing an extraordinary efficiency of movement. When we see the poise of many traditional peoples, perhaps carrying heavy loads on their heads, we are seeing perfection in movement. Or when we see the focussed mastery of a skilled martial artist totally committing herself to the execution of a technique, again we see the kind of efficiency in which there is no unnecessary muscular action, where neither too much nor too little energy is spent; nothing detracts from the coordinated action of the whole.

Many who work in the somatic field have this appreciation of the aesthetic in movement and wish this inherent grace and efficiency for themselves and for their clients. Structural bodyworkers have long noticed that as their work unfolds – as they free up the soft-tissue restrictions in their clients and assist them in bringing more awareness to the quality of their movement – their movements become more fluid and generous. There can be more presence, poise, rhythm and delicacy of balance in the client's movement, which of course means less stress on their body. Encouraging this kind of efficiency and harmony in movement is one of the chief aims of any somatic work.

FASCIA AS THE ANTAGONIST

Biomechanical research is beginning to paint a picture of human movement that is rather different to the somewhat robotic model of early kinesiology. The early model sees movement purely in terms of the coordinated action of antagonistic or synergistic muscle groups. Now fascia itself is seen as an antagonist to muscular action, and movement is seen less as the coordinated action of opposed muscles and more in terms of the dynamics of the elastic and oscillatory properties of the myofascial network as a whole. In this view of rhythmic movement, muscular action works primarily to maintain oscillatory patterns with an occasional and timely input of energy each movement cycle (Gracovetsky 1988, Novacheck 1998).

Work in the field of vertebrate biomechanics has demonstrated how animals utilize the springiness of their tendons and ligaments in locomotory behaviour such as hopping, walking and running, and how they have found some very efficient ways of recycling some of the energy of movement through their connective tissues (Alexander 1975, 1988). More recent work, however, is even challenging the basic kinesiological assumption that muscles need to shorten against resistance in order to propel the organism forward. Once the animal is in rhythmic motion and has established a forward momentum, then some muscles work purely *isometrically*, that is, they work to maintain a constant length against resistance as if they are trying to turn their tendons (and by implication their myofascia) into springs – by holding the ends of the 'spring' rigid, as it were (Pennisi 1997).

It was mentioned in Chapter 8 that the human body can be partially understood as a tensegrity structure and that one of the essential features of tensegrity structures is that they are able to absorb external forces, distributing them throughout the whole system, and thus avoiding an excessive loading on any one part. These forces are absorbed and dampened by the stretch and elastic recoil of the tensile elements of the structure, and communicated throughout the whole. In fact a tensegrity structure will bounce or oscillate in a dance of exchanging kinetic and potential energies. In the human body fascia is the tensile element, and it is becoming increasingly apparent that the inherent rhythmicity of much of our movement arises from the mechanical properties of the totality of the fascial network. A clever body would surely find a way to harness the rhythmicity inherent in our structure to find more economy in movement. From an evolutionary perspective it makes sense that animals should have discovered the efficiency of energy expenditure that arises from sensing and capitalizing on the pendular, oscillatory behaviour of their own bodies.

Many of our most important activities are essentially rhythmic – breathing, walking and running. They have a repetitive, cyclical, periodic quality. There is an emerging perspective around such movement that sees the sensory-motor intelligence utilizing the elastic recoil of the connective tissues by recycling it into the next movement cycle. In breathing for instance, muscles of inspiration actively work to expand the thoracic cavity, creating a pressure gradient that induces air to be pushed into the lungs. The expansion of the thoracic cavity is resisted by the elasticity of all the fasciae of the thorax, so part of the kinetic energy supplied by the muscles of inspiration is stored as potential energy in the stretched fascia. As the muscles of inspiration release, the elastic recoil of the fascia can then be recycled, restoring the thorax to its resting state, and in the process inducing the expiration of air. This is an example of how the body can intelligently harness this stored elastic energy of the connective tissues. The same principle can be seen in the design of fusiform muscles themselves. The collagen fibres in the epimysium of muscles tend to encircle the muscle belly, running perpendicular to the long axis of the muscle. Again, as a muscle actively contracts and shortens, it swells in the middle, against the elastic

resistance of these fibres, which on relaxation will squeeze the muscle belly back in and assist the muscle in returning to its resting length. However, it is the oscillatory tendency of the fascial system as a whole that most concerns somatic therapists (Fig. 10.1).

Physics tells us that all complex elastic structures have their own resonant frequencies, whether they are structures such as bridges and buildings, guitar strings or even human bodies. Engineers need to know the resonant frequencies of the bridges and tall buildings they design. This information is vital since it is quite possible for such structures to be shaken apart during high winds of specific velocities; they can literally resonate to their own destruction. The human body, however, is much more complex than a bridge or building, and unlike these mechanical constructions has the remarkable ability of being able to vary the pattern of its internal tensions, meaning that its resonant frequencies can also be varied by the states of tension in the various body segments. If we recall the anaesthetized spaceman in Chapter 8 (Fig. 8.9, p. 54), where we had a pure structural body with no muscular activity whatsoever, we can easily visualize that a body in this condition could be induced to undulate in various ways. For example flexion–extension, lateral flexion (left and right) and transverse undulation around the long axis of the body would be possible, and the actual frequency of these undulations would be quite specific to the mass and proportions of the body, as well as to the tensile structure of the fasciae of that body. This would change of course in gravity and in full function; however, it may be surmised that being able to tune in to the inherent resonant qualities of one's body would greatly assist in movement

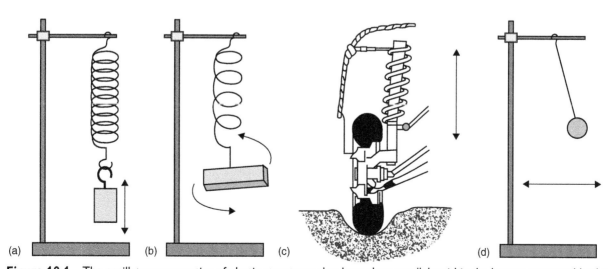

Figure 10.1 The oscillatory properties of elastic structures that have close parallels within the human structural body: (a) a spring in tension; (b) a torsional pendulum; (c) a spring in compression; and (d) a pendulum.

efficiency, and there is now evidence that supports this view.

Some observers have been amazed at the ability of porters throughout the world to carry considerable loads on their heads with little apparent effort. Studies of Kenyan women have shown that they routinely carry up to 70% of their own body weight on their heads, yet they are not particularly fit by ordinary standards of physical fitness. In his review of the research in this area, Samuel (2001) concludes that this ability arises not through muscular strength but through the women's sensitive use of the inherent periodicity of walking, the pendular motion of their hips.

Treadmill experiments measuring oxygen uptake show that these women can carry up to a fifth of their body weight before their breathing even becomes affected, such is their efficiency under load! They were found to be more efficient porters than extremely fit, trained soldiers. It was speculated that their extraordinary efficiency arose from the pendular motion of their hips and the seemingly effortless transfer of weight from foot to foot during each gait cycle. The aspect of the women's timing that differed from soldiers', however, was too subtle for the observers to notice. Samuel suggests that gait works on similar principles to the pendulum clock, which requires a minimal input of energy in each cycle to maintain the momentum of the pendulum. The efficiency of the gait of these women is seen as arising from their use of their hips as an 'inverted pendulum'. Only at the beginning of each gait cycle is an input of muscular energy required. The author makes no specific reference to the spring-like qualities of tendons and fascia; however, it may be surmized that in this instance the iliotibial tracts could act as springs to absorb the energy of the hip's lateral translation and then recycle the stored elastic energy to assist the return of the hips to the midline.

What the author did not mention is that these women are obliged to be economical in movement as a matter of survival. Carrying heavy loads for long distances is part of their everyday existence and their bodies would soon break down if they did not discover the most efficient way to do this work. They have the capacity to 'listen' to their bodies and sense which movements do, and do not, cause strain. This 'listening' is perhaps a skill that we have largely forgotten in the West, a skill that we as somatic therapists can awaken in our clients.

However, the undulatory movement of the hips in walking is more complex than this simple 'inverted pendulum' model would suggest. Gracovetsky has shown that the spine, coupled with the pelvis, has a complex motion that has elements of flexion–extension, side flexion–extension and rotation, which all combine into a complex motion that actually forms the basis of efficient gait. Even the motion of the legs is partly driven by this complex motion of the spine (Gracovetsky 1988). In the assessment section of Chapter 14 it will be suggested that one way of assessing gait is to analyze it into the above three components; this can prove an invaluable means of seeing where structural or functional work is required in our clients.

Part of the work of somatic therapists, therefore, must be in helping people listen more carefully to the inherent rhythmicity of their structure. In the practical section of this book we will look at the three main elements of pelvic undulation in walking, how they combine into a complex movement, and how this can be enhanced by appropriate bodywork.

REFERENCES

Alexander R M 1975 Biomechanics. Chapman and Hall, London

Alexander R M 1988 Elastic mechanisms in animal movement. Cambridge University Press, Cambridge

Gracovetsky S 1988 The Spinal Engine. Springer, Vienna

Novacheck T 1998 The biomechanics of running: review paper. Gait and Posture 7. Elsevier Science

Pennisi E 1997 A new view on how leg muscles operate on the run. Science 275: 1067–1070, 21 February

Samuel E 2001 Walk like a pendulum. New Scientist 169(2272): 38

CHAPTER

11

THE MUSCULAR SYSTEM

In Chapter 8 it was stated that the connective tissues and muscle cells were two major outflows of the mesoderm during embryogenetic development and they were called the *yin* and *yang,* or the passive and active, aspects of the mesodermic system. These outflows, the muscle fibres with their fascial environment, form an inseparable unity, the musculature, which under the control and coordination of the central nervous system provides the orchestrated pattern of tensions that enables the structural body as a whole to move within the gravity field. In this chapter we will take a brief look at the kinds of muscular dysfunction that can arise through direct trauma, underuse and overuse – all of which will in time contribute to creating and maintaining structural imbalances.

Structural bodywork training traditionally requires a detailed working knowledge of the action of muscles; however when it comes to the practical application of this approach, there is less emphasis on the musculature than in other ways of working with posture. It has already been stated that it is an artificial distinction to talk of the fasciae and musculature as if they were independent of each other, yet, when strategizing their work, structural bodyworkers often think almost in dressmaking terms of which areas of the body need to be 'opened up'. So that although a general knowledge of the action of the underlying muscles is essential and remains in the background awareness of structural bodyworkers, it is often secondary to a more global sense of which areas need more 'length' or resilience. And in practical terms, the techniques of structural bodywork are aimed less at isolating particular muscles than in working on the overlying superficial and deep fasciae, as well as the most superficial aspects of the myofascia.

What happens when a muscle changes length?

Through repetitive usage, muscles may adaptively lengthen or shorten from a baseline resting length, and whenever there is such a change in length it is a change more in the fascia than in the contractile cells. Remember that muscle tissue is 50–60% fascia. Essentially it is the fascia that has lengthened or shortened. Nevertheless, when muscles do adaptively shorten, over time some muscle cells that were organized in series will be lost. This is not irreversible however; it is now apparent that if a muscle *lengthens* from its average resting length, then muscle cells can be generated to 'fill the gap' (Alter 1996). This suggests that there is a greater potential for structural change in the musculature than was once thought to be the case.

MUSCLE SUBCLASSIFICATION

Muscles can be subclassified in a number of different ways. Two that are important in the field of structural bodywork are the tonic–phasic and genetic flexor–extensor classifications. We will look at tonic–phasic classification now, and in the section on Janda in Chapter 13. In that chapter we will also look at the genetic flexor–extensor distinction in the section on Schleip's postural model.

Phasic and tonic musculature

There are two broad functional categories of muscle types: *phasic* and *tonic*. Essentially this classification depends upon the overall predominance of either 'fast-twitch' or 'slow-twitch' muscle fibres within the muscle.

All skeletal musculature contains both kinds of fibre and there will be varying proportions of each; one type, however, will predominate. This leads to a full spectrum of functional muscle types. And just as muscles are able to adapt to different working lengths through usage, so also are they able to change their tonic–phasic tendency. In other words, the balance of fast-twitch and slow-twitch fibres can be modified through usage to a certain extent. Various approaches to classifying individual muscles within the tonic–phasic distinction have been proposed, leading to a number of different 'lists' of tonic and phasic muscles (Schleip 1995).

Tonic muscles

Tonic muscles (sometimes called postural muscles) are those that have predominantly a postural, a maintaining, or a stabilizing function, while phasic muscles are more active in making big, powerful or 'willed' movements. Tonic muscles have a predominance of slow-twitch fibres, work anaerobically, and can usually work for longer periods at low intensity without tiring. Think of your jaw for instance, which can remain closed all day against the pull of gravity by the action of the masseter and temporalis muscles, both tonic muscles, and yet they do not seem to tire from this sustained work. Tonic muscles work at a subconscious level, beneath our everyday awareness, and are continuously making minute adjustments to our posture, even when we are stationary. They maintain our upright stance within gravity and stabilize distal parts of the body.

Phasic muscles

Phasic muscles on the other hand have a predominance of fast-twitch fibres, work aerobically and tend to tire after explosive use. Unlike the tonic muscles, which are constantly working to maintain our posture beneath the level of our conscious awareness, phasic muscles are 'doers'. In other words, they operate at a more conscious level and respond whenever we *decide* to perform a movement. Of course, the tonic muscles are obliged to cooperate with these 'willed' movements athough, as Godard (2000) suggests, subconscious emotional attitudes can be expressed through the tonic musculature and may even oppose or 'sabotage' willed movements. In some postural imbalances phasic muscles are obliged to do the work of tonic muscles, and vice versa. Performing work that they are not designed for can lead to fatigue and inflammation, and also contribute to the onset of overuse syndromes (Key 1993).

Research has suggested that postural and phasic muscles respond differently to stress, with postural muscles responding by shortening, but phasic muscles becoming inhibited neurologically and thence weakening. This behaviour will have structural outcomes in the longer term. In Chapter 13 we will look at a number of postural syndromes proposed by Janda that can arise from the differential behaviour of postural and phasic antagonist groups (Chaitow 1996).

THINGS THAT CAN GO WRONG WITHIN THE MUSCULATURE

In Chapter 1 it was suggested that the soft tissues of the body will gradually conform to the average patterns of daily usage and that these structural changes will then reinforce the neuromuscular habits that led to them in the first place, regardless of whether those habits are ultimately healthy or unhealthy (see Figs 1.2 and 1.3, pp 8 and 9). We will now look in more detail at some of the physiological mechanisms by which the process of structural adaptation may occur, and particularly the body's response to overuse, underuse and the results of direct insult or trauma to the soft tissues.

Overuse

There is a great deal of current interest in overuse syndromes, since in recent times there has been a spate of insurance claims for overuse injuries, resulting in payouts that have imposed a heavy burden on industry. The heavier burden perhaps has been upon the sufferers themselves who, despite their considerable discomfort, have sometimes been accused of malingering. Overuse syndromes have variously been called *repetitive strain injury* (RSI) and *cumulative stress disorder*; however they might more accurately be described as a '*cumulative and constant tension complex*' (Damany and Bellis 2000).

These syndromes have been reported as affecting smaller muscle groups, in the wrist, arm, neck and shoulder, and have been attributed to repetitive muscle use over extended periods of time, often involving a large degree of distal stabilization. A number of factors have been blamed, including repetitive work with poor ergonomic support, or certain sports that have a large repetitive component. However, many structural bodyworkers would broaden the scope of this perspective significantly and affirm that virtually any function performed repetitively under adverse biomechanical conditions will in time lead to some kind of cumulative stress dysfunction. Even 'harmless' functions such as carrying a bag over one shoulder, standing with hyperextended knees, jogging on hard surfaces, sitting in low soft fur-niture, playing computer games, gardening in a flexed position, practising on a musical instrument, carrying a baby on one hip, lounging in front of the TV, or simply the heightened muscular tension that accompanies habitual anxiety, can all lead to the same kind of dys-function through the gradual modification of the soft tissues. From this perspective, even postural syndromes such as the head forward syndrome can be seen as a form of repetitive strain dysfunction.

In Chapter 9 we outlined how increased mechanical demands on soft tissues can lead to an increase in fibros-ity within that tissue, and how this can then contribute to structural dysfunction. Another possible pathway to structural imbalance is through the formation of trigger points within the musculature.

Simons and Travell have carried out some extraordin-arily detailed and definitive work on the study of trig-ger points – how they arise and how they can be treated. They define a *trigger point* as 'a hyperirritable spot in skeletal muscle that is associated with a hypersensitive palpable nodule in a taut band' (Simons and Travell 1999). These points are said to arise from the overuse of cer-tain muscles, either through repetitive movements with incomplete relaxation between cycles; through pro-longed contraction, say in stabilizing a distal part, or in the unnecessary co-contraction of antagonistic muscles (what Feldenkrais has called 'parasitic' muscular tension).

Simons and Travell propose an *energy crisis hypothe-sis*, which suggests that when muscles work under such unfavourable conditions they effectively cheat them-selves of oxygen and metabolic fuel. They do this by compromising the efficiency of their own circulation, while at the same time retarding the timely removal of the by-products of their own cellular respiration: car-bonic and lactic acids, for instance. These and other by-products can act as irritants that maintain the elevated tonus within the muscle and, in a vicious cycle, work to further compromize circulation. Muscles are being asked to do more and more with less and less – hence the 'energy crisis'.

We know that the musculature acts as an indirect cir-culatory pump that mechanically squeezes venous blood towards the heart. For this to occur harmo-niously the muscle must *actually pump*, that is, it must contract and fully relax in a cyclic manner in order to maintain this throughput of fluids. If muscles are work-ing for too long or too continuously then they will mechanically restrict the arterial and venous flows within their own tissues, creating a localized ischaemia. This can be illustrated by the simple analogy that a squeezed sponge will always hold less water than an open and expanded one.

In time this energy crisis leads to a dysfunction of the motor end-plates in certain muscle fibres, such that they do not respond to efferent nervous impulses but instead maintain a state of constant contraction. These fibres can be palpated within the body of the muscle as taut bands. Trigger points normally occur at the sites of motor end-plates, and when pressed give rise to a char-acteristic distribution of referred myofascial pain. Trigger points can precipitate further satellite trigger points in nearby muscles, starting a chain reaction of effects by reflexively inhibiting the action of related muscles. This all occurs subconsciously; many clients do not know they have trigger points until you press them! These points are therefore constraining the clients' movements without their even being aware of it.

Many somatic therapists, both mainstream and com-plementary, have been turning their attention to repeti-tive strain disorders and trying to find ways of dealing with them. These disorders are often attributed to the changes in work habits that came with the computer revolution, especially in the use of keyboards designed with little regard to sensible ergonomics.

RSI is seen as a cumulative disorder that arises from the complex interaction of many factors. It develops gradually, perhaps over many years, and may go unno-ticed until there is a rapid onset of symptoms triggered by some relatively minor stressful episode that often seems out of all proportion to the discomfort caused (Damany and Bellis 2000).

These authors suggest two common 'trauma paths' that can lead to RSI: through muscular inflammation and through nerve entrapment. Muscular inflammation they see as arising as in Simons and Travell's model, that is, through localized ischaemia, congestion, irritation and so on. Nerve entrapment is seen as arising from myofascial constriction along the pathways of periph-eral nerve trunks. Such indirect pressure on nerves can lead to paraesthesia, numbness or pain, which again will force the sensory-motor intelligence of the body to avoid movements that stress such tethered nerves. It is interesting that both Simons and Travell and Damany and Bellis recommend myofascial release techniques as an important aspect of treatment.

Underuse

Prolonged immobilization of tissues will encourage a chaotic build up of collagen fibres, which may then attract fat deposits and increase the possibility of mineralization within the tissues. Such 'haystacking' is particularly evident in the periarticular connective tissues around joints. Immobilization can be deliberate, for instance in the therapeutic use of splints or plaster casts to immobilize broken bones. However, it is apparent that many people simply *immobilize themselves*: they slow down and move less and less, and this is not only among the aged. This process can start quite early in life, particularly for those in sedentary work. This kind of immobility can also arise from muscular holding patterns that create a general heightening of tonus levels. This leads to a widespread pattern of low-level co-contraction that can give a 'rigid' appearance to clients and constrain all movement. At the end of Chapter 9, two 'armoured types' were mentioned: those with a congenital tendency to dense connective tissues, and those with a generalized elevation in muscular tonus. In either case, whole areas of the body may be missing the movement required for basic tissue health, and this underuse in some areas will inevitably lead to overuse in others that are obliged to take on a heavier share of the work.

Trauma

Trauma to any part of the body will set in motion a massive and complex healing response. The response in the soft tissues, such as the fascial and myofascial tissues, nerves and the viscera, is very similar to that in skeletal tissue. There is an inflammatory response consisting of a mobilization of the cells of repair, the synthesis of collagen fibres by fibroblasts, the formation of a connective tissue scaffolding for the construction of new tissue, and a period of fibrous reorganization that may result in scar tissue being formed. Scar tissue tends to be debrided of redundant collagen as healing progresses, but depending on the severity of the trauma some may remain as keloid tissue which, like the biblical new cloth used to repair the old cloak, will tend to tug on all the surrounding tissue during movement. Ida Rolf's image of the 'snagged cardigan' illustrates how a localized restriction can have effects throughout the whole body, far from the actual site of restriction, and can influence all movement (see Fig. 9.17, p. 74).

The kinds of trauma suffered by tissues can vary considerably in its intensity. It is not only 'one off' injuries that lead to this healing response. It is common for clients to suffer repeated microtrauma, low-level strain, which may not lead to significant pain at the time, however the cumulative effects of such repeated microtrauma can produce marked structural changes in the longer term.

If the trauma is considerable, then at the same time as the inflammatory response is proceeding, the sensory-motor intelligence of the body will do its best to immobilize the injured part by a coordinated muscular splinting around the injury. This is a protective *spasm*, usually accompanied by pain. Like any of the short-term measures taken by the body, if it persists too long it will leave a lasting influence on movement, and lessons learned in pain tend to be learned very deeply. A by-product of the formation of scar tissue is the increased possibility of adhesions between adjacent structures. If nerve trunks happen to be in the vicinity of the injury they may become enmeshed within the local process of fibrous infiltration, resulting in a tethering of the nerve, which normally should slide through the tissue like string through a ball of wool. Additionally, other structures may become tethered in this process, potential spaces within the musculature for instance.

AN OVERVIEW OF THE PROCESSES THAT CAN LEAD TO STRUCTURAL DYSFUNCTION

Figure 11.1 is an expansion of Figure 1.2 (p. 9). It is an attempt to bring together in diagrammatic form some of the different physiological mechanisms that have been proposed as giving rise to structural dysfunctions. The diagram is not meant to be definitive in any way but summarizes proposals from various sources, all of which are mentioned in this book. Although Figure 11.1 is presented in a linear or flow-chart format, the web of causation is almost certainly far more complex and interrelated than this 'simple' diagram would suggest.

Central to this diagram is a 'black box' consisting of what throughout this book has been referred to as the *sensory-motor intelligence*. This refers collectively to those aspects of the central nervous system that:

- integrate proprioceptive information
- store movement 'programs'
- orchestrate whole body patterns of movement (via efferent outflows)
- initiate novel movements
- find real-time solutions to immediate movement problems.

This black box can be conceptualized as the repository of all our learned movement behaviours. It receives afferent information from sensory and proprioceptive receptors, and constantly modifies the efferent symphony of its movement 'programs' in response to this incoming information. This kind of real-time modification

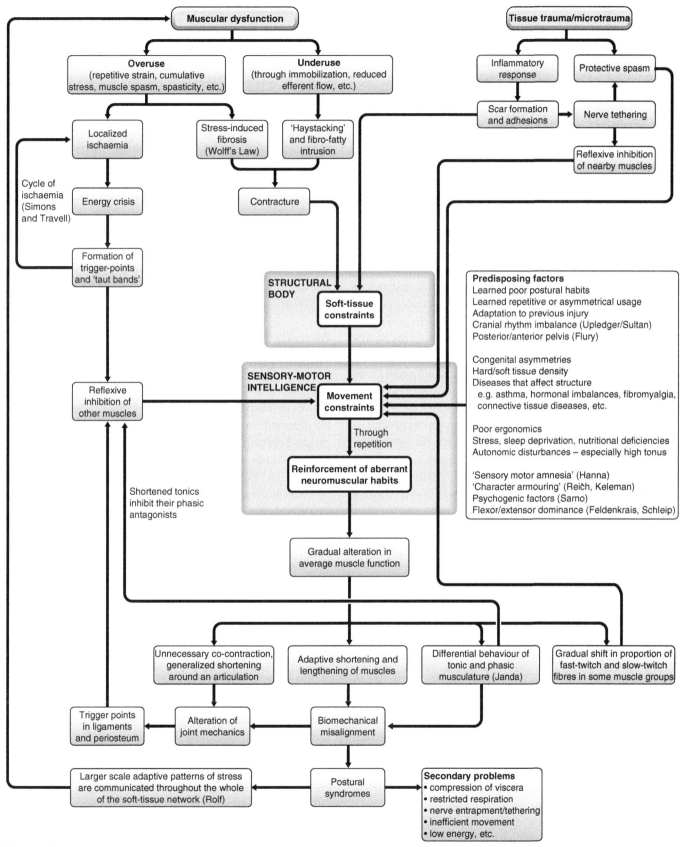

Figure 11.1   An overview of the physiological mechanisms regarded as contributing to structural dysfunction.

to movement programs can be a short-term response to the immediate environment of our organism or, if there is sufficient rehearsal and repetition, the modification can become ingrained as a learned pattern by the process we usually refer to as sensory-motor learning. The sensory information comes from the external environment and the proprioceptive information flows from the internal environment of the structural body, especially from the mechanoreceptors within the myofascial network. Figure 11.1 shows that movement constraints can arise from: pre-existing learned patterns; tendencies; 'complexes' and states of the organism; the short-term results of muscular spasm and reflexive inhibition, and from soft-tissue constraints.

The structural body is shown as another 'black box': one source of input for the sensory-motor intelligence. Soft-tissue constraints are just one of several sources of afferent information to which the sensory-motor intelligence must respond. It is bound to take into consideration these genuine mechanical constraints as it organizes movement.

The heart of Figure 11.1, like Figure 1.2, suggests that structural dysfunctions essentially arise from restricted movement. Through repetition, restricted movement patterns become learned. These learned patterns will in time lead to compensatory adaptations throughout the whole of the soft-tissue network, and these adaptations will tend to maintain those learned patterns. Habit becomes fixed in the tissues, and then fixed tissues reciprocate by supporting the habit.

Soft-tissue constraints stem from two basic sources: from the results of dysfunctional muscular usage and from tissue trauma. Muscular dysfunction can arise through the gradual process of fibrotic contracture, induced by over- or under-use of musculature, or from the scar tissue and adhesions that arise from direct trauma. All these constraints become superimposed on the core of learned movement patterns.

The diagram suggests that there are a number of predisposing factors that may exist in the background of any individual that will hasten the onset of structural dysfunction; they include *historical* and *congenital factors*, current *environmental stressors*, and perhaps certain *emotional, behavioural or psychological tendencies* or complexes. These factors will make the arising of structural imbalances much more likely without necessarily being sufficient or prime causes in themselves.

Historical factors

These include aspects of individual history, such as the postural and movement habits learned within the socialization process, particularly the imitation of parents and peers; the results of ill-advised postural advice ('Shoulders back, chest out, stomach in'), and learned patterns of repetitive or asymmetrical usage. These factors also include broad cultural influences; for instance, most people in the world squat, while in the West we use chairs. Many 'traditional' peoples are actually taught to move with more fluency than Westerners; in many parts of Africa children are actively taught efficient rhythmic movement through games, and so on. There is also a 'trauma history' for each individual. Ida Rolf spoke often of childhood diseases and accidents, and the effect that these could have on the development of posture and movement patterns. All such developmental episodes require an adaptive response in the short term, and often the resulting adaptations are never fully relinquished (Feitis 1978, Rolf 1977, Schultz and Feitis 1996).

Congenital factors

These include such things as: a constitutional tendency towards the extremes of soft-tissue density, that is, too hard or too soft; skeletal asymmetries such as a leg length discrepancy or hemipelvis; the tendency towards heightened or depressed autonomic activity, and the predisposition to diseases that can affect structure. The latter include asthma, fibromyalgia and connective tissue disease. Perhaps there may also be inherited features of form, for instance a tendency to an anterior or posterior tilt of the pelvis, which can often be seen strongly expressed within some families.

Immediate environmental stressors

These include such factors as sleep deprivation, emotional stress and nutritional deficiencies. Prolonged periods of stress can lead to a shift in autonomic tone towards extremes of either sympathetic or parasympathetic activity, which can have a major effect on tonus throughout the entire musculature.

Behavioural, emotional and psychological patterns

These have been proposed by some authors as being factors that may affect structure in the longer term. The whole somatic psychotherapeutic movement starting from Reich has proposed that the musculature can 'hold' and express certain emotional tendencies (Keleman 1985).

Coming from a more Freudian perspective, Sarno (1998) proposes that repressed emotion can lead to muscular pain and a host of other psychosomatic disorders. He suggests that the physiological mechanism

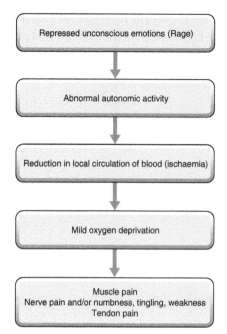

Figure 11.2 Sarno's proposed pathophysiology for tension myositis syndrome (TMS).

by which the subconscious mind can affect the body in this way is through the limbic system's influence on the autonomic nervous and immune systems (see Fig. 11.2). Sarno cites some research evidence that support some aspects of this proposed mechanism. It is known that the autonomic nervous system has the ability to adjust the amount of blood flowing through any part of the body by control of the smooth muscle of arteries and veins – the process known as vasodilation. During sympathetic activation, for instance, the blood is partially shunted away from the visceral space to the surface layers of the body, where the musculature is in more immediate need; similarly during parasympathetic activation, blood can be directed more towards the core space, to aid in digestion. Sarno takes the bold step of saying that repressed emotions can evoke the same kind of response in the body. He suggests the autonomic nervous system can be induced to provoke very specific areas of ischaemia, which then give rise to mild oxygen deprivation and to expressed physical symptoms. If this is indeed a valid mechanism then it must be assumed that there must be structural consequences in the longer term.

In Chapter 6 we discussed Hanna's concept of 'sensory motor amnesia', in which whole aspects of our soma may be 'anaesthetized' to proprioceptive information; even to mild pain signals. If this proprioceptive information is not being fully received by the central nervous system then we can expect aberrant patterns to increase, since the corrective power of pain is not even being received.

A number of different authors in the somatic field have speculated about the tendency of some clients to have an exaggerated flexor or extensor tone. In Chapter 13 various structural–postural models will be discussed that use this as an explanatory concept. One model developed successively by Feldenkrais, Hanna and Schleip suggests that such a neurological imbalance will have significant structural outcomes in the longer term.

SUMMARY

In Section 2 we have explored many of the background concepts and maps used within the structural bodywork tradition, especially the mutual influence of structure and function, and the adaptive, mediating role played by the connective tissue network. We have looked at some of the mechanisms by which functional patterns give rise to structural patterns, and how structural patterns feed back into the functional patterns that gave rise to them. In Section 3 we will look more specifically at the kinds of structural dysfunctions that can arise and at ways that a structural bodywork approach addresses them.

REFERENCES

Alter M J 1996 Science of flexibility. Human Kinetics, Champaign, p 40

Chaitow L 1996 Muscle energy techniques. Churchill Livingstone, New York, pp 15–46

Damany S, Bellis J 2000 It's not carpal tunnel syndrome: RSI theory and therapy for computer professionals. Simax, Philadelphia, p 3

Feitis R (ed) 1978 Ida Rolf talks: about Rolfing and physical reality. The Rolf Institute, Boulder

Godard H 2000 Notes from Bodywisdom Conference. Coromandel, New Zealand

Keleman S 1985 Emotional anatomy: the structure of experience. Center Press, Berkeley

Key S 1993 Body in action. Bantam Books, Sydney, pp 104–115

Rolf I 1977 Rolfing: the integration of human structures. Harper and Rowe, New York

Sarno J 1998 The Mindbody prescription: healing the body, healing the pain. Warner Books, New York

Schleip R 1995 Tonic/Phasic muscles. Online. Available: http://www.somatics.de

Schultz R, Feitis R 1996 The endless web: fascial anatomy and physical reality. North Atlantic Books, Berkeley

Simons D, Travell J 1999 Myofascial pain and dysfunction: the trigger point manual. Vol 1. Upper half of body. Lippincott, Williams & Wilkins, Baltimore

PRACTICAL MANUAL

CHAPTER 12

A CATALOGUE OF SOME COMMON POSTURAL DYSFUNCTIONS

Structural bodyworkers are vitally interested in their clients' posture and how they move in the world, but recognizing such patterns is one thing, discovering how efficiently these patterns are regulated is another. So it may be useful here to recall Rolf's distinction between posture and structure:

Posture is holding your structure as well as you can. When the structure is properly balanced, good posture is natural. A man slouches not because he has a bad habit but because his structure doesn't make it easy for him not to slouch.

It has been a theme repeated throughout this book that functional patterns will over time consolidate into structural patterns. *Our moving and postural habits create the structural body.* The structural body then becomes an underlying, unconscious influence on all our postural and movement patterns – a relatively constant background constraint that our sensory-motor intelligence must continually allow for in organizing movement. In this section we will examine the more common kinds of postural dysfunction that structural bodywork attempts to address, realizing that beneath these overt postural patterns there are hidden structural patterns that sustain them.

Ida Rolf used a 'block model' as a simplified means of demonstrating the relationship between the major elements of the human structure such as the head, chest, pelvis, and upper leg (see Figs 8.4 and 8.5, pp 52 and 53). This is a useful, though limited, means of viewing the body and visualizing its gross postural dynamics, and has the practical advantage of giving an approximate idea of where the individual segments need to be 'taken' in order to normalize the structure. Postural dysfunctions, according to this model, are seen as the horizontal displacement of bodily segments from the vertical midline,

or as the various rotations and counter-rotations of segments around this midline. However, the body can also be viewed as having many structural levels (Flury 1987), and underlying this gross segmental description of structure are skeletal configurations. So, in this section we will examine the most common postural dysfunctions that form the 'bread and butter' of structural bodywork, and we will define them in terms of skeletal organization, even though it is largely the soft tissues that determine the patterns and the soft tissues that we seek to reorganize when working with our clients.

THE ARTHROKINEMATIC PERSPECTIVE OF MOVEMENT AND POSTURE

When we look at the extraordinary complexity of a body in motion, one crucial aspect of what we are observing is the movement of bones relative to other bones. And similarly, when we analyze someone's stationary posture (which is a function as surely as any gross movement), we are observing the static spatial relationships between contiguous bones. This *arthrokinematic* perspective is a fundamental aspect of scientific kinesiology. It views movement as the movement of contiguous bones away from the 'home' of anatomical position to the degree that the ligamentous and myofascial environment of each joint will permit. It defines movement in terms of angles and velocities, using its specialized terminology of 'flexion', 'extension', 'abduction', and so on. Similarly, when it describes static positions, or postures, it does so again by describing the skeletal configuration relative to anatomical position. Even though no-one ever habitually stands in anatomical position, this convention remains a precise and convenient means for describing movements and postures. It is an essential tool in the tool-bag of the structural bodyworker, allowing them to define gross patterns and to communicate with other somatic professionals.

The skeletal definition of posture allows us to make judgements such as: the head is too far forward (or the neck too protracted), or there is potential for this shoulder girdle to settle more comfortably down on the thorax, or that this pelvis would be more balanced if there were more posterior tilt. It helps us recognize that there is more potential for hip extension in a client's gait. When we make such judgements we are essentially describing skeletal relationships. Recognizing these patterns is a vital first step in understanding the structure of our clients, although ultimately such descriptions say very little about the structural dynamics and tonus patterns required of a real body; nor is this anatomical language particularly useful for describing subtle or rhythmic movement, for which a more metaphorical vocabulary may be needed – for instance the evocative language of dance.

Many aspects of our clients' functionality will be missed if we focus on their skeletal organization alone. However, when making an initial assessment of our clients, the first step is to look for segmental displacements (which are ultimately defined by their skeletal configuration) without necessarily focussing on whether perceived misalignments are postural (i.e. functional) or structural.

Poor postural–structural organization can arise in many ways, and some of the physiological mechanisms have been discussed already in Chapter 11. However, even a seemingly balanced or 'aligned' posture may mask an underlying structural imbalance, with a 'balanced' posture sometimes being maintained only with great effort. This could either be through a widespread pattern of unnecessarily elevated muscular tonus, or perhaps through an over reliance on the powerful sleeve muscles when deeper tonic muscles could do the work more efficiently. For instance, the apparently aligned posture of a student of yoga or dance may conceal a subtle holding pattern: an effort to find 'form' that may mask some underlying structural dysfunction, and which reveals itself only when they relax a little. One also finds clients who appear classically aligned in standing (see Fig. 2.2, p. 16) yet maintain a widespread pattern of elevated tonus, of unnecessary co-contracture, which compresses their structure generally and may only become apparent from the quality of their movements. Most clients, when having their posture/structure evaluated tend to 'hold to form' rather than allowing themselves to drop into a habitual, comfortable posture. It is common for clients to suck in their abdomen in a vain attempt to meet the Western aesthetic ideal of the flat belly, or to retract their shoulders because they do not like to feel them rounding forward.

Regardless whether a posture is balanced or dysfunctional, it is the spatial relationships between the bones that define it and alert us to potential structural problems. All of this emphasizes the fact that the language of anatomy and kinesiology is very useful for recognizing the basic postural patterns of our clients, but that this is never sufficient for a more complete understanding of their structural organization. So, in our evaluation of our clients we examine their posture, making a preliminary assessment based on the organization of the skeleton; then we see what is revealed by the quality of their movement and refine these impressions as we use touch in working with them.

It was suggested in Chapter 8 that it is the fascia that creates the unified skeleton because it spans the bones and defines the range of possible spatial relationships between them. Although it is the fasciae that maintain the postural arrangement, and the fasciae that we seek to change in structural bodywork, when we come to describe postural dysfunctions and syndromes it is easier to follow the conventions of anatomy and to define them skeletally. In the following section we will describe the most commonly presented postural–structural dysfunctions by their skeletal configuration. We will also make some reference to the tonic patterns required to maintain such configurations, as well as the typical patterns of fascial shortness that arise from them.

THE SKELETAL SYSTEM

The skeleton is the densest aspect of the connective tissue continuum, the densest form of 'the one fascia'. Bones are a bone-salt–collagen composite, consisting approximately of 75% bone-salts and 25% collagen and ground substance. They are surrounded by their own fascial 'bag', the periosteum, which serves to connect the skeleton to its tendinous muscle attachments and making the skeleton entirely continuous with the fascial network.

If we look at the body as a tensegrity system then bones are the lightweight compressive beams. They are strong in compression, torque and shear, but are also slightly flexible through their long axis. The long bones are marvellously constructed of an outer shell of dense or compact bone that encloses a network of canals and trabeculae: the cancellous bone (Fig. 12.1). The trabeculae

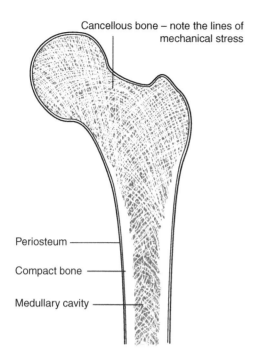

Figure 12.1 Compact and cancellous bone.

Cancellous bone – note the lines of mechanical stress

Periosteum

Compact bone

Medullary cavity

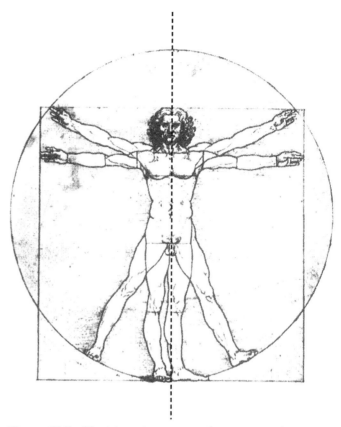

Figure 12.2 The bilateral symmetry of our structural organization (after da Vinci).

are arranged precisely along the lines of mechanical stress as predicted by Wolff's law. In the skeletal system the bones articulate but do not touch; they are kept apart either by a resilient and shock-absorbing cartilage and a film of synovial fluid, or else by fibrous matter.

STRUCTURAL OVERVIEW OF THE HUMAN DESIGN

Like all vertebrates, the grand structural plan of the human body is based on bilateral symmetry around the mid-sagittal plane (Fig. 12.2). However, the bilateral symmetry of the human body is of a particular kind; it is not the perfect mathematical symmetry of a snowflake. Most of the musculoskeletal units that are recognized in anatomy exist in pairs, and although in general each is close to being a mirror image of the other, the reflection is never perfect. Biological entities tend not to have the symmetry of crystals. All elements of the musculoskeletal system are subject to a wide range of developmental pressures, many of which are asymmetrical in nature.

There is a strong tendency in humans to develop lateralized functionality; that is, left- or right-handedness, 'leggedness' and 'eyedness', and often even different sensitivities to the left or right side of the perceptual field. Because of this tendency, perfectly symmetrical function and symmetrical growth are highly unlikely in any aspect of the connective tissue network. As was

mentioned in Chapter 9, Wolff's law operates throughout the entire connective tissue network, and if any aspect of our structure *can* adapt, then it *will* adapt, and probably in an asymmetrical fashion.

If we divide the body through the mid-sagittal plane we observe individual (i.e. non-paired) bones only along this plane. These bones include the frontal, occipital and mandible bones of the skull; the hyoid; the individual and the fused vertebrae of the spinal column, and the sternum. All other bones are paired, somewhat symmetrically, on either side of the mid-sagittal plane, including the parietal and temporal bones of the skull, the clavicles, the scapulae, the ribs, the innominates and all the bones of the limbs (Fig. 12.3).

There are left–right differences even at birth, and these differences may diverge even further during development. For instance, the ribs are shaped partly by the underlying viscera; the liver on the right and the aorta on the left cause deviations in the shape of the ribs. The ribs will also respond to the torsional forces within a scoliotic structure and will, in time, flatten in some areas, become more rounded or angular in others, close up in some areas and spread apart in others. The

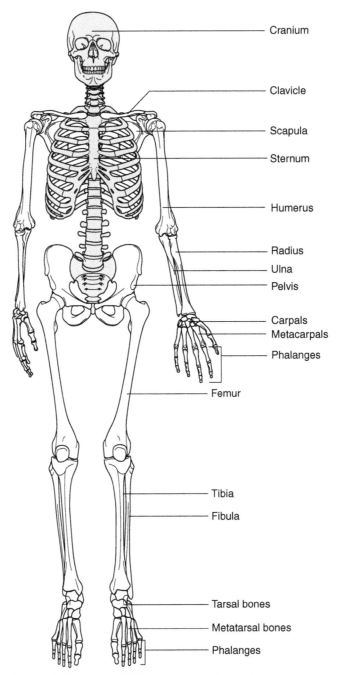

Figure 12.3 The axial skeleton – anterior and posterior aspects.

innominates vary in shape and can be of variable lengths, a condition known as hemipelvis, and legs are commonly of unequal length. Laughlin in his review of the radiological research into leg length discrepancy (LLD) reports that half the subjects surveyed had a length discrepancy of 5 mm or more (Laughlin 1998).

This 'near-bilateral symmetry' is found also within the muscular system. Most somatic musculature exists as paired muscles on either side of the midline, with the diaphragm, sphincters and some facial muscles being the only exceptions. Muscles are even more immediately responsive to usage patterns than the skeleton. And again, because of our lateralized functionality and asymmetrical usage, it is very common to have muscle pairs that differ in mass, length and other adaptive characteristics, such as degree of fibrosity. This is obvious for the superficial and more easily palpated muscles, but ultrasound investigations have confirmed this now for deeper muscles such as the psoas and multifidus (Richardson 1998) – the psoas being the least symmetrical of all muscle pairs.

Within our core space, the thoracic and abdominal cavities, there is even less symmetry. The lungs have two lobes on the left side and three on the right. The liver is to the right and stomach is normally to the left. The heart is usually left of centre. The alimentary canal, being a long tube, has to be folded to remain within its confining peritoneal bag and cannot be symmetrically arranged. The pattern of visceral connective tissue, the supportive mesentery and suspensory ligaments of organs, are not symmetrical and this, it has been argued, is another reason why absolute bilateral symmetry is impossible.

Segmental standard rotation

Flury (1991) observes that there is an almost universal pattern of rotatory asymmetry in the human body, which is independent of handedness. In this pattern, the various bodily segments are rotated relative to each other around the longitudinal axis of the body (see Fig. 12.4). For the axial components: the head is rotated right, the thoracic segment left and the pelvic segment right. For the appendicular components: the left leg as a whole is externally rotated to the left, while the right leg is more conflicted, having the right femur internally rotated compared to the left, while the right lower leg and foot are more externally rotated relative to the femur above. Variations from this pattern, he states, are rare, and although there may be reversals in some aspects, in Flury's clinical experience he has not found a single instance in which there has been the complete reversal of this pattern. He suggests that asymmetrical tensions within the mesentery may be a factor. He also suggests that this rotational pattern may be related to a common pattern of skeletal asymmetry, described as ilial torsion, in which the right ilium tends to rotate forward and out relative to the left ilium.

Flury does not draw any practical conclusions from this finding; however, it does seem to have important implications for the structural bodyworker. The near universality of this pattern does suggest that any attempt to 'correct' it may be futile as there may be genuine limits to how much bodywork can achieve in bringing a body towards greater symmetry. Here, the advice 'Don't fix what ain't broke' may be salutary. So perhaps the pattern of segmental standard rotation is best seen as a baseline: as the best one can achieve in creating symmetry.

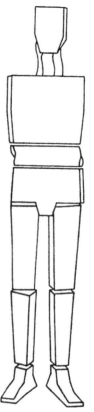

Figure 12.4 Segmental standard rotation. (With the kind permission of Dr Hans Flury.)

Asymmetrical usage, injury and other factors will tend to push the body further away from this baseline towards asymmetry, and these are the adaptations that can be addressed fruitfully by the structural bodyworker. Judith Aston, student of Ida Rolf and developer of the Aston Patterning movement system, affirms from her extensive clinical experience that if the outer structure is made too symmetrical it can give rise to somatic conflict: 'If the body has asymmetry on the inside and you hold symmetrically, you create what I call "micro-whiplashes," shear patterns which over time create scar tissue' (Pare 2002).

The axial–appendicular design

The basic pattern of structural organization for all mammals is a central axis defined by the axial skeleton and two appendicular systems – the superior and inferior girdles and their associated appendages. In humans these are the shoulder and pelvic girdles with their attached limbs. In the human being the axial system consists of: the skull, a vertebral column of seven cervical vertebrae, twelve thoracics with their attached ribs and sternum, five lumbar, the five fused sacral vertebrae and the four fused segments of the coccyx. The sacrum belongs to the axial skeleton but is ligamentously bound to the two innominates, forming the relatively stable unit of the pelvic bowl. Appended to the axial skeleton are the shoulder and pelvic girdles, from which issue the upper and lower limbs.

POSTURAL–STRUCTURAL DYSFUNCTIONS DEFINED SKELETALLY

In the following analysis we will look at postural–structural dysfunctions that:

- relate specifically to the organization of the axial skeleton
- arise from dysfunctional relationships between the girdles and the axial skeleton
- arise from the relationship between the girdles and their attached limbs.

A fuller analysis of dysfunctional patterns would also look in detail at dysfunctional relationships within limb complexes themselves.

What does it mean to say that a postural–structural pattern is dysfunctional? It means at the very least that the pattern is not an optimal arrangement in a bio-mechanical sense; it is not the most efficient possible. It means that gravity will in time tend to exaggerate the pattern and that, *of itself*, will give rise to undue stress to soft tissues, ultimately causing tissue damage and degenerative changes. Practical constraints will not allow us to examine all the postural–structural dysfunctions that structural bodyworkers typically deal with. Instead we will limit ourselves to the most common ones that arise in practice that can be addressed through soft-tissue work alone. Resolving these patterns will be an excellent 'first approximation' in normalizing the structure of our clients.

We will examine in most detail:

- dysfunctional patterns within the axial skeleton
- dysfunctional relationships between the pelvic girdle and the axial skeleton
- dysfunctional relationships between the shoulder girdle and the axial skeleton
- dysfunctional whole body patterns such as excessive shift of the pelvic segment

and, of the whole possible range of dysfunctional limb patterns, we will only consider

- the pattern of externally rotated legs (which is one of the most common gross structural dysfunctions of the lower limbs).

We will not examine intersegmental or intrasegmental dysfunctions either of the limbs or of the pelvis, with their conditions such as inflare, outflare and other torsional patterns that are traditionally the domain of osteopaths and chiropractors, although these are definitely amenable to change through soft-tissue work (Maitland 2001).

AXIAL OVERVIEW

From a structural bodywork perspective, the main structural themes associated with the axial skeleton relate to:

- the form of the spinal curves
- the placement of the head on top of the spine
- the relationship between the rib cage and the thoracic spine.

In the sagittal plane we are interested in the overall pattern of curvature of the spine (Fig. 12.5), that is, the

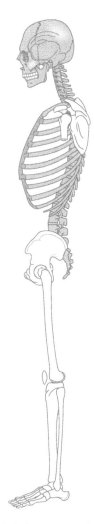

Figure 12.5 The axial skeleton, sagittal view.

relationships between the primary and secondary curves, while in the frontal plane it is scoliotic curvature with its inevitable rotatory compensations. We will look at the biomechanical importance of the curves of the spine in more detail later, but briefly, the spinal curves serve many important functions, which may be compromised if they are either too curved or not curved enough.

Being the bearer of our main orienting sense receptors, it is critical that the head be placed efficiently on top. Misalignment of the head and neck can have a disproportionately large influence on our moving efficiency. Conversely, any small refinement in the alignment of the head and neck will be keenly sensed by the client as an improvement. In the traditional Rolfing 10-series, the neck, like the back, is generally addressed each session, although it is not until the seventh session that there is a serious intent to 'get the head on top' as the whole spine and thorax needs to be prepared before the head can be stabilized around a new, more balanced home position.

In the thoracic region, the rib cage plays a large part in determining the movement possibilities of the thoracic spine. For any movement through the thoracic spine, the attached ribs will necessarily participate and constrain the kind of movement possible in the thoracic segments. It is important to see how our clients maintain elevation through the front of the ribcage when there is no bony support from below; often there is a tendency either to overcompensate and struggle 'to keep the chest up' or to allow the ribs to collapse down the front. It is a problem that has arisen from our bipedal existence and how a client approaches this problem often becomes a major theme in their ongoing structural work.

The spinal curves

At birth there is only one primary spinal curve in the sagittal plane since the foetus has usually developed in a fully flexed position within the uterus. However, segmental rotations around the midline may be evident even at this stage as it is not uncommon for the foetus to be non-symmetrically flexed within the uterus, with the shoulders rotated relative to the pelvis and with the head turned to one side (Schultz and Feitis 1996). Such rotations may predispose individuals to scoliotic patterns later on (Fig. 12.6).

The secondary spinal curves are developmental. At birth, reflexive flexor tone predominates over extensor tone, and much of the early development of movement

is concerned with bringing the head under control and bringing extensor tone into balance with flexor tone (Fiorentino 1981). The cervical lordosis develops in response to the child's drive to orient its head (and its full complement of teleceptors) out into the sensorial world. At about two months the tonic neck reflex emerges. This is an activation of the neck extensors to allow visual tracking (of the mother in particular) and the ability to orient the eyes and mouth to the horizontal. An increase in extensor tone gradually progresses inferiorly until it includes all the spinal extensors; this eventually allows upright sitting, supported standing and finally unsupported standing. The lumbar lordosis develops in response to the child's persistent efforts to stand upright. The curve develops as the child activates the lumbar extensors to bring the trunk more erect, against the resistance of the hip flexors that are still shortened from their term of full flexion in the womb (see Fig. 12.7).

Sagittal organization of the spine

In the sagittal plane, certain deviations of the spinal curves from a normal range can be problematic. The curves may be too exaggerated or (and this is not often acknowledged), too flat. What 'too curved' or 'too flat' actually means for any individual is difficult to determine

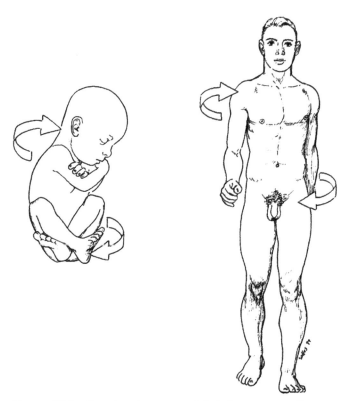

Figure 12.6 Rotations in utero and their longer term effects. (Schultz and Feitis 1996.)(With the kind permission of R Schulz.)

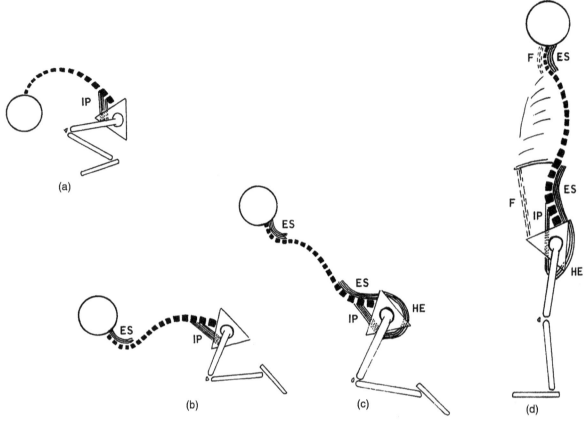

Figure 12.7 The development of the secondary spinal curves showing the gradual lengthening of the iliopsoas and shortening of the hip extensors. Abbreviations: ES, erector spinae; F, weak flexors; HE, hip extensors; IP, iliopsoas. (From Cailliet R 1981 Low back pain syndrome. F A Davis Company, Philadelphia).

exactly; it depends on many factors including body mass, bodily proportions, and distribution of fat, and it can vary throughout life depending on usage. However, the more exaggerated or extreme forms are easily recognized, and structural bodyworkers consistently find that when they resolve these extreme forms and the spinal segments become re-aligned, then clients feel better, function more efficiently, and usually find that many of their postural discomforts will resolve of themselves.

We should have stayed in the trees
Conventional scientific wisdom for many years has suggested that humans are essentially quadrupeds that have not yet fully adapted to bipedal existence. There is a widely held view regarding the sagittal curvature of the spine that 'the flatter the better'; this is just another aspect of the 'somatic Platonism' mentioned in Chapter 2. In this view, the lumbo-sacral junction is seen as inherently unstable, with the toboggan of L5 resting on the slippery slope of S1. The greater the lumbo-sacral angle, the more unstable the L5–S1 junction becomes, and the greater the tendency for shearing forces to stress the

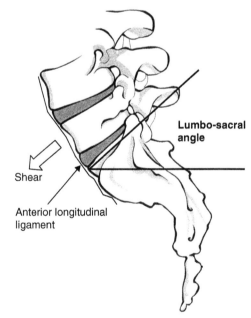

Figure 12.8 The lumbo-sacral angle.

disc and the supporting anterior longitudinal ligament (Cailliet 1981) (see Fig. 12.8). The practical implication normally drawn from this view is that we need to decrease the lumbo-sacral angle, reducing the spinal

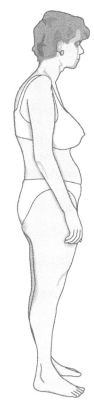

Figure 12.9 Tuck the tail under – appropriate advice?

curvature as much as possible; and the advice usually given is to 'tuck the tail under'. Actually, this effort of tucking the tail under, which is a lumbar flexion, usually realized through a contraction of the abdominal and gluteal muscles, does have an immediate effect of reducing the lumbar lordosis. It will be argued strongly, however, that this advice is usually misplaced. Any postural advice that involves asking someone to maintain a continual holding pattern is doomed to failure; in any case, the experience of many structural bodyworkers suggests that having too flat a spine can be equally problematic. Giving advice such as 'Tuck your tail under' is always dubious anyway because we are asking people to wilfully assume a posture that cannot be assumed naturally, that is, unconsciously (Fig. 12.9). This advice seems doubly inappropriate in that for about half our clients this advice will tend to exaggerate their pattern, and has the potential to *dis*organize them even further.

An alternative view is that problems arise from the extremes of curvature – too much or not enough. Among the spine's many functions is the gross biomechanical function of shock absorption. Mechanically, a curved spine acts as a spring that can absorb and dissipate the constant waves of compressive forces passing upwards through the skeleton in standing postures or through

the impact of heel-strike in walking or running (Alexander 1975, 1988). It is suggested that very straight spines are less able to absorb these 'ground forces' and are more likely to incur a thinning of the discs in the longer term. It is known for instance that marathon runners can lose several centimetres in height during a race; the constant pounding of heel-strike on a hard surface sends waves of compression through the legs, pelvis and spine that will extrude water from the discs. In fact we all tend to lose height during the day and are normally tallest (and our discs juiciest) in the morning when we rise. We always recover our height in the short term; however, it may be reasonably conjectured that a lifetime of inefficient shock-absorption will cause undue wear and tear on the spinal discs. Feldenkrais, who prior to his period of somatic invention was an engineer and physicist, makes the interesting point that

Force that is not converted into movement does not simply disappear, but is dissipated into damage done to joints, muscles and other sections of the body

(Rolf 1977)

Ida Rolf, too, realized the importance of disc health:

Discs constitute one-fourth to one-fifth of the spinal structure. Therefore, establishing or maintaining a good fluid balance in the discs is important in maintaining healthy spinal performance

(Rolf 1977)

Many elderly clients with a flat back are more likely to have a rigid, even fused, lumbar spine, thinning discs and secondary problems like sciatica that arise from such compression.

In addition, if we look structurally at a straight back, we note that it is at a mechanical disadvantage when compared with a lordotic back in its ability to support the cantilevered rib cage; in crude terms, it is much harder to keep you chest up if you have a flat back. A lumbar lordosis does tend to bring the lumbar spine closer to the midline of the body. Having a flat back means that the thoracic erectors (working synergistically with the scalenes) have to work harder to prevent the chest collapsing down the front. This fact goes a long way to explaining why flat-backed clients so often report muscle pain between the shoulder blades; it is because the thoracic erectors are overworked and strained in their effort to keep both the head and the chest up.

In Chapter 13 we will examine a postural model that has arisen from the Rolfing community, which is known as the *internal–external model*. Briefly, this model looks at the sagittal organization of the pelvis and spine and suggests that the sagittal tilt of the pelvis can be too extreme in either an anterior or posterior direction. Here, *pelvic tilt* is defined as the movement of the superior aspects of the pelvis away from a neutral or 'home' position around an axis that passes through both acetabula. An anterior tilt means that the anterior superior iliac spine (ASIS) has moved to the anterior and inferior, a posterior tilt means that the posterior superior iliac spine (PSIS) has moved to the posterior and inferior. Pelvic tilt is synergistically related to certain patterns of spinal curvature, having most effect on the form of the lumbar lordosis. Figure 12.10 is a simplified model showing the two basic patterns of tilt of the pelvic segment: the anterior tilt of the internal arrangement and the posterior tilt of the external.

Additionally there are *shift patterns* of the pelvis, in which the pelvic segment as a whole translates in an anterior or posterior direction over the feet. Tilt patterns combined with shift patterns will result in characteristic patterns of soft-tissue contracture. The internal–external model suggests that it is the extremes of these patterns that need to be addressed when we try to promote a more balanced structure. This view means that as somatic therapists we need to know our client's structural tendencies, whether towards an anterior or posterior tilt in pelvic organization.

There are many practical reasons why therapists need to know if their clients' spines are too curved or too straight, and this kind of information should be known not just by structural bodyworkers but by personal trainers, yoga teachers, Pilates teachers and physiotherapists. The 'tuck the tail under' advice seems to be almost universal and unquestioned; indeed this crude form of somatic Platonism is extremely widespread, and was never ever confined to Ida Rolf alone. Even massage therapists would benefit from some rudimentary ideas about structural variation, since a knowledge of their clients' tendencies can help them position them more comfortably on the table. Internal (lordotic) clients for instance are often more comfortable in a prone position with a pillow under their abdomen, and clients with an exaggerated 'head forward' posture cannot be comfortable with the face-hole of the conventional massage table.

If spines are deemed to have too much curvature, we can do the soft-tissue work that will tend, indirectly, to reduce that; and likewise if they are too straight we can do the soft-tissue work that will encourage more curvature. Inducing more curvature to a spine is more problematic than reducing it, and in general the changes are less dramatic visually than when we try to reduce curvature; however, the work is rarely wasted and will always remove some of the strain from the system, giving a sense of lift and giving more 'spring' to the structure. Figure 12.11 shows drawings from before–after Rolfing photos demonstrating how in these cases lumbar lordosis may be diminished or augmented by this work.

Figure 12.12 demonstrates the synergistic relationships between the primary and secondary curves – the general tendency for them *to increase or decrease together*.

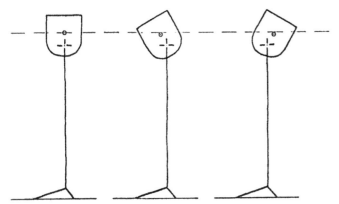

Figure 12.10 The patterns of anterior and posterior pelvic tilt. Note how the centre of gravity of the pelvic segment is superior to the axis of the acetabula, meaning that gravity will tend to exaggerate these patterns unless opposed by muscular action. (With the kind permission of Dr Hans Flury.)

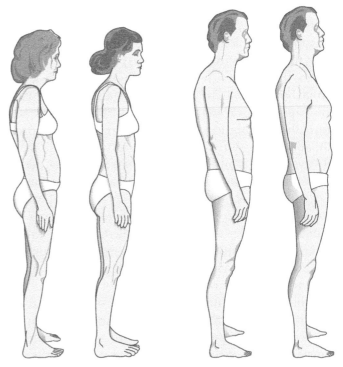

Figure 12.11 Reducing curvature, augmenting curvature.

However, this is hardly a comprehensive selection of profiles; spinal curvature can be very idiosyncratic, and it is common to find spinal organizations that do not fit these profiles at all. This diagram does suggest, however, that the spine is an integrated system, that there are mutual influences between the primary and secondary curves. If we bring a more holistic perspective to bear, it would suggest that it makes no sense to try to reorganize the contour of one curve without allowing for the reorganization of the others. Hence the conventional wisdom among structural bodyworkers that the lumbar and cervical lordoses need to be treated together.

Figure 12.13 illustrates the complex system of ligamentous support for the spine in the sagittal plane; the lateral ligaments connecting the transverse processes are not shown. Looking at this diagram it becomes apparent that ligaments, including the one-segment ligaments, will probably have a larger structural influence in maintaining spinal curvature than the investing fasciae of the spinal musculature, owing to the fact that they are denser and can more powerfully bind adjacent vertebrae together. In practical terms it means that if

we are intending to influence spinal curvature then working with the superficial fascia alone may not be sufficient to bring about the intended change; some way of influencing the deeper ligamentous structure of the spine needs to be found. In the practical section of this book (Chapter 16) some indirect stretches will be shown which are powerful means of influencing the spinal curves at a ligamentous level. These stretches will then support the more superficial fascial work.

Frontal organization of the spine

In the frontal plane scoliotic patterns may be apparent as lateral deviations of the spine from the midline, inevitably associated with rotatory patterns in the transverse plane that will always be accompanied with alterations to the symmetry of the rib cage. Scoliosis is a structural dysfunction that has received much attention from physical medicine. There are clearly many factors that contribute to scoliosis, many different reasons why a spine will adapt in this rather ingenious way. Some of the factors include: neurological developmental problems, proprioceptive insufficiency, postural reflex problems at a spinal cord level, and degraded collagen metabolism (Larson 2000). Idiopathic (i.e. of unknown cause) scoliosis is often of adolescent onset, particularly in young women, and has been attributed to a mismatch between the growth of the skeleton and the tardier growth of the supporting soft tissues. Possibly the most common form of scoliosis seen by structural bodyworkers, however, is that induced by a leg length

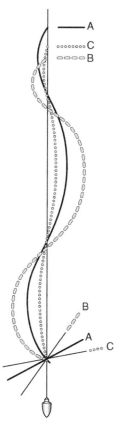

Figure 12.12 Different forms of the spinal curvature in the sagittal plane. A, B and C show different degrees of spinal curvature associated with different degrees of lumbo-sacral angle. (After Cailliet R 1981 Low back pain syndrome. F A Davis Company, Philadelphia).

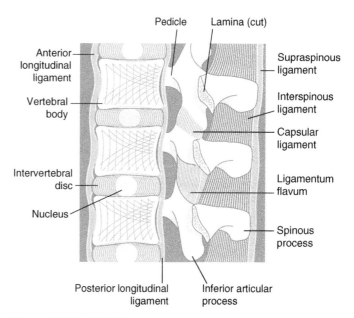

Figure 12.13 The ligamentous structure of the spine. (After Gorman.)

discrepancy (LLD). In this case a scoliosis can be seen as the body's ingenious solution to solving the problem of LLD. It was mentioned in Chapter 5 that structural bodywork is very effective in reorganizing fascia; bones however adapt over a much longer time span. If a scoliotic pattern is maintained too long during early life then the vertebral bodies may become wedge-shaped and asymmetrical. For many, however, the vertebral bodies maintain their shape and the scoliotic curves are taken up in the asymmetrical deformation of the discs themselves; for the latter group there is more possibility of lasting change through soft-tissue work.

The head

Evolutionary biologists point to the major evolutionary trend known as *encephalization*, which is the tendency for the brain, the sense receptors and the mouth to cluster towards one end of the organism. In humans the head is the bearer of most of our major exteroceptors: the ears, eyes, olfactory receptors, taste buds, and also the vestibular apparatus. In the human structure the neck too has a crucial role in this regard; its job is to orient the head to optimize its sensorial contact with the environment, allowing the head to scan more efficiently for sensory impressions. Additionally there is a concentration of proprioceptors in the sub-occipital muscles, some of the most densely innervated muscles of the body. Our sense of balance, in fact our whole orientation in space, depends largely upon the coordinated proprioceptive input from the eyes, the sub-occipital muscles and the vestibular apparatus.

Many somatic pioneers have stressed the importance of the balance of the head, and the role of the neck in organizing our overall movement patterns. Alexander spoke of *primary control*, the notion that it is the neck that chiefly organizes our movements. Human beings have an intricate orienting response that operates when we negotiate any complex terrain, whether in the bush, playing a team sport or traversing a busy supermarket. This deeply habitual orienting sequence is: the eyes glance and fixate, the sub-occipitals orient the head in that general direction, the larger neck muscles join in, and then the trunk orients itself in the desired direction. This orienting response forms very early in our development and is vital for efficient interaction with the environment. The neck must be delicately poised if it is to support this orienting sequence in an efficient way.

It has been reported that Feldenkrais, too, believed in the critical importance of the neck in organizing our movement (Wildman 1993). Feldenkrais worked with

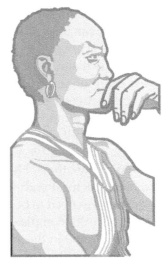

Figure 12.14 The poise of the head. (From M Gelb 1981 Body learning: an introduction to the Alexander technique. Henry Holt, NY, p. 46.)

some of the top sports-people of his day and expressed the opinion that although top athletes have extremely well organized necks, the best organized necks he ever worked with belonged to top business people and military officers, and he offered the suggestion that the ability to make quick decisions, as it were, on the run, requires a delicate poise of the head (see Fig. 12.14). Many authors have pointed to the extraordinarily poised head posture seen in less Westernized cultures: Nubian tribesmen, Australian aborigines, the Balinese, and in traditional representations of the Buddha. We instantly ascribe to a balanced head posture expressions of nobility, containment, poise, balance and mastery (Von Dürkheim 1977, Gelb 1981).

The positioning of the skull on top of the spinal column is critical in achieving postural balance. This is problematic, however, since even with the most balanced upright posture the skull itself is inherently *unbalanced* – its centre of gravity being anterior to the fulcrum of the atlanto-occipital (AO) junction (Fig. 12.15). Therefore, the cervical extensors are inevitably obliged to work all the time, whenever we are upright. It is a first class lever (the fulcrum lying between the effort and the resistance) and is a hangover from our quadrupedal past. The reason why your head drops forward to your chest when you 'nod off' is that the cervical extensors simply turn off, and gravity asserts itself. So, in normal upright stance, the tonic extensor muscles of the neck are bound to work *non-stop all day*; however, as true tonic muscles they are well adapted to do this. If the head is not carried too far forward, these

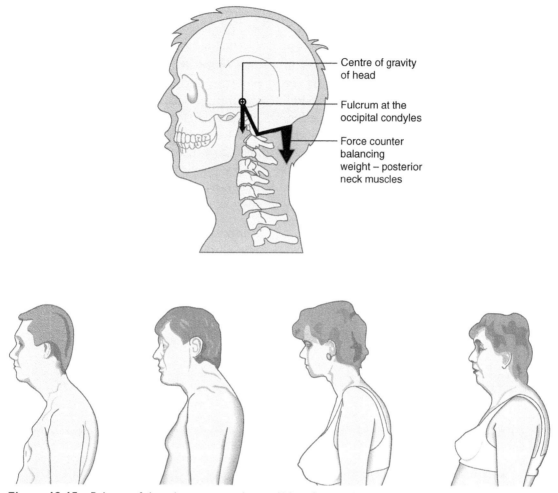

Centre of gravity of head

Fulcrum at the occipital condyles

Force counter balancing weight – posterior neck muscles

Figure 12.15 Balance of the atlanto-occipital joint. (After Gorman.)

muscles, being tonic or slow-twitch, are easily capable of working continuously throughout the day without tiring. It is only when the centre of gravity of the head is habitually held too far forward that these muscles exhibit signs of strain. The 'head forward syndrome' is very common in our culture, with nearly all of our work requiring us to look forward and down.

The head forward syndrome

Whether cutting vegetables, typing at a desk or working over a bench, the head tends to be drawn forward and to look down. There is a recognized reflexive relationship between the oculo-motor muscles, the suboccipital muscles and our trunk flexors and extensors; when we look down it facilitates the action of the flexors and when we look up it facilitates our extensors. Therefore, having our work tasks always below eye-level will always tend to encourage both head and trunk flexion. It has been estimated that for every 2.5 cm the

head moves forward, the workload of the cervical extensors is doubled; hence the ropy, fibrotic feel of these muscles so often found in our clients and their common complaints of muscle pain between the scapulae.

Forward head syndrome is accompanied by a chain of compensatory adaptations. It is probably more accurate to see this syndrome as a whole body pattern in which the forward head is the most conspicuous aspect. This pattern typically includes a depressed rib cage and shoulder girdles that protract and elevate, with scapulae that rotate and abduct giving the typical 'up and over' appearance of the shoulder girdle.

One major consequence of the head forward position is that the AO junction becomes compromized in a number of ways. Tonic neck reflexes operate to keep our face vertical and our eyes oriented towards the horizon. There is a habitual relationship between our eyes and the angle of our face: the sensed 'home position' of the eyes within the orbits. To change this would require different tonus patterns in the oculo-motor muscles of the eyes, a completely different proprioceptive feel, which we will try to avoid if at all possible. Hence, as the head translates forward, neck reflexes operate to keep the face relatively vertical. This can only be achieved through cervical flexion and capital extension, and this action closes the AO joint posteriorly (see Fig. 12.16). If this pattern becomes habitual many neural and vascular structures that congregate in the AO area may be compromised. Additionally, the delicate sub-occipital muscles themselves are placed under strain. We now know that the sub-occipital muscles, although minimal movers and initiators, have an important proprioceptive function. Neurologically they are very much related to the functioning of the oculo-motor muscles and to the proprioceptors of the inner ear, thereby helping us orient ourselves in the world, telling us the

direction of 'up', 'down' and where the horizon is. As mentioned earlier, somatic pioneers such as Alexander and Feldenkrais have emphasized the critical importance of this region in organizing our overall movement patterns, and subsequent research has confirmed their intuitions (Garlick 1982). So, if the AO junction is compromized in this way we may expect it to adversely affect how we move around and function in the world. You just need to put on a restrictive neck brace for a while to realize how much we rely on neck mobility to organize our movements from moment to moment. Figure 12.17 shows further examples of the head forward syndrome.

Importance of the sub-occipital muscles
The sub-occipital muscles (Fig. 12.18) are minimal movers of the head; they can initiate a little nod 'yes', or

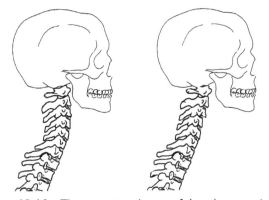

Figure 12.16 The posterior closure of the atlanto-occipital joint as the head shifts forward.

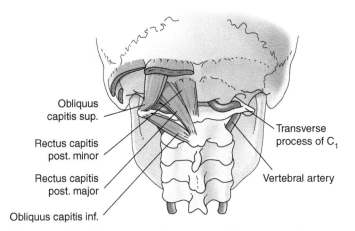

Obliquus capitis sup.

Rectus capitis post. minor

Rectus capitis post. major

Obliquus capitis inf.

Transverse process of C₁

Vertebral artery

Figure 12.18 The sub-occipital muscles. (After Gorman.)

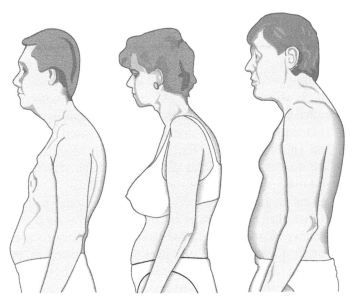

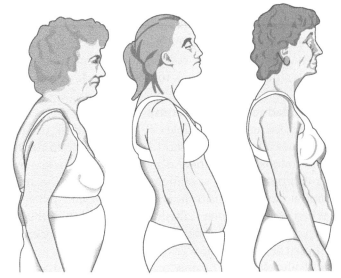

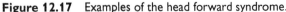

Figure 12.17 Examples of the head forward syndrome.

a little 'no' and the little circle that combines both these movements. Like all of the deepest spinal muscles they have a vital proprioceptive role, acting as movement sensors for the head (Abrahams 1982). They are densely innervated, densely populated with motor units, and have many mechanoreceptors that provide information about the angle of the head. This input, when coordinated with related input from the oculo-motor muscles and the vestibular apparatus, provides vital information to the central nervous system concerning where the head is in space and how it relates to the horizon (Berthoz 2000). Experiments in which the sub-occipitals are disabled with local anaesthetic show that subjects will have a staggering gait, as if drunk. If the injection is one-sided then the subject will have an irresistible sensation of listing to that side (Abrahams 1982).

The sub-occipitals are small muscles and definitely not prime movers and, like the deeper, smaller spinal muscles, they can easily be inhibited by the larger overlying musculature. In the forward head posture the more superficial musculature will of necessity be called upon to stabilize the head. To work with their inherent delicacy the sub-occipitals must not be overwhelmed by the sheer power of these more superficial neck muscles. So a vital aspect of structural bodywork is what Ida Rolf called 'getting the head on top', that is, bringing the head into a more posterior position without strain, and giving the deeper muscles more freedom to act. She emphasized the critical importance of activating the deeper muscles of the neck to achieve poise:

> When the head functions incompetently, movement of the head is initiated and largely executed by the superficial muscles that attach to the shoulder girdle. Thus in the random individual, the head or neck turns with little or no participation of the deep-lying intrinsics
>
> (Rolf 1977)

Ida Rolf also emphasized the importance of working around the jaw and the important relationship between the jaw and the base of the skull. The jaw is often slung asymmetrically, particularly for clients with scoliosis. Interestingly the whole face including the line of the nose tends to conform to the general winding curvature of scoliosis. This can lead to the habit of one-sided chewing. As structural bodywork reduces the curvature of scoliosis it is often necessary to deal with the myofascial asymmetries around the jaw to assist it to sit more symmetrically.

Secondary aspects of the head forward syndrome

The head forward tendency will be exacerbated if there is a tendency for the chest to collapse down the front (into what will be described later as an *expiration fix* pattern). The ribs will tend to angle down more in the front, and this means that the thoracic outlet may be compromised. If to this is added some shoulder girdle depression, this may result in the compression of the neurovascular bundles that run beneath the clavicle producing a condition known as *thoracic outlet syndrome*. The brachial plexus is the neurological telephone exchange for the arms, and consists of an interconnected complex of the cervical nerves emerging from C5 to T1. The plexus exits between the anterior and mid scalene muscles before diving beneath the clavicle and entering the arm. Like most nerve bundles it shares a pathway with other plumbing, in this case the brachial artery. Localized compression can exert pressure on the nerve and vascular bundles, and can arise from tight, overworked scalenes; elevated tonus in the upper trapezius and other neck muscles, or from excessive shoulder girdle depression in which the pectoralis minor is often involved. This pattern is often connected with *repetitive strain syndromes* in which myofascial impingement on the brachial plexus can give rise to numbness, pain or 'pins and needles' sensations in the arm and hand and reduced circulation at the extremity.

Often the collapse of the chest will lead to breathing restrictions and a compression of the abdominal contents. This overall pattern has long been recognized by somatic therapists, with Janda, for instance, calling it the 'upper crossed syndrome' (Chaitow 1996), and it has been explored in some of the earliest literature about posture (Todd 1937). For people with a 'straight back' tendency this often results in the so-called Dowager's hump, a fibro-fatty pad that builds around the spinous processes of C7 and T1. It seems to be the body's attempt at bracing those segments of the spine to prevent a further translation of the head forward. It is more common in women, but can appear in either sex, particularly among those with a flattened thoracic spine.

Thoracic spine

The rib attachments in the thoracic spine makes this part of the spine the least flexible, so that any attempt to reorganize the thoracic curvature here will require parallel work with the structure of the rib cage. If the thoracic spine is 'too flat', it will produce an unfavourable angle of action for the neck extensors, which are consequently overworked and liable to form trigger points and fibrotic adaptations between the shoulder blades. The thoracic erectors have a mechanical advantage when they pull around a curve, and become stressed if this curve is absent. However, if the thoracic spine is too curved, or kyphotic, then it will feed into patterns such as the expiration fixed chest or a shortened ventral aspect of the trunk, so there will inevitably be a corresponding shortness on the anterior chest wall. But as is often the case with the spine, the chief contributors to the spine's form are the long spinal ligaments rather than the fascia. The thoracic aspect of the anterior longitudinal ligament is obviously not amenable to the application of direct techniques so, although direct myofascial work to the ventral aspect of the trunk will assist in ameliorating a kyphotic pattern, it is probably only through 'counter-curve' stretching that this deep, strong ligament can be significantly affected. In Chapter 16 several stretches will be shown that can influence this ligament in the thoracic area.

The lumbar spine

There is a widespread misconception among the general public (and even among some somatic professionals) that a lumbar lordosis is not a good thing. Additionally, the lordosis is often confused with a *sway back*, which is probably best described as an anterior shift of the entire pelvic segment and can be accompanied with either an excessive or a diminished lumbar lordosis. Hence, many new clients will insist that they have too much lordosis when in fact they have very little. The view of many structural bodyworkers, however, is that having either an excessive or diminished lordosis can be equally problematic.

Excessive lordosis is normally associated with an anterior tilting pelvis, shortened hip flexors and lumbar erectors, and internally rotated femurs. At a ligamentous level there is a shortening of the posterior longitudinal and interspinous ligaments of the lumbar spine, and often a tension in the ilio-femoral ligament that severely limits hip extension. An exaggerated lordosis tends also to be linked with an exaggerated kyphosis and a cervical lordosis. On the basis of a meticulous mathematical modelling of the spine, Gracovetsky (1988) suggests that a lumbar lordosis is absolutely necessary for lifting and, in general, for the transmission of power through the skeleton in trunk flexion and extension. Other investigators have emphasized the shock-absorption potential for the lumbar lordosis because it can act as a spring, somewhat like the old-fashioned car suspension, and can dampen the shock of compressive ground forces coming up through the skeleton (Alexander 1975, 1988). So the common practice of attempting to reduce this lordosis uncritically is often shortsighted.

The flattened lumbar spine is typically associated with a posterior tilting pelvis, shortened hip extensors (particularly the hamstrings), obliques, and the lower rectus abdominus, as well as a tendency towards flaccid gluteals and external rotation of the femurs (what later we will call the 'external' pattern). At a ligamentous level, it is the anterior longitudinal ligament in the lumbar spine that has shortened (though it is more likely the case that it has never lengthened). Because of the widespread use of chairs in Western societies, there is a common tendency to slump in sitting, and even to develop lumbar kyphosis in the seated posture. This can be deleterious for those whose lumbar lordosis is diminished anyway, and especially deleterious for soft-tissued types whose lax ligaments will tend to even greater laxity through slumped sitting. Biomechanically there is less shock absorption in the flat lumbar spine and therefore a greater tendency towards compression problems in later life. In the elderly one often sees this typical pattern of collapse where there is an extreme posterior tilt of the pelvis, which combined with a growing thoracic kyphosis leads to a compressed abdomen and the habit of sitting on the coccyx or even the sacrum instead of the 'sit bones'. It is also common for flat-backed clients to develop non-specific knee pain, and it might be conjectured that this is another consequence of inefficient absorption of compressive ground forces.

The rib cage

The common term 'rib cage' is actually a misnomer since there is little of the rigidity that 'cage' might suggest; the ribs are usually quite springy and compressible and have synovial connections with the thoracic vertebrae and discs, but also at the cartilaginous connections around the sternum.

The ribs can be visualized as a series of cantilevered rings of bone connected to the spine at the back, to the sternum at the front, to adjacent ribs by the intercostal fasciae, and unified internally by the endothoracic fascia. The ribs are 'hinged' at their synovial attachments at the spine and have quite a complex movement during respiration that involves rising and falling in a 'bucket-handle' fashion, but also twisting as they rise and fall. During respiration the rib cage expands in all directions, including backwards and downwards, but is stabilized by the quadratus lumborum against the pull of the diaphragmatic crura.

If we consider the structural environment of the rib cage as a whole we note that the skeletal support is entirely posterior; the anterior aspect, the space between the xyphoid process and the pubic bone, is spanned by soft tissue alone. This does suggest a potential design problem – since there is no skeletal support down the front, just how do we prevent the front of the chest from dropping towards the pubis, compromising breathing and pressing on the contents of the abdominal cavity? This is actually one of the most common postural dysfunctions of all. There are two main ways of preventing this collapse:

- by tightening the erector spinae, which in synergy with the scalenes can lift the chest from above (no doubt assisted by other accessory breathing muscles)
- through a valsalva manoeuvre – a general increase in the tonus of the abdominal muscles, which turns the visceral core into a hydraulic balloon that can support the rib cage from below (what has more recently been termed *core support*), or
- through a balanced combination of both of the above.

It has been suggested already that the erector spinae–scalene solution is less favourable for those with diminished spinal curvature, so it is quite common for 'flat back' clients to mobilize the scapular retractors as well in an attempt to lift the chest, which leads to the military-squared shoulders seen in so many of them.

Rolfers talk of two extremes of rib adaptation: *inspiration fix* and *expiration fix*. Since we rarely use our whole lung capacity for most activities in daily life our breath can habitually hover around the point of maximum capacity or minimum capacity, or anywhere between, and this will in time modify the fascial and ligamentous structure of the chest. Those who tend towards maximum capacity are called 'inspiration fixed' and have the 'pumped chest' look of bodybuilders; those towards minimum capacity are called 'expiration fixed' (see Fig. 12.19). According to many in the field of somatic psychology, there are definite emotional tendencies associated with these patterns of chest organization, and the breathing patterns that go with them (Keleman 1985).

These patterns also tend to reflect the solutions people have found to counter the collapsed chest. Inspiration fix is often associated with the above-mentioned pattern of an elevated tonus in the thoracic erectors, scalenes and shoulder girdle retractors. Expiration fix can be the result of several factors: the tendency just to collapse and 'let go' into our fascial and ligamentous slings, or as a result of a constant low level of elevated tonus in the trunk flexors, which is what Feldenkrais

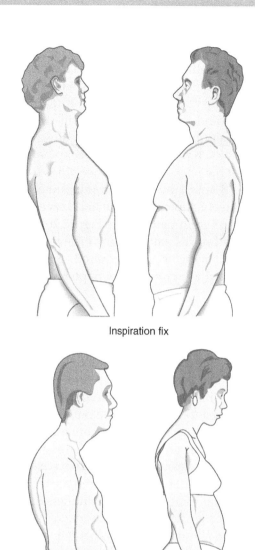

Inspiration fix

Expiration fix

Figure 12.19   Inspiration and expiration fixation of the chest.

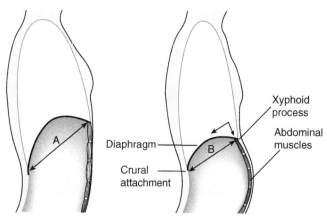

Figure 12.20   Expiration fix and the shortened diaphragm.

called 'the body pattern of anxiety' (see Schleip in Chapter 13). Both of these tendencies may also be exacerbated if there is insufficient tonus in the deep abdominals, the transversus in particular. In either case, the costal arch and xyphoid process will not only drop closer to the pubis but will also angle inwards towards the crural attachments of the lumbar spine. One might expect that the *internal* fascial connections from front to back, the diaphragm and visceral connective tissue, will adaptively shorten in time and serve to maintain the collapsed chest pattern (see Fig. 12.20). So, in order to fully address this pattern some means of lengthening the internal fascia is also required. Some stretching approaches will be covered in Chapter 16.

Shoulder girdle

The shoulder girdle is the clavicle–scapula complex from which the arms are suspended (see Fig. 12.21). Its function is bringing the hands into contact with as much of the immediate tactile environment as possible. It is connected to the axial skeleton chiefly by soft tissues, since the only ligamentous connection to the axial skeleton is at the sterno-clavicular joint. Because of the extensive musculature connecting the axial skeleton to the shoulder girdle and other muscles crossing the gleno-humeral joint, the mutual influence of the neck and shoulder girdle can be quite marked. So work on the neck and shoulder girdle go hand in hand.

Embryologically, the shoulder girdle is related to the pelvic girdle since the limb buds appear about the same time; however, functionally it does not have the stability or weight bearing function of the pelvic girdle, but is adapted more to positioning the hands in as wide a sphere as possible. And in one of the typical compromises in our somatic organization, mobility is gained at the expense of stability. The shoulder girdle is designed to allow free movement via the sterno-clavicular and acromio-clavicular joints, and the scapulo-thoracic articulation. As a unit the shoulder girdle should ideally rest snugly on top of the superior, conical apex of the rib cage, yet we continually find the girdle shifted from this natural 'home' position and displaced in a number of ways.

Through habitual usage, the shoulder girdle may be displaced in elevation, depression, retraction, protraction, or more likely in some combination of these directions (see Fig. 12.22). And since the girdle rests on the top of the rib cage it will naturally conform to the shape of the upper ribs, whether lifted above the 'pumped' chest or dropping forward and down onto the collapsed

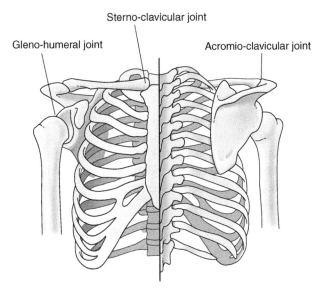

Figure 12.21 The shoulder girdle.

chest. Elevated and protracted shoulders are particularly implicated in 'the body pattern of anxiety', while retracted (or military squared) shoulders are statistically related to what we later call the external posture, involving a flat back and a posteriorly tilted pelvis. Less frequent is the depressed shoulder girdle, which tends to be found mostly among those we have called the soft-tissued types. The elevated–protracted pattern is produced by the synergistic operation of the shoulder girdle elevators and the pectoralis minor, and is usually an aspect of the forward head syndrome.

The shoulder girdle will inevitably adapt to a scoliotic pattern of the spine and tend to sit approximately perpendicular to the upper thoracic spine, leading to the common postural pattern of one shoulder sitting higher than the other (Fig. 12.23). Even if the scoliotic client has cleverly managed to maintain horizontal shoulders there will be a left–right asymmetry in the rhomboids and trapezius.

The pelvic girdle

The pelvic girdle is the central exchange for the mechanical forces in the body. It mediates the trunk above and the lower limbs below, transmitting compressive vectors down through the lumbo-sacral junction, the sacroiliac joints, the pelvic arches and into the legs via the acetabula. Compressive ground forces travel upwards by the same route. The pelvic girdle serves as the attachment for a great many very powerful muscles and therefore responds to tensional vectors from many directions; and it must also withstand the wedging action

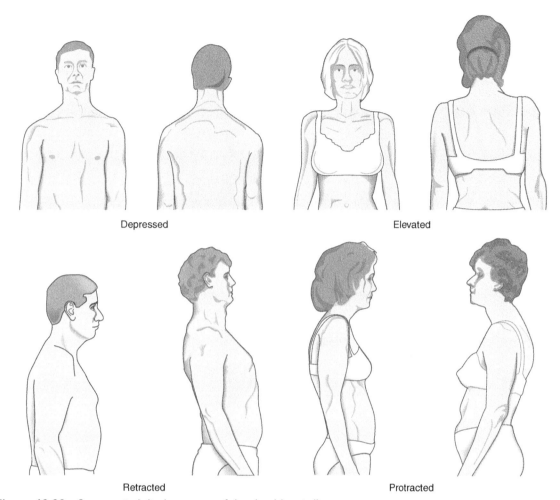

Depressed   Elevated

Retracted   Protracted

Figure 12.22 Some typical displacements of the shoulder girdle.

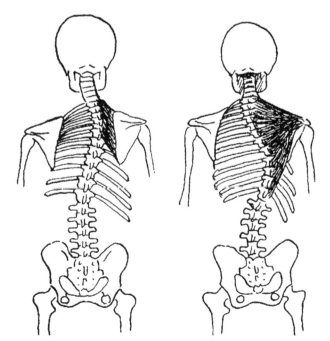

Figure 12.23 The relationship between the shoulder girdle and thoracic spine in the scoliotic client. (Dalton 1998.)

of the visceral mass above. During gait there is a shearing moment through the pubic symphysis and sacro-iliac joints as weight shifts from one side to the other. In all, there are a great many vectors to deal with. However, the pelvic girdle is able to harmonize these forces because of its extraordinary structural design. The innominates and sacrum are stitched together and unified by an intricate network of ligaments that either reinforce the points of articulation or else act like pliable cables by uniting the bony superstructure of the pelvis from the inside and creating a tensegrity structure of great strength (see Fig. 12.24). All the ligaments work together to make for a strong yet yielding structure that can safely transmit all the distorting mechanical forces that pass through it.

The pelvic segment can habitually be shifted anteriorly or posteriorly in standing such that the weight of the upper body falls in front of or behind the hip joint, requiring different muscles to stabilize the pelvis in standing. Flury notes that the different combinations of pelvic tilt and shift tend to set up fairly predictable

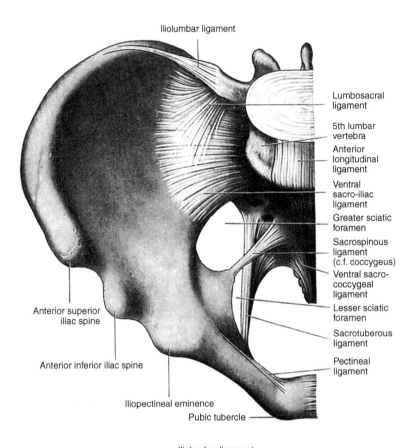

Iliolumbar ligament

Lumbosacral ligament

5th lumbar vertebra

Anterior longitudinal ligament

Ventral sacro-iliac ligament

Greater sciatic foramen

Sacrospinous ligament (c.f. coccygeus)

Ventral sacro-coccygeal ligament

Lesser sciatic foramen

Sacrotuberous ligament

Pectineal ligament

Anterior superior iliac spine

Anterior inferior iliac spine

Iliopectineal eminence

Pubic tubercle

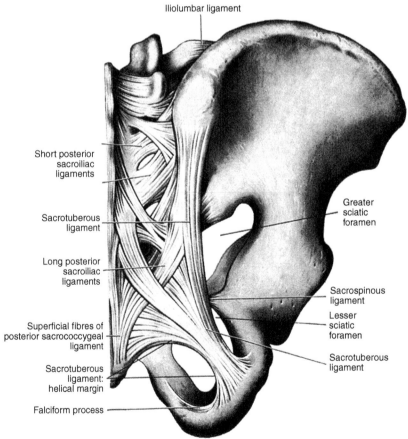

Iliolumbar ligament

Short posterior sacroiliac ligaments

Sacrotuberous ligament

Long posterior sacroiliac ligaments

Superficial fibres of posterior sacrococcygeal ligament

Sacrotuberous ligament: helical margin

Falciform process

Greater sciatic foramen

Sacrospinous ligament

Lesser sciatic foramen

Sacrotuberous ligament

Figure 12.24　The ligamentous structure of the pelvis. (After Gorman.)

patterns of fascial strain and contracture that may need to be addressed through soft-tissue work (Flury 1989). The myofascial adaptations related to these patterns will be examined in more detail in Chapters 13 and 14.

There may also be asymmetries in the frontal plane, side-shifted patterns, in which left–right imbalances of the hip abductors and adductors arise. These side-shifts may be due to asymmetrical usage, or through a difference in leg lengths.

Leg length discrepancy (LLD)

Radiological research has shown that:

- 17% of people have a leg-length discrepancy of more than 10 mm, and
- 35% of people have an LLD of between 5 and 10 mm (Laughlin, 1998).

Hence more than 50% of the population have a true discrepancy in leg length of 5 mm or more (see Fig. 12.25). Laughlin argues that, depending on other interacting factors; an LLD of this seemingly small magnitude can have serious ramifications in terms of postural balance and its attendant pain, depending on usage factors. For example, a 10 mm LLD is more significant if you teach four aerobic classes a day than if you sit all day at a desk. In their review of the research into LLD, Simons and Travell (1999) note that this condition can:

- promote muscular imbalances that will perpetuate trigger points in the affected muscles, especially in the quadratus lumborum
- cause back pain (which is frequently relieved by a compensating heel-lift).

It was also noted that if an LLD is artificially induced with a heel-lift, then normal subjects will begin to experience back pain within a few days, They also make the interesting point that if children are given compensatory heel-lifts then leg lengths will equalize within 3–7 months (Simons and Travell 1999).

An LLD will inevitably result in pelvic obliquity, an induced scoliosis and altered gait biomechanics that can cause stress around the lumbar-thoracic junction. LLD may also result in other postural patterns such as ilial torsion or rotatory displacements around the midline. It should not, however, be confused with a unilateral contracture of the adductors, which can mimic its outward appearance.

If we look at the geometry of LLD in standing, the first obvious fact is that the different heights of the femoral heads will cause the tops of the ilia to stand at different heights, setting up the pelvic obliquity in the frontal plane (see Fig. 12.26). A factor often missed by researchers in this area is that the width of the hips is a confounding factor here. The larger the distance between the

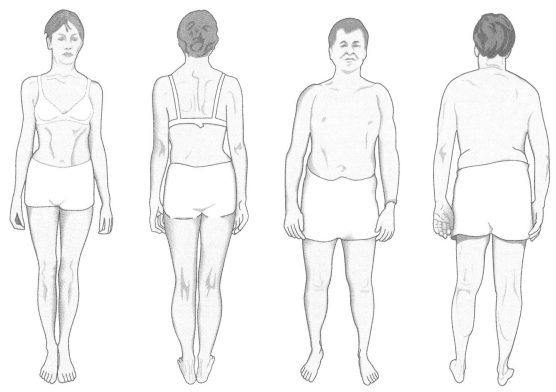

Figure 12.25 Some examples of leg length discrepancy.

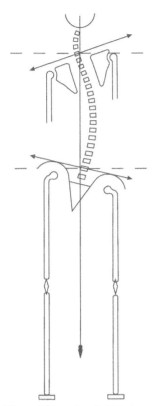

Figure 12.26 The pelvic angle of obliquity.

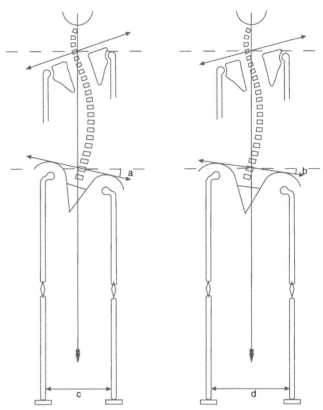

Figure 12.27 How the angle of obliquity is influenced by hip width (distance c < d, angle a > b).

femoral heads, the smaller the angle of the pelvic obliquity caused by an identical LLD (see Fig. 12.27). In crude terms, the wider your hips the less the effect of an LLD. This factor is not considered in most studies, which implicitly assume that a 10 mm difference will be the same for all.

In all cases of LLD the sensory-motor intelligence of the body is obliged make some kind of adaptive response, and there are essentially two main avenues open to it:

1. To accept the height difference at the acetabula by adapting through the upper body
2. To minimize the height difference at the acetabula by adapting through the hips and legs.

Or, of course, it can try a little of both.

If the height difference at the acetabula is accepted then inevitably the sacral base will tilt from the horizontal in standing, setting up an induced scoliosis. With a sacral base tilting from horizontal in the frontal plane, the lumbar spine will list from vertical. An intelligent body is then obliged to bring the centre of mass of the upper body back towards the midline, setting up a side-bending adaptation in the lumbar spine with further compensating side-bends in the thoracic and cervical spine – forming the common 'C' or 'S' curve adaptations of scoliosis – or sometimes curves even more complex than this. These side-bendings are accompanied by rotatory compensations in which the anterior aspects of the vertebral bodies tend to rotate towards the side of the concavity at that level.

If the sensory-motor intelligence of the body opts to minimize the effects of LLD by trying to level the pelvis, it can achieve this by:

● keeping the longer leg continuously flexed
● externally rotating the longer leg (which will tend to pronate the foot, collapse the medial arch, bring the calcaneus more valgus and thereby shorten the leg on that side: a 10 mm difference is achievable by pronation alone)
● rotating the hip of the longer leg forward or back (usually forward), circling around the vertical axis of the shorter leg (which means that the longer leg is then constantly maintained at a more acute angle to the ground in the sagittal plane and one hip will be rotated forward)

or more likely some combination of the above.

The adaptations of the rib cage and shoulder girdle are not entirely predictable from the longer leg as a 'C' curve adaptation will usually lead to a low shoulder on the side of the longer leg (see Fig. 12.26), while an 'S' curve adaptation will often lead to a low shoulder on the side of the shorter leg. Laughlin (1998) notes that, in his clinical experience, the complexity of scoliotic patterns seems to be largely associated with how adaptable people are in the upper chest. Those with little ability to adapt here tend to develop a simple 'C' curve scoliosis. Those with cleverer bodies tend to develop the 'S' or even more complex curvatures.

There are two ways that the structural bodyworker can address the LLD-induced scoliosis: to relieve the system in the short- to medium-term by releasing the shortened fasciae and allowing the system to lengthen generally, or to suggest an orthotic, a simple heel-lift, to partially compensate the shorter leg. In either case the myofascial work is virtually identical.

Clients that have been given heel-lifts by podiatrists often report annoying settling discomforts and even emotional irritation; this is probably because the body is being asked to make a lot of quick adjustments to a new postural regime. The approach of structural bodywork is first to perform general lengthening and balancing, and then to prepare the client for the orthotic by making the soft-tissue adjustments *in advance* of their wearing it. The body is then prepared and can easily 'slot into' the new postural arrangement.

In physiotherapy circles, this pattern is known as *the short-leg syndrome*. Key (1993) describes the common pattern in which the longer leg is slightly advanced in standing, leading to a flexion contracture, a reduced stride length in the shorter leg that alters gait pattern. There is an asymmetrical pattern of rotation around the longitudinal axis during walking that results in stress at the lumbar-thoracic junction because the lumbars, having very little rotation in themselves, will conduct the rotatory aspect of gait directly to the lumbar-dorsal junction, thereby stressing it asymmetrically. The asymmetrical stresses around the hips can lead to mild sacroiliac disorders and back pain.

Legs

Apart from length discrepancies between the lower limbs, legs can exhibit internal or external rotations that may emanate from the hip (which are readily addressed

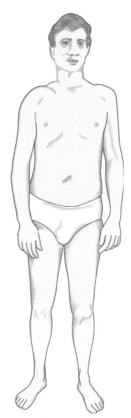

Figure 12.28 The externally rotated leg.

through the myofascial approach), or there may be intersegmental rotations such as tibial torsion or eversion of the feet (which are less readily addressed, being fixated at a ligamentous level).

Ida Rolf spoke a great deal about the pattern of externally rotated legs, the 'toes out' posture that is an aspect of the 'first position' in ballet, and regarded it as a particularly stressful habit (see Fig. 12.28). In the internal–external model of structure (see Chapter 13), the external rotation of the leg is more commonly found in the 'external' (flat-backed) form of organization. Myofascially it is the external rotators of the hip that will adaptively shorten. The anterior adductor mass will present forward and will be positioned to work more like hip flex ors. The gait pattern of this 'toe out' position leads to a swaggering gait (try it), like an inverted pendulum. Because of the external rotation of the foot, the 'toe off' phase of walking will bring more weight to bear on the inner arch of the foot encouraging pronation and, in the longer term, the stressing of the ligaments that support the medial arch, ultimately encouraging the medial migration of the navicular and the tendency to big toe adduction or bunion formation.

REFERENCES

Abrahams V 1982 In Garlick D (ed) Proprioception, posture and emotion. Committee in Postgraduate Medical Education, Kensington, NSW

Alexander R M 1975 Biomechanics. Chapman and Hall, London

Alexander R M 1988 Elastic mechanisms in animal movement. Cambridge University Press, Cambridge

Berthoz A 2000 The brain's sense of movement. Harvard University Press, Cambridge, Massachusetts

Chaitow L 1996 Muscle energy techniques. Churchill Livingstone, New York

Fiorentino M R 1981 A basis for sensorimotor development–normal and abnormal. Charles C Thomas, Illinois, Chapter 1

Flury H 1987 Structural levels at the pelvis. Notes on Structural Integration 1: 25–34

Flury H 1989 Theoretical aspects and implications of the internal/external system. Notes on Structural Integration 1: 15–35

Flury H 1991 The line, the midline, the postural curve, and problems of stance. Notes on Structural Integration 1: 22–35

Garlick D (ed) 1982 Proprioception, posture and emotion. Committee in Postgraduate Medical Education, Kensington, NSW

Gelb M 1981 Body learning: an introduction to the Alexander Technique. Henry Holt, New York

Gracovetsky S 1988 The spinal engine. Springer, Vienna

Keleman S 1985 Emotional anatomy. Center Press, Berkeley

Key 1993 Body in action. Bantam Books, Moorebank, pp 116–130

Larson J 2000 Central nervous system processing in idiopathic scoliosis. Rolf Lines 28(4): 21–22

Laughlin K 1998 Overcome neck and back pain. Simon and Schuster, New York

Maitland J 2001 Spinal manipulation made simple: a manual of soft tissue techniques. North Atlantic Books, Berkeley

Pare S 2002 An interview with Judith Aston, Part III. Rolf Lines 30(1): 8–11

Richardson C 1998 Therapeutic exercise for spinal segmental stabilization: in lower back pain. Churchill Livingstone

Rolf I 1977 Rolfing: the integration of human structures. Harper and Rowe, New York, pp 277, 184, 232

Schultz R, Feitis R 1996 The endless web: fascial anatomy and physical reality. North Atlantic Books, Berkeley

Simons D, Travell J 1999 Myofascial pain and dysfunction: the trigger point manual. Vol 1. Upper half of body. Williams & Wilkin, Baltimore, pp 179–182

Todd M 1937 The thinking body. Princeton Book Company, Princeton

Von Dürkheim K 1977 Hara: the vital centre of man. George Allen & Unwin, London

CHAPTER 13

SOME USEFUL MODELS FOR WORKING WITH STRUCTURE

Having catalogued some of the most common postural dysfunctions in the last chapter, we will now look at some different ways of visualizing and understanding whole body patterns. In this chapter we will examine a number of important models that can help us perceive aspects of our clients' postural–structural organization:

- The internal–external model, which has evolved within the Rolfing community as a means of differentiating different kinds of sagittal organization.
- Janda's identification of the muscular patterns involved in common postural dysfunctions, particularly the different responses of tonic and phasic musculature to stress.
- Feldenkrais' contribution to our understanding of how emotional complexes can have a postural outcome – particularly through 'the body pattern of anxiety', a pattern of exaggerated flexor tonus.
- Hanna's extension of Feldenkrais' ideas to include a postural pattern based upon exaggerated extensor tonus.
- Schleip's extension of Hanna's typology to include a collapsed pattern.
- Myer's anatomy train concept – a detailed map of the longitudinal fascial lines of the body.

THE INTERNAL–EXTERNAL MODEL

The internal–external model is a way of looking at structural dysfunctions that are most evident in the sagittal plane. It looks at the broad tendency for the body's extremities to rotate internally or externally and how this tendency relates to other segmental displacements in the body, for instance, the organization of the chest, pelvis, legs and the form of the spinal curves. It looks

particularly at how pelvic tilt and shift can interact to influence the curvature of the spine and how the muscular dynamics of these different aspects of postural habitus can lead to fairly predictable patterns of strain within the fascial network. The model was originally inspired by a relatively minor observation made by John Upledger in his classic text on craniosacral therapy (Upledger and Vredevoogd 1983). Upledger noticed a pronounced postural habitus that correlated with two kinds of disturbance to the craniosacral rhythm – towards the 'flexion' or 'extension' phase (at the sphenobasilar junction). He observed two polar postural types: (1) the 'flexion lesion' type, who are externally rotated at their extremities, have a broad cranium and a 'waddling quality' to their gait; and (2) the 'extension lesion' type, who have internally rotated extremities and a narrower cranial vault. Craniosacral therapists of the Upledger school call them flexion or extension types. This model, however, has been considerably augmented and extended within the Rolfing community.

Jan Sultan, a senior Rolfing instructor, became interested in this correlation observed by Upledger and sought to clarify this typology within his own clinical practice (Sultan 1986). When palpating the cranial rhythm of his clients he found about a 90% correlation between the pressure preference (towards the extension or flexion phase of the rhythm) and the tendency towards internal or external rotation of the femora. For the most part, however, he discovered people were of mixed types, rather than being one of the 'pure' types in Upledger's schema. Sultan took the pure types as extremes on a spectrum calling them *congruent types*, while those with mixed characteristics he called *conflicted*. From his clinical observation of the two congruent types he arrived at the broad set of tendencies shown in Figure 13.1.

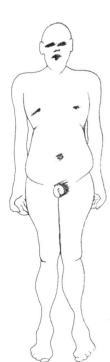

External congruent		Internal congruent
Vault broad, prominent frontalis, 'retracted' mandible, 'flat' occiput	Head	Long narrow vault, jaw delineated, prominent occiput
Primary and secondary curves diminished	Spine	Spinal curves augmented
Inspiration fixed, wide chest, narrow back	Thorax	Expiration fixed, wide back, narrow chest
Drawn posterior-medial (back)	Shoulder girdle	Drawn anterior-lateral (forward)
Ilia tilted posterior on axis through acetabula, narrow tuberosities, broad across crest	Pelvis	Ilia rotated anterior on axis through acetabula, wide tuberosities, narrow crest
In external rotation referenced to sagittal plane, 'valgus', X-legs	Femurs	In internal rotation referenced to the sagittal plane, 'varus', O-legs
Short, anterior	Calcaneus	Long
Arches fixed high, often rigid	Sub-talar foot	Low to flat

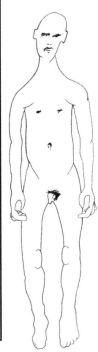

Figure 13.1   Sultan's congruent types.

He also noticed a broad correlation with personality characteristics, externals tending to be more 'outgoing' and internals more 'reserved'.

Sultan suggests that each type will tend to present with characteristic patterns of fibrous density within the myofascial network: 'In each of the polar types then, there is a predictable imprint on the myofascial web that is demanded by the habitual use of the structure'. This imprint consists of lines of increased fibrosity within the myofascial network which arise from the increased mechanical stress that follow these lines during everyday usage, and is determined by the different biomechanics of each type. It can be thought of as a three-dimensional pattern of increased collagen density within the structural body.

Although there are some people who clearly are congruent types, that is, they display all the listed characteristics of the type, in practice most will have mixed tendencies, being incongruent, or in Sultan's terminology 'conflicted'. All, however, will tend to show a preference towards one end of this structural spectrum (Sultan 1986). In practical terms, knowing the client's tendency, whether towards the internal or external organization, has major consequences in strategizing the subsequent bodywork. He suggests that the first aim should be to take the client towards more congruence

with their underlying type, that is, to try to resolve the conflicts within their structure. Then the work should be to ease any exaggerated segmental displacement in the now more congruent structure.

Figure 13.2 shows some typical profiles of internals and externals. Subjectively, we sense the difference expressed. Note the stolid groundedness of externals and the springiness of internals.

Flury's internal–external model

Hans Flury is a Swiss Rolfer and physician who has delved deeply into the biomechanics of the internal–external typology and has published extensively his musings and findings. In his prolific writings he has attempted to elucidate the biomechanics of structure, exploring key functions such as standing, sitting, folding and breathing from a structural point of view. He has also made an extensive semantic analysis of the meaning of key concepts such as 'structure', 'integration' and 'normal' in an attempt to clarify their meaning, and hence lead the way to a clearer discourse within the structural bodywork community. Also, he has contributed to our understanding of efficiency in movement with his theory of *normal movement*. Briefly, his movement work is concerned with the initiation of

Figure 13.2 Typical internal and external profiles.

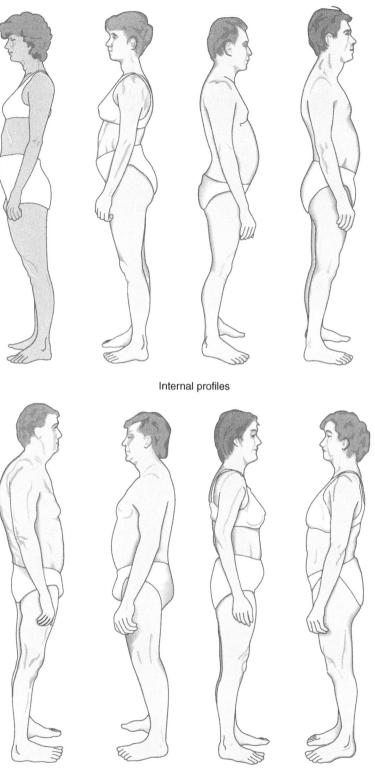

Internal profiles

External profiles

movement, whether through a relaxation of the antagonists, or an increased tonus in the agonists, which is a distinction that bears considerably on movement efficiency. One of his major achievements, however, has been to describe the different muscular dynamics of different structural types. It has been mentioned before that there is a widespread, unacknowledged assumption in the world of somatic therapy that there is only one best kind of posture and one best way of trying to achieve it. Flury shows that there are qualitatively different kinds of organization of the pelvis and that to treat them as if they are the same means risking taking some clients further into an unbalanced pattern.

His approach is based on the strict application of Newtonian physics and especially the rotatory effect of gravity on the various segments of the human body. The structural model is developed in great detail in his *Notes on Structural Integration* (Flury 1986–1993). He takes the primary structural unit to be the fascial net and sees the integration of structure as balancing the fascial net such that the musculature supplies the least force necessary to counteract the bending and shifting effects induced by gravity.

The expression 'fascial net' has been widely used in the field of structural bodywork to give an impression of the three-dimensional organization of the 'organ of structure'. Flury states, however, that the more appropriate metaphor is a system of:

> *balloons inside balloons, with the characteristic that the balloon wall has a certain tension and the contents (the filling) a certain pressure. The tension of the balloon wall (a passive tension) is modified by the active tension from muscle tissue or fibers, something like the basic frequency of a radio station that always remains the same but is modulated in order to produce music.*
>
> (Flury, personal communication 2002)

This inherent passive tension in the fascia perhaps explains why muscles immediately shorten if a tendon snaps or becomes detached.

In Chapter 8 we touched upon Flury's elucidation of structure. He states that we cannot see structure but can only infer it. When we look at someone standing still, we see a coordinated pattern of muscular tonus, superimposed upon a three-dimensional tensile pattern within the fascial web. Different tensile patterns within the fascial network can lead to various degrees of efficiency in standing and in movement. A poorly balanced fascial network will require a greater expenditure of physical and nervous energy, whereas a more organized fascial network will require less. Therefore he regards structure, abstractly, as the pattern of passive tension within the fascial network *minus* the effects of the current tonus pattern of the musculature.

In this analysis of standing posture, the average midline of the body can be visualized as composed of the centres of mass of each horizontal section of the body, what Flury calls the 'zig-zag' line. It may be recalled that 'the Line', in Rolfing terminology, is a plumb line through the body's centre of gravity, and the average midline can be closer to or further from 'the Line'

depending on the organization of the fascial net (see Fig. 13.3). The greater the divergence between the zig-zag line and 'the Line', the more the muscular energy is required to stabilize the segments or 'blocks' of the body, and therefore the less efficient the standing organization (see Fig. 13.4). He sees structural improvement

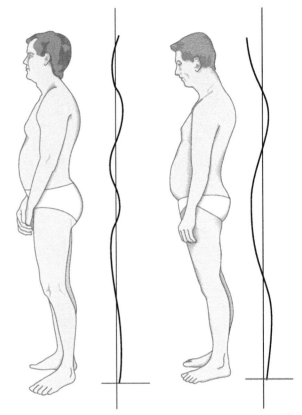

Figure 13.3 Two sagittal profiles showing the average midline and 'the Line' (adapted from Flury).

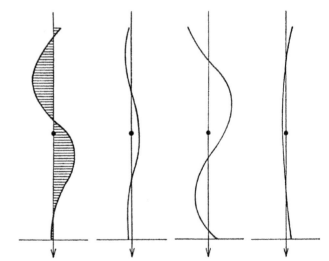

Figure 13.4 'Various midlines and their relationship to the Line ... The shaded area on the *left* and *right* of the line are equal and indicate how much energy must be spent to hold up the "body" against gravity' (Flury 1991).

as bringing the zig-zag line closer to 'the Line' in a way that allows maximum muscular efficiency. For various reasons there can never be an exact correspondence between the zig-zag line and 'the Line'.

Whereas Sultan takes femoral rotation to be the key factor in determining the structural type, Flury uses the degree of tilt of the pelvic segment. Flury makes a critical distinction between the structural 'pelvic segment' and the anatomical pelvis, noting that the pelvic segment has a rotatory axis higher than the axis connecting the acetabula (Flury 1989). He has extended some aspects of Sultan's model by focussing on the different kinds of organization of the pelvis. His postural–structural typology is based upon four different organizations of the pelvic segment in standing, four different combinations of sagittal tilt and shift, and each having a fairly predictable pattern of fascial elasticity or rigidity that determines the shape of the whole. These structural patterns, however, may evolve differently in both the cranial and caudal directions, and they are overlaid by permanently changing functional patterns of active tension. Some people may habitually have 'collapsed' and given in to gravity while others may have actively 'overcompensated' and struggled against it, and each of these tendencies in the longer term will leave a definite imprint in the fascial net.

Tissue that has adaptively shortened is described by Flury as being in 'primary shortness'. For instance, in cases where the shoulder girdle is habitually protracted the pectoral fascia is actually shorter in a geometric sense. In contrast, in his terminology, he says tissue is in 'secondary shortness' when it has lengthened geometrically and adapted to continuous functional demands by stretching and rigidifying, for instance the erector spinae group over a strongly kyphotic back. In both cases the tissue has become less resilient, less able to lengthen.

The practical aspect of this model is that by knowing the areas of primary shortness in the fascial net we are informed of where we need to work. It is the tissue that is in primary shortness that needs to be lengthened or made more resilient. This then removes the functional burden from the 'antagonist' tissue in secondary shortness.

The structural types

Adopting the basic terminology of Sultan, Flury calls the pattern of an anterior tilting pelvis 'internal', while that with a posterior tilt 'external' (see Fig. 13.5). Here *pelvic tilt* is defined as the movement of the superior aspects of the pelvis away from a neutral or 'home' position around an axis through the centre of gravity of the pelvic segment (which is actually higher than the axis

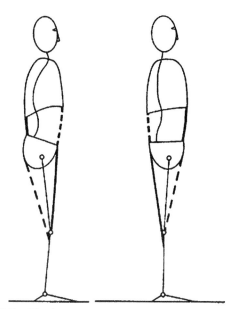

Figure 13.5 The basic internal and external pattern. The *dense lines* show shortened tissue, the *dotted lines* show lengthened tissue (with the kind permission of Dr Hans Flury).

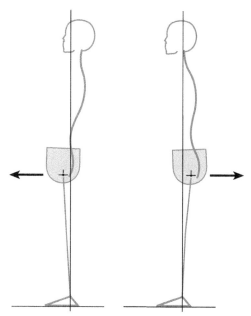

Figure 13.6 Anterior and posterior shift patterns of the pelvis (with the kind permission of Dr Hans Flury).

through the acetabula). An anterior tilt means that the ASIS has moved anterior and inferior, a posterior tilt means that the PSIS has moved posterior and inferior.

The other major variable Flury considers is *pelvic shift*, the sagittal shift of the pelvic mass, either forward or back of 'the Line' (Fig. 13.6). Of shift, Flury notes that this tendency can be more difficult to determine than tilt, simply because most of us at times slip into an anterior shift as a posture of relaxation. Flury calls this a 'sleeve supported stance' because it is a stance in which we rest into the 'sling' or 'sleeve' of all the superficial anterior fasciae (the abdominal fasciae, the iliofemoral ligament, and the anterior aspect of the fascia lata).

Thus, when we combine the two aspects of pelvic tilt with the two aspects of pelvic shift we have four basic structural types, as shown in Figure 13.7.

The four types are characterized as follows:

Regular internal
– anterior tilt, posterior shift

- The hip joint is behind 'the Line'; the weight of the upper body comes down in front of the hip joint, the thorax tilts back to maintain balance.
- A constant tonus in the hip extensors is required in order to prevent further anterior tilting of the pelvic segment – a 'tensional' dynamic.
- The hip extensors are spared overwork by a slight flexion of knees, which may lead to hypertrophy of the vasti group.
- The upper thorax often sags through the front, there is often a strong kyphosis at back, thoracic inlet slopes forward.

The tissues that are in primary shortness are: the groin; the hip flexors, especially the psoas; the lumbar erectors; the neck extensors, and the pectoral fascia.

Locked knee internal
– anterior tilt, anterior shift

- The anterior pelvic tilt is less obvious than in regular internals (however when they are brought back into a normal stance by shifting the pelvis back to the midline, the anterior tilt is usually enormous).

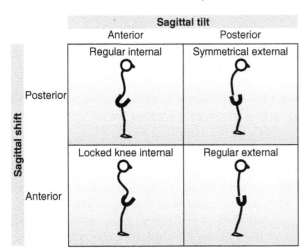

Figure 13.7 The four structural types of the Flury internal–external model (with the kind permission of Robert Schleip).

- The anterior shift is quite pronounced.
- There is a tendency to 'rest' in the ligaments and fascial slings, resulting in secondary shortness in this tissue.
- The knees are always hyperextended.
- The lower legs are shifted posteriorly in relation to the thigh.
- The biggest curvature is in lumbar area, with the mid-back usually kyphotic.

Since this stance is considered habitual (because it is quite economical in a way), postural education is strongly indicated, with less work required in lengthening the areas of primary shortness.

The tissues that are in primary shortness are: the lower lumbar erectors and thoracolumbar fascia, the chest, the hip flexors, the distal quadriceps and the tibialis anterior.

Symmetrical external
– posterior tilt, posterior shift

- The posterior tilt is pronounced, with the upper body weight coming down behind the hip joints.
- Shift is usually of secondary importance to tilt and, when tired, such individuals can often allow an anterior shift into a 'sleeve supported stance'.
- The upper body 'hangs' rather than 'bends' forward, and there is a tendency for the thorax to sag through the front.
- The knees are flexed or extended but rarely hyperextended.
- The whole back tends to have a long C-curve kyphosis in secondary shortness – the 'clearest expression of symmetrical externals'.
- There is sometimes a lumbar lordosis of small radius.
- Lateral rotation of legs often brings the adductor mass forward.

The tissues that are in primary shortness are: the hip extensors (hamstrings and gluteals) and the whole ventral surface of trunk.

Regular external
– posterior tilt, anterior shift

- The shift element is considered more important and there is a slight tilt.
- Support is 'compressional' (i.e. maintained less through tissue tension and more through the more vertical stacking of the skeletal elements).
- The pelvis sits almost on top of the femora.
- The knees are extended.
- There is often a hyper erect spine, sometimes with short lumbar lordosis.
- There is a characteristic 'banana' profile.

The tissues that are in primary shortness are: hamstrings, gluteus maximus, posterior gluteals, deep hip rotators and the lower part of abdominal wall.

Figure 13.8 shows the typical profile of Flury's types.

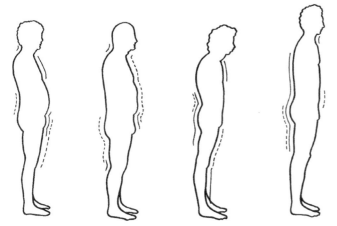

Figure 13.8 Profiles of a regular internal, symmetrical external, locked knee internal and regular external showing areas of primary shortness. The *bold lines* show shortness resulting from pelvic shift; the *dotted lines* show shortness resulting from pelvic tilt (with the kind permission of Dr Hans Flury).

JANDA'S APPROACH – THE BEHAVIOUR OF THE TONIC AND PHASIC MUSCULATURE

Whereas the internal–external model focuses on patterns of shortness within the myofascial network, Janda's approach is more concerned with the aberrant muscular patterns that can arise from and then maintain postural syndromes, although he appears to be describing patterns virtually identical to those in the internal–external model. Janda's work is based on an extensive amount of research that has established the different responses of tonic (postural) and phasic musculature to stress (see Fig. 13.9). Under stress tonic musculature will respond by shortening, while phasic muscles respond by weakening and showing signs of neurological inhibition (Chaitow 1996).

The tonic muscles that will shorten under stress include: gastrocnemius, soleus, hamstrings, short adductors of the thigh, hamstrings, iliopsoas, piriformis, tensor fasciae latae, quadratus lumborum, the spinal erectors, latissimus dorsi, upper trapezius, sternocleidomastoid, pectoralis major and the elbow flexors. Others could include the oblique abdominals, the lateral hamstrings and the anterior and posterior tibialis.

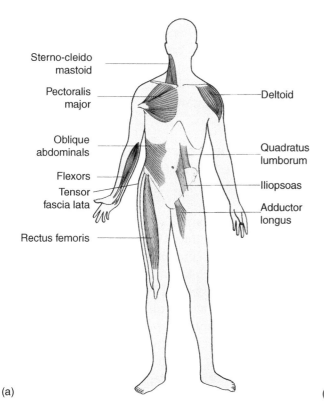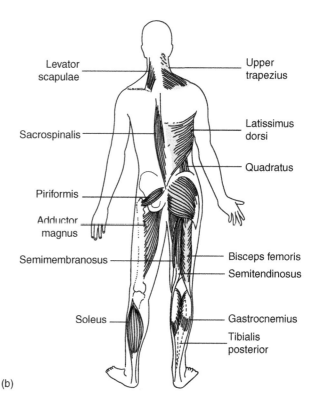

(a)

(b)

Figure 13.9 The tonic musculature (from Chaitow 1996).

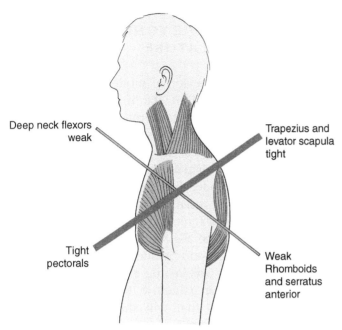

Figure 13.10 The upper crossed syndrome (from Chaitow 1996).

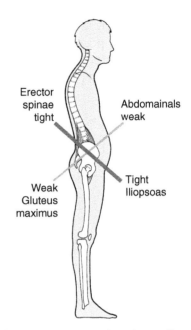

Figure 13.11 The lower crossed syndrome (from Chaitow 1996).

Janda suggests that the main task of the therapist is to lengthen the shortened postural muscles, and emphasizes that it is not necessary to strengthen the weakened antagonists. This is an important departure from the widely practiced 'stretch and strengthen' protocol. He suggests that as the shortened muscles lengthen they lose their inhibitory effect on their already lengthened antagonists; hence these antagonists will spontaneously become more easily recruited and will therefore strengthen through normal usage and without any need for specific strengthening exercises.

He described a number of common whole-body adaptations that have characteristic patterns of muscular shortness and weakness as the upper and lower 'crossed' syndromes. Treatment is based on lengthening the shortened structures, followed by postural re-education.

The upper crossed syndrome

This pattern (Fig. 13.10) is very close to what we have already referred to as the forward head syndrome. In the upper crossed syndrome a number of muscular adaptations will occur, some tightening and shortening and others lengthening and weakening. The muscles that tighten and shorten are: the pectorals (major and minor), upper trapezius, levator scapulae and the sternocleidomastoid. Those that become weakened are: the lower and mid-trapezius, serratus anterior and the

rhomboids. Typically the occipital area will hyperextend and the upper cervicals become compromised.

The lower crossed syndrome

This pattern (Fig. 13.11) is essentially the same as an extreme internal pattern in the internal–external model. In this syndrome the muscles that typically become tightened and shortened are: the hip flexors (especially the psoas and rectus femoris), tensor fasciae latae, quadratus lumborum, and the erector spinae in the lumbar region. The muscles that weaken are: the abdominals and gluteals.

FELDENKRAIS – THE 'BODY PATTERN OF ANXIETY' AND THE WORK OF HANNA

Feldenkrais coined the phrase 'the body pattern of anxiety' (Feldenkrais 1949). He was one of the first to suggest that our emotional habits and tendencies can be intimately correlated to patterns of muscular organization. He suggested that negative emotions are associated with a muscular response in the flexors of the body, while emotional patterns such as 'interest', 'outgoingness', 'assertiveness' and 'exploration' are associated with a response in the extensors. Thomas Hanna, one of Feldenkrais' protégés, developed these ideas further and looked at known whole-body reflexes such as the 'startle' or 'withdrawal' response, and the Landau

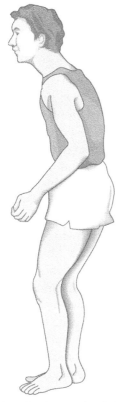

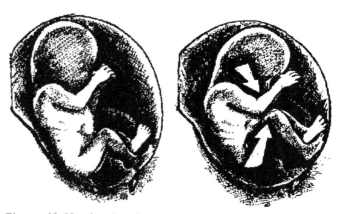

Figure 13.13   Startle reflex in the human embryo (with the kind permission of Robert Schleip).

- The knees flex.
- The pelvic floor tightens.
- The feet pronate and evert.
- The toes lift.

Schleip notes that in human embryos the startle response is apparent at as early as twelve weeks. A sharp sound will cause the foetus to flex even further (see Fig. 13.13) (Schleip 1993). Hanna suggests that the startle response may still be operating even when there are relatively low-levels of stress; in this case the body's response will be essentially the same as for more severe stress, although to a less obvious or dramatic extent. Basically, flexor tone will tend to override extensor tone, leaving people with a slightly flexed look that we often recognize as a sign of stress. This tends to explain the key areas of muscular soreness that arise from stress, the areas people like to have massaged after work: the occipital area and the back of the neck, the upper trapezius and levator scapulae, and the solar plexus area.

The Landau response

The Landau response is regarded as a developmental milestone that appears between the 5th and 7th month in babies. When the prone baby is lifted from beneath its belly it will arch its trunk backwards, extending its neck, trunk and hips by actively engaging its extensor musculature, especially the erector spinae (see Fig. 13.14). It seems to be a genetically programmed function that enables the child to orient more into the external world and is a necessary prerequisite for functions that appear later such as crawling, standing and walking. Fiorentino (1981) suggests that in the early stages it is more about orienting the mouth and eyes into the world.

Hanna argues that for some people this muscular pattern becomes a chronic habit that then shapes their

Figure 13.12   Startle reflex in man (with the kind permission of Robert Schleip).

reflex. He noted that elements of these responses could become relatively fixed and consolidated into our everyday postural organization (Hanna 1988).

The startle reflex

This reflex is universal throughout the animal kingdom and is a primitive reflex of survival. With a stimulus such as a sudden loud noise there is an extremely rapid wave of muscular contraction, mostly in the flexors, that starts at the head and works down to the feet (see Fig. 13.12). Some authors, however, suggest that the flexion phase of the response is preceded by a brief extensor response (Keleman 1985).

In response to a sudden threat, the following will happen in rapid succession:

- The jaws contract, then the eyes and forehead.
- The neck flexes and capitally extends.
- The elevators of the shoulder girdle contract – lifting the shoulders and drawing the head forward and closer to the trunk.
- The arms abduct, the elbows flex and the hands pronate.
- The abdominals contract – both inhibiting deep breathing and flexing the hip.

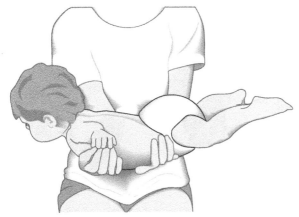

Figure 13.14 The Landau response (from Fiorentino M R (1981) A basis for sensorimotor development: normal and abnormal. Charles C Thomas, Ill.)

overall posture and movement patterns. He describes this as the 'Green Light Reflex' to indicate the psychological state of preparedness or readiness for active interaction with the environment. He writes:

The Green Light reflex is assertive; its function is action. If somebody's posture is dominantly shaped by this reflex – or one could say by this attitude – it will become a chronic feature and show in a shortening of the genetic extensor muscles.

(Hanna 1988)

It seems likely that the extremes of these emotional tendencies will result in structural imbalances and inefficiencies in the overall postural organization and, furthermore, that these postural tendencies may serve to maintain the emotional tendencies that led to them in the first place. What can be termed a *postural–emotional complex* can develop. Just as the internal–external model and Janda's approach lead us to expect certain patterns of myofascial shortness, so does this model. The green and red light responses lead to definite patterns of myofascial shortness. So, if our clients present with these kinds of pattern, we can address them directly and thereby help them towards biomechanical integrity, and indirectly perhaps towards more emotional balance.

SCHLEIP'S EXTENSION OF HANNA'S TYPOLOGY

Robert Schleip is a Rolfing instructor who, through his cross-training in the Feldenkrais work and his interest in neurology, brings his functional insights to bear upon many issues of structural bodywork. In his writings he often challenges the long held maps and concepts of structural bodywork, particularly the more mechanical views of structure. He emphasizes the role of the central nervous system, suggesting that many so-called myofascial restrictions actually disappear when aspects of the nervous system are 'turned off'. He and others have observed that under general anaesthesia some myofascial restrictions seem to disappear, while the soft tissues cease responding to the direct form of myofascial manipulation used by structural bodyworkers. He believes that the nervous system must be engaged in the process for this work to be effective.

He is interested in the development of postural habits and how these can lead to structural adaptations in the longer term. Following the models of Sultan and Flury, Schleip proposes a 'third model' for the use of structural bodyworkers, a model that was inspired by the thinking of Feldenkrais and Hanna. Whereas Sultan perceived the cranial system as driving our structural tendencies, and Flury saw the fascial organization around the pelvic segment as central to structural organization, Schleip focuses on three major *functional* determinants of postural patterns: the tendency towards an exaggerated flexor or extensor tone in the musculature, and the tendency to postural collapse.

As discussed previously, Hanna proposed two broad postural–emotional tendencies based upon a predominance of one of two primary reflexes: the Landau response and the startle reflex. He suggested that the Landau response in the longer term could lead to a chronic shortening of the genetic extensor musculature, while the startle reflex could lead to a chronic shortening of the genetic flexor musculature – patterns that Schleip calls *the short extensor pattern* and *the short flexor pattern*. However, he extends Hanna's typology by suggesting that the short flexor pattern can be divided into two subtypes, depending on whether the ventral side has shortened through an exaggerated flexor tonus, as in 'the body pattern of anxiety', or through a postural collapse through the front induced by a 'giving up' of the trunk extensors (Schleip 1993, 1995).

The genetic extensors develop on the dorsal side of the developing embryo, the flexors on the ventral side, and due to the lateral migration and rotation of the limb buds during embryological development, there is a loose 'cross-over' at the hips. In crude terms, the flexors are found on the front of the trunk and on the back of the legs, while the extensors are found on the back of the trunk and on the front of the legs (see Fig. 13.15).

In order to understand the different postural effects of the genetic flexors and extensors Schleip examines the characteristics of these two groups of muscles.

In differentiating the genetic extensors and flexors, he notes that this distinction is not quite the same as the tonic–phasic distinction of the musculature that was discussed in Chapter 11, although there are close parallels. The genetic extensors have a high proportion of slow-twitch fibres (type I, slow oxidative fibres) and are innervated from the ventral part of the anterior horn of the spinal cord. They are located on the dorsal side of the trunk and arms, the ventral side of the legs and the plantar side of the foot. The genetic flexors, on the other hand, have a high proportion of fast-twitch fibres (type IIb, fast glycolytic) and are innervated from the dorsal part of the anterior horn of the spinal cord. They are located on ventral side of the trunk and arms, the dorsal side of the legs and the dorsal side of the feet.

Schleip categorizes the genetic flexors and extensors as primary, secondary and associated, as can be seen in Table 13.1.

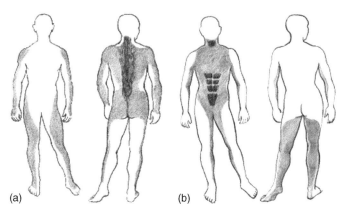

Figure 13.15 The genetic extensors (a) and flexors (b) (with the kind permission of Robert Schleip).

The short extensor pattern

A generalized increase in the tonus of the trunk extensors will favour an extension of the spine and an inspiration fixated pattern of the chest. An increase of tonus of the dorsal musculature around the pelvis will tend to open the innominates anteriorly into an outflare pattern, which involves narrowing the space between the ischial tuberosities and widening the space between the ASIS. The spiral orientation of the leg extensors will tend to rotate the femora externally.

Other postural features that would tend to arise from a generalized heightening of extensor tonus are:

- a posterior pelvic tilt (due to increased activity of the hip extensors)
- shoulder girdle retraction
- a pronation of the feet
- abducted and internally rotated arms
- abducted legs
- valgus knees.

In extreme examples of this pattern you may find the rigidity of what Ida Rolf called the classical military posture of shoulders back, chest out (see Fig. 13.16).

The short flexor pattern

A generalized increase in the tonus of the trunk flexors will lead to trunk flexion. In other words, there will be a kyphotic thoracic spine and the expiration fixated pattern of the chest manifested in the very common pattern of the collapsed or sunken chest. There will be less of a tendency for the femora to rotate externally,

Table 13.1 Schleip's categories of genetic flexors and extensors

	Genetic extensors	Genetic flexors
Primary	Erector spinae (including head and neck extensors) Levatores costarum	Rectus abdominis Infrahyoids
Secondary	Sartorius Rectus femoris Tensor fasciae latae Neck extensors	Short foot muscles Oblique and transverse abdominals Abdominal aspect of pectoralis major Serratus anterior
Associated	Extensor digitorum longus and brevis Extensor hallucis longus Peroneals Latissimus, teres major and subscapularis Deltoid Triceps, brachioradialis, supinator and all wrist and hand extensors	Tibialis posterior, flexor hallucis longus, flexor digitorum longus (the three deep flexors of the lower leg) The long adductors and the obturator externus Internal intercostals and transversus thoracis Pectoralis minor and subclavious Sternocleidomastoid

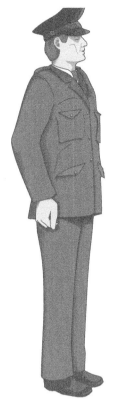

Figure 13.16 The short extensor pattern – the classic military posture (after Schleip).

and shoulder blades will tend to be protracted. The pelvis will tend towards an inflare pattern, that is, a narrowing between the ASIS in front and a widening of the ischial tuberosities.

Other features could include:

- an anterior pelvic tilt (from hip flexor activity)
- a high arch in the feet
- elevated shoulder girdles
- adducted arms and legs
- varus knees.

However, Schleip distinguishes two subtypes within the short flexors category: a contracted and a collapsed type. For the contracted type the flexor muscles are overactive and shortened, and this seems quite close to what Feldenkrais described as 'the body pattern of anxiety'. However, some have a shortening on the ventral side to the trunk not so much through overactive flexors but through trunk extensors that have 'given in' to gravity and allowed the front to collapse. In both cases there is a lengthening of musculature of the dorsal side of the trunk resulting in a kyphotic back. Schleip suggests that neurologically this pattern may be more closely related to what has been called 'postural collapse', a typical primate reaction to early deprivation of

touch and maternal care. He suggests that a want of emotional/tactile 'nourishment' might form the basis for this slumped pattern.

There are obvious parallels between Schleip's model and the internal–external model. The short extensor pattern shares many of the features of the external pattern, and the short flexor pattern looks very much like an internal pattern, the main difference being in how the feet are organized. But since these typologies are predicated on different driving forces, one can imagine perhaps examples that cross this divide, for instance someone with a genetic tendency towards an external pelvis but dominated by flexor tone. Schleip even suggests that the Landau and startle reflexes are not mutually exclusive but can overlay each other, resulting in a trunk tightened both front and back. It is not unusual to find clients that are armoured through the trunk in this way.

MYERS' ANATOMY TRAINS

Rolfer and somatic educator, Thomas Myers has over a number of years developed an extraordinarily vivid and useful metaphor for describing the chief, three-dimensional fascial–skeletal linkages throughout the structural body. Following a line of enquiry that was inspired by the holistic vision of many thinkers within the somatic tradition, he has developed a series of 'fascial maps' that can assist greatly in assessing the deep structure of our clients, seeing where specific fascial restrictions to functional patterns exist, and in practical terms, knowing where specific releases are required. He describes a number of longitudinal 'trains', or fascial continuities, throughout the structural body: the superficial back and front lines, the lateral lines, spiral lines and arm lines, but also lines that run deeper within our core space (Myers 2001).

Ida Rolf stressed that local restrictions in the fascial network will have global repercussions throughout the entire structural body and her 'snagged cardigan' image demonstrates in a simple way the directional spread of a strain pattern (see Fig. 9.17). Myers' anatomy train maps (Fig. 13.17) can give much more precise information about how such restrictions and patterns of strain spread throughout the structural body; so, in using these maps as a tool for visualizing our clients' structure, there is an implicit demand that we take a more holistic perspective and move away from the 'fixing' mentality of a more remedial approach.

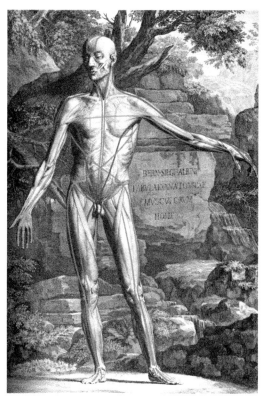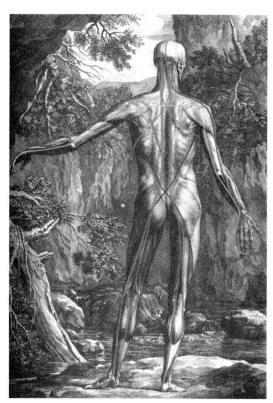

Figure 13.17 Myers' anatomy trains (Myers 2001).

REFERENCES

Chaitow L 1996 Muscle energy techniques. Churchill Livingstone, New York

Feldenkrais M 1949 Body and mature behaviour: a study of anxiety, sex, gravitation and learning. International Universities Press, New York

Fiorentino M R 1981 A basis for sensorimotor development – normal and abnormal. Charles C Thomas, Illinois, Chapter 1

Flury H (ed) Notes on structural integration. Zurich, Switzerland, May 1986, March 1987 December 1988, November 1989, August 1990, September 1991, December 1993 [*Obtainable through the Rolf Institute.*]

Flury H 1989 Theoretical aspects and implications of the internal/external system. Notes on Structural Integration 1: 15–35

Flury H 1991 The line, the midline, the postural curve, and problems of stance. Notes on Structural Integration 1: 22–35

Hanna T 1988 Somatics – Reawakening the mind's control of movement, flexibility, and health. Addison-Wesley, Reading, Massachusetts

Keleman S 1985 Emotional anatomy. Center Press, Berkeley

Myers T 2001 Anatomy trains: myofascial meridians for manual and movement therapists. Churchill Livingstone, Edinburgh

Schleip R 1993 Primary reflexes and structural typology. Rolf Lines 21(3): 37–47

Schleip R 1995 The flexor-extensor typology: in a nutshell. Rolf Lines 23(3): 10–11

Upledger J, Vredevoogd J 1983 Craniosacral therapy. Eastland Press, Seattle, pp 108–110

PRACTICUM: ASSESSMENT, TECHNIQUE AND STRATEGY IN STRUCTURAL BODYWORK

In this section we will look at some practical aspects of structural bodywork: making a structural assessment of our clients, strategizing a structural session and series of sessions, and looking at some of the technical approaches to working with structure.

ASSESSMENT

An essential feature of structural bodywork is that it is *a process*; it does not consist of isolated or stand-alone sessions; it needs its time. It can take a while to get a clear idea of a person's structure, and what seems obvious from an initial visual assessment of the client may need to be modified as the work progresses. The human being is an extraordinary 'system of systems' and we need to adopt a holistic perspective if we are to understand the structure at all. Taking a linear or 'fixing' approach to understanding structure can be useful only in the very short term. This means that even the best structural work has an exploratory, provisional flavour, as work with any complex system must have. Things are rarely as predicable as one would wish, and it takes time to understand the complex dynamics involved in standing and moving in gravity. This means being prepared to modify conclusions as new information comes to light. Ida Rolf expressed this dilemma as 'working in a quicksand'. Hence, this kind of bodywork does sometimes lead to surprises (though not necessarily unpleasant ones!), and occasionally, after doing everything that your experience tells you to do, you still do not obtain the expected result.

Working with such complexity requires a willingness to engage in a process of *continuous assessment*: always checking on the outcomes of any particular structural or functional intervention. A certain kind of humility can result as we realize that structural bodyworkers are facilitators rather than doers. Therefore, it is important not to come to premature conclusions about what clients need and never to force an issue, but instead engage in a genuine ongoing dialogue with them.

There is no absolute distinction between assessment and ongoing work; one is continually assessing the client, and asking them to assess themselves. They need to sense the changes in their body, feel the results of an intervention, sense how it is integrated, how it 'ripples through' their system. Constant checking in this way also keeps clients challenged into listening to their bodies.

As therapists we have the advantage of an external perspective of our clients; we can see them from behind, above and from the side; we can see how they move in a way that they cannot. The clients, on the other hand, have the advantage of the somatic perspective into their own situation – what it feels like to be in their particular body. We can never experience that for them. So both kinds of information need to come together and this is only possible through dialogue, though this need not necessarily be verbal.

Essential background information

In the initial sessions, it is important to get a sense of:

- their hopes and expectations from this work
- aspects of their daily routines of movement and work activities that may affect structure
- any significant musculoskeletal injuries or surgery in the past
- acute and chronic conditions that may affect the ongoing work, and
- their exercise regimen, if any.

It is necessary first to uncover what clients would like to achieve through somatic work and how they 'frame' it: do they believe they have a 'problem' or not? Here it is important to realize that clients may have all sorts of erroneous beliefs about their posture/structure and unrealistic expectations about what can be achieved through somatic work. They may have embodied many old wives' tales about what is 'good posture'; they may have a confused terminology (confusing lordosis and 'sway back' for instance), or believing that their 'hip' is their 'pelvis', or even not knowing that they have scapulae. It is quite common to find that clients have a very incomplete somatic map, with misplaced perceptions of themselves, which can be seen in its extreme forms in conditions such as body dysmorphism, and often it is only the direct knowledge that something hurts that brings them to a practitioner in the first place.

In gathering aspects of their medical history it is important to know if the client has any conditions that may affect the connective tissue network. Structural bodywork has much the same list of contra-indications as massage, so without medical advice to the contrary, you would not normally work on clients with active cancer, active inflammation or really acute problems. You would also need to weigh up carefully whether to work with women who are in the last trimester of pregnancy, although with experience (and the agreement of the client's medical practitioner) it is possible to do some relieving work around all the above conditions.

It is important to know of any musculoskeletal injuries, impact traumas, and any other physical trauma, including surgery, the client may have undergone. Trauma can cause internal adhesions or nerve tethering that can become inflamed if you work too deeply in the area. It is vital to know their employment and the postures and movements required of it. You also want to know about any movement regimen they may have: physical activities, yoga, sport, or stretching, and whether

their preference is for a strict regimen or a playful and exploratory one.

It is then necessary to examine how the client stands and walks. This is very different from normal massage practice in which the client, after the initial gathering of information, is immediately invited to lay face down, bypassing the opportunity to see their stance or movement.

Standing assessment of posture

For the visual assessment, the client should ideally be disrobed to basic underwear, although a skilled eye can detect what is happening beneath clothing. This assessment is often referred to as 'body-reading' and is a vital skill that is taught in structural integration training. It involves simply taking as much time as necessary to 'take in' the details of a body, but also seeing the body as a whole. This is, of course, quite confronting to clients and they may need to be introduced to the idea gently. It is also traditional in structural bodywork to take photos at this initial stage so that clients can see themselves from a different perspective.

The first and most obvious problem at this stage is how to get beneath the client's automatic posing, 'holding to form', or trying to present as well as possible. Clients can be asked to stand 'naturally' without trying to correct anything, but it can also be useful to ask them to slump into a too-relaxed posture, to 'let go' into what they feel is a habitual posture; this can give essential information about how this body responds to fatigue. You can also ask them to move back and forth slowly between these extremes; this is vital proprioceptive learning that can help them experience new postural options in a new way.

This visual assessment should take in the three planes of standing posture: from the front to see left–right asymmetries; from behind to check on scoliotic patterns and how the scapulae are organized; from the sides to check on segmental displacements in the sagittal plane, and from above to note any segmental rotations. The latter can be done standing on a stool behind the client and looking down the full length of the body (see Fig. 14.1). The degree of internal or external rotation of limbs can be assessed from in front. At this stage other important impressions can be taken in, for instance, noting whether their basic body type is ecto-, meso- or endomorphic.

Chapter 12 detailed some of the more important postural–structural dysfunctions that interest structural bodyworkers, so in this section they will only be mentioned briefly. When assessing the axial organization it is important to look at the form of the spinal curvatures,

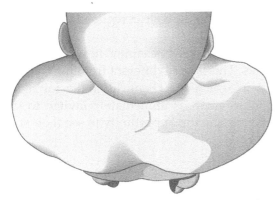

Figure 14.1 The view from above to assess segmental rotations in the transverse plane.

the tilt of the pelvic segment, the placement of the head on top, and rib cage adaptations. The relationship between the pelvic segment and the spinal curves should be appraised both in the sagittal plane, noting if there is an obvious internal or external tendency in the organization of the pelvis, and in the frontal plane to see if there is any scoliotic tendency or obliquity in the pelvis, either through a unilateral contracture or an adaptation to a leg length discrepancy. With a fuller training one might then go on to assess any intrasegmental distortion of the pelvis, inflare, outflare, up- and down-slip and sacro-iliac torsions, though these are not covered in this introductory book, and in any case such patterns would probably not be dealt with until some of the more basic structural issues have been resolved.

When assessing the legs note:

- any internal or external rotation of the femur
- the degree of 'toe out'
- whether the knees are valgus or varus, and
- whether there is any tendency to pronation in the feet.

A simple test to determine any asymmetry in external rotation of the legs is to have clients lie supine on the table with feet together. Ask them to press the toes together then release. As the feet drop laterally note the degree of external rotation, and if one hip rotates out more than the other, remembering the *segmental standard rotation* pattern and that some degree of asymmetry is normal.

Then look at the shoulder girdle, its relationship with the axial skeleton (especially the neck and thorax), and then how it relates to the upper limbs.

Palpatory assessment

It is important to get a general sense of the level of muscular tonus throughout the entire standing arrangement.

For this it is helpful to palpate key areas of the body very softly, using what Godard (2000) has called 'gamma touch' – a light, non-directive kind of touch. Simultaneously palpate the abdominals and the lumbar erectors. Trace the erectors the whole length of the spine, noting the general tonus and any ropy areas. From behind gently palpate the scalenes to see how hard they are working. Simultaneously palpate the quadriceps and the hamstrings to sense which have the higher tonus. It should be realized that the very act of palpation can induce an increase in tonus, particularly in the abdominal region, which is why an unobtrusive 'gamma touch' is essential.

If you have sports massage or physiotherapy training it may be useful to supplement this information by employing some of the standard tests for myofascial shortness, such as the Ober test, the straight leg raise, trunk flexion–extension, side flexion, and so on.

A simple test for internal or external pelvic organization is valuable here. To do this, sit on a stool beside the client and gently align the major segments of the body, bringing them as close to 'the Line' as possible in the sagittal plane; then ask the clients to become taller by reaching up through their crown. How they perform this will usually show where their segments actually need to be taken in order for them to become taller in fact. Internals will usually flatten their lumbar region to become taller; externals will usually take the lumbar spine further into lordosis. It is not a foolproof test since some clients who have good awareness of their body have several options for lengthening up, while some clients with poor awareness will have no idea at all how to lengthen – and may do things like lifting the shoulders to become taller! This information must be coordinated with other visual cues about their pelvic organization; Flury has also proposed some more detailed tests for this (Flury and Harder 1988).

A more advanced kind of postural–structural analysis would look closely at spiral patterns of shortness throughout the structure, but this is probably best learned in a formal training situation.

From all of the above assessments an abstract picture of the total pattern of myofascial shortness within the client's structure begins to emerge. Then, after working with the client for a while, other aspects of their somatic organization become clearer: whether they are hard- or soft-tissued, what their overall level of 'body intelligence' might be, and their autonomic tone. Hard-tissued types have a recognizable rigidity in 'feel', a lack of differentiation in movement, and when you press into them on the table they have the tendency to roll 'as one piece'. With practice one can get a sense of whether such restrictions are in the fasciae, the ligaments or the nervous system. Soft-tissued types will have a discernible laxity in the ligaments and often a hypermobility of their spinal segments. Those with a generally elevated tonus are often 'sympathetically tuned' (Cottingham 1987) and this can manifest as an inability to relax, a tendency towards constant internal vigilance and control throughout the sessions, and an inability to fall into a light alpha state.

Assessment of gait

It is important also to see how a client walks. This can give valuable information not only about the client's general level of moving intelligence but also which areas are moving easily and which are not – remembering that long-term functional patterns will inevitably be reflected in fascial adaptations. So, if an area does not move much it is likely that there is a degree of fascial contracture that underlies that pattern.

When observing a client's gait it is important to have enough working space to allow them to walk without too much interruption, even if it is just down a passageway. As they walk, notice the degree of movement in the following planes:

- the lateral sway of the pelvis in the frontal plane
- a rocking of the pelvis in the sagittal plane
- the counter-rotation of the shoulder and pelvic girdles in the transverse plane – a slight twisting and untwisting through the longitudinal axis of the body.

There are many other more subjective aspects to focus upon, including the degree of coordination, the general sense of the connectedness of the movement, whether the movement is organic and how it flows.

The perceptual skills needed for this kind of assessment are usually developed in structural integration training; however, you can learn a great deal by just being interested in movement and observing the gait of people in the street. One then begins to acquire a 'vocabulary' of movement, and to see what is average and what is 'normal'. Without this baseline information it is very difficult to make reliable judgements.

The totality of the information gathered from the postural and gait analyses will begin to give a sense of the unique structure of a client and some preliminary ideas about which areas are in particular need of being opened up or given more resilience. For most clients the work is bound to take a number of sessions; it simply

cannot be done all at once. This means a certain choice on your part and you need to ask yourself, what am I going to do today, and what will I do next? Sequencing is important, so now some initial ideas will be offered to help determine how you strategize a series of sessions as well as deciding on the content of any particular session.

STRATEGIZING A SERIES OF SESSIONS

Most schools of structural bodywork will teach some variation on the classic ten-session 'recipe' of Ida Rolf. For beginning structural bodyworkers, this does remove some of the need for a detailed evaluation of the clients' posture and gait. In Rolfing training, the principles for strategizing structural interventions are also taught, alongside this relatively fixed beginners' protocol. What follows here, however, is neither an exposition of the Rolfing principles nor a procedural recipe, but rather some 'rules of thumb' that can be of assistance in guiding the initial stages of structural bodywork, in working towards what previously has been called 'a first approximation' in balancing structure.

Having already gathered some initial impressions about the client's structure you know which areas of fascial shortness need addressing but not necessarily the order in which to address them. Experience has shown that the rules of thumb given in Box 14.1 are very useful in guiding the progress of structural bodywork.

Box 14.1   Some 'rules of thumb' for strategizing structural bodywork sessions

- Work superficially at first and later work to affect deeper layers
- Then work on front–back balance (in the sagittal plane)
- Then as the work progresses further, begin gradually to work on left–right balance (in the frontal plane)
- Then work on axial and limb de-rotations (in the transverse plane).

These steps should not be taken as strictly sequential and mutually exclusive. They refer to the focus of the work at any stage of the process. Any session will probably address the organization in all three planes but will tend to concentrate more on one of them. So it does not mean that when you work on sagittal balance you cannot also work on frontal symmetry, simply that as front–back balance progresses it facilitates the later work of left–right symmetry. Earlier sessions are often aimed at generally lengthening and decompressing the system, with less of an intention of achieving balance of any kind. Then sessions will tend to address front–back balance rather than left–right balance, and the emphasis gradually reverses. Experience has shown that as both front–back and left–right work progresses, many of the rotational patterns apparent early on will tend to resolve and unwind of themselves, so it is natural to deal with them later in the sequence of sessions.

There is a real wisdom in Ida Rolf's original recipe, in which the first three sessions concentrate on the most superficial layers only, aiming for a general decompression of the system and an overall lengthening. It is certainly safer in most cases to begin in this way since it is not asking too much of an adaptive response from the body in the early stages. The body then becomes more prepared to receive deeper work, and practitioners have time to familiarize themselves with their clients' structure. How long this superficial work should last, or even whether it is necessary at all, will depend on many factors. Clients who have a high level of sensory-motor intelligence are more able to integrate greater changes and can receive deeper work sooner. Clients who are deemed to be 'rigid' or 'armoured' should definitely receive only *superficial work to begin with*, even if it seems they are crying out for a deeper kind of work. It is a common mistake to work too deeply, too soon with such clients, and often they will report pain later, and usually not in areas that have been worked; it is as if suddenly they have a new range of movement in certain areas of their body to which their sensory-motor intelligence is unable to adapt, so strain is thrown elsewhere and 'settling pain' results. So if there is any doubt, do less, then deepen the work by degrees.

Strategizing a session

Figure 14.2 is a more detailed schema of the three-level model of structural intervention that was shown in Figure 7.2 (p. 46). It outlines one possible sessional format (among others) for any individual session, once the main theme or themes of the session have been decided. At the start of each session it is important to know where you are within the overall progress of the sessions you have envisaged, for example whether you intend focussing on front–back, left–right or rotational issues. Then decide on which areas you wish to address. Then use the three levels of interventions to guide the process: first, soft-tissue releases to a particular area, then neuromuscular releases followed by some small-scale integration work. Towards the end of the session, include some broad back and neck work, and at the end of a session always

include some kind of larger-scale integrating movement work, even if only by helping clients to 'ground' themselves by tuning in to their standing posture or exploring new options in walking, or maybe just asking them to walk with awareness.

Sometimes it is useful for clients to have some specific 'homeplay' to maintain areas that have been 'opened'. This could include traditional stretches, but very often clients have not been taught to 'feel' or 'breathe' into a stretch; they can be too brutal with themselves and will

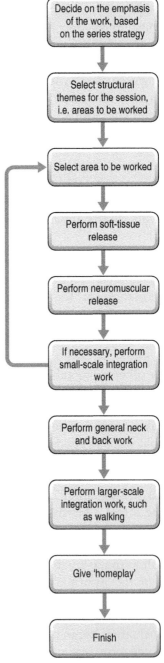

Figure 14.2 An outline for a possible session structure.

therefore tend to avoid stretching. It is preferable to teach them the self-applied contract–relax (C–R) style of stretching that will be described later in this chapter. Virtually all traditional stretches can be creatively transformed into a safe C–R type of stretch.

TECHNIQUES OF INTERVENTION IN STRUCTURAL BODYWORK

It was suggested in Chapter 7 that the complete structural bodyworker requires at least three levels of technique:

1. Soft-tissue releases
2. Neuromuscular releases
3. Integrative techniques.

In this practical section we will look at myofascial release as the principal approach to soft-tissue release used within structural bodywork, and C–R stretching as a highly effective neuromuscular release technique. The scope of this book will not allow even a sketchy exposition of the various integrative methods as it is simply too vast a field. Instead a few key examples will be demonstrated to give a general idea of how to proceed and the interested reader can look at the many possible avenues to movement training in Appendix 1. Additionally, some self-applied C–R stretches and some passive stretches have been included for homeplay.

Myofascial release (MFR)

Myofascial release is an extraordinarily versatile technique that can be used within a wide range of somatic and therapeutic contexts. It can be used within an integrative context to create a better balance within the human structure, but it may also be effectively used within a corrective or remedial context for treating connective tissue fixations in the short to medium term. It is one way among many of bringing more resilience to selected areas of tissue. There are several styles of MFR, some soft and indirect, some firm and direct. The approach outlined in this book is a direct approach that originated in the Rolfing tradition. It has been characterized by its use of very slowly applied, deep sliding pressure into restricted tissue combined with an appropriate assisting movement from the client to enhance the practitioner's input of energy. This technique is to be distinguished from the myofascial approach popularized by John F. Barnes (PT), which is also called myofascial release (Barnes 1990). In Box 3.1 (p. 22) the Barnes approach has been grouped with the listening-touch systems. These systems use very little force in their

application, involve a lower intensity and longer duration of contact, and are based on the premise that the body will respond with a subtle unwinding if 'listened to' in this way. A form of this technique is taught within osteopathic circles; Greenman, for instance, demonstrates many such techniques for releasing superficial tissue (Greenman 1996), while Stanborough (2004) provides an excellent detailed exposition of the more direct approach that derived from the Rolfing tradition.

The direct technique of MFR involves the manual application of controlled mechanical stress into areas of restriction within the myofascial network, thereby changing the mechanical properties of the tissue and allowing new possibilities of movement in the surrounding structures and to the organism as a whole. There has been no definitive research into the effects of this kind of myofascial release. In Chapter 9 various theories about how it works were proposed: Ida Rolf took thixotropy as the likely explanation, emphasizing the colloidal nature of the connective tissue complex; Schleip conjectures that it is neurological feedback into the local tissue that produces the effect, while others believe that the collagen fibres are realigned by the mechanical stress applied to the tissue, which breaks cross-linkages and hydrogen bonds. That it does work is not disputed by anyone who has ever applied it or received it. It can easily be tested in a minor way by pre-testing for a range of motion (ROM) with any of the standard myofascial length tests (the Ober test for instance), applying the technique and then post-testing the range. One virtually always finds an immediate increase in ROM. The important thing is that it actually works (see Box 14.2).

Box 14.2   The myofascial release technique

Having selected the area in which you wish to work, you decide which is the most appropriate tool – finger chisel, knuckles, soft fist, forearm blade and so on. Then:

- gently contact the surface (too rapid or deep an entry will provoke a reflexive, protective response)
- sink to an appropriate depth – more or less, depending on your intent
- hook into the appropriate layer by changing the direction or vector of application (usually away from you)
- using your weight and gravity alone, slide/drift *very slowly* through the tissue, controlling the drift by changing the angle of application rather than changing the amount of effort you use
- ask the client to make small assisting movements that introduce a lengthening vector through the area of tissue receiving the work.

From a somatic perspective the technique is also a valuable means of bringing more sensation, vitality and biological energy to an area. Proprioceptively it 'awakens' the tissue in areas that may be only vaguely sensed, and as such is a valuable tool in cases of what Hanna has termed sensory motor amnesia, and like the sensory awakening techniques of Feldenkrais, this technique can help fill in the hazy areas in the client's internal body map. More than superficial massage techniques, MFR greatly enhances local circulation. The redness in the skin after this work is the result of the release of local histamines which dilate the superficial capillaries and bring a greater volume of blood to the surface. It is likely that an identical histamine response is occurring deeper within the tissue. This makes it an ideal technique for treating localized ischaemic conditions.

It is possible to influence relatively deep layers within the body using this form of MFR. There are ways of achieving deep penetration quite naturally, into muscular septa for instance, or by introducing unusual vectors of force one can indirectly reach into deeper layers. However, it is probable that this technique has most of its effect in the more superficial layers. Stretching techniques have the potential to reach deeper layers after the more superficial layers have been opened with a MFR approach, so the two techniques can work synergistically.

How the technique is applied in a particular situation depends on many factors: the area of tissue being worked, the client's tolerance to pressure, the mass of the underlying muscle tissue, the general collagen density, the client's tonic status at that time in the session (as the client relaxes more it is possible to go deeper without evoking a protective response), and their general tonic habitus.

If the client is unable to relax then the approach will be less effective as it becomes difficult to achieve an adequate penetration into the correct layer; this simply results in stretching the skin and superficial fascia alone. Very occasionally one finds clients who are deeply conditioned to hardening themselves. Any pressure into their tissue will provoke a resistance to entry, completely unconsciously of course. For these clients it may be necessary to try a completely different approach that seduces them into muscular relaxation, such as the Trager approach.

This technique is inherently slow. All the research on the 'creep' and 'flow' behaviour of connective tissue suggests that it is the duration of the intervention that is the most important factor in producing change. The viscoelastic properties of fascia mean that a quick stretch and return will not affect the tissue's resilience, the underlying properties of the material will remain unchanged; a longer duration of stretch allows for plastic deformation to occur, and for any 'slow flow' effects in the colloidal matrix. Hence watching the technique performed is highly unexciting. Yet the experience of the client is very different. Clients experience the technique as strong. There is strong sensory input, which is not to say that this is experienced as painful. There is an implicit sense of safety in the slow speed of the technique; the client is able to anticipate the progress of the work at all times, which gives ample time for feedback, for instance if there are some tender spots ahead that need lighter work. The application can be quicker if you wish to use it as a warm-up, preparing the tissue for deeper work. The sense of safety in the technique can be gauged by the fact that most clients soon fall into a light alpha state during this work.

Varying the vector of application

In general, control of the strokes comes from altering the body's position rather than using arm muscles to push through the tissue; the arm muscles are then reserved for a stabilizing function and the energy of the stroke comes from the whole body, using the floor as a fulcrum. Looking at the vector diagram in Figure 14.3 it is evident that the force delivered through this technique

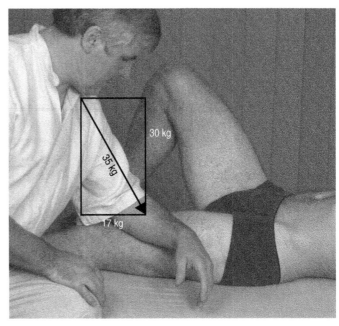

Figure 14.3 Vector diagram showing the direction of forces involved in the application of the direct myofascial release technique.

can be decomposed into its component vectors. Any force directed into the tissue will have a vertical or penetrating component, and a transverse or sliding component; in this instance, 35 kg of pressure applied in a direction directly through the long axis of the humerus (at this angle) will provide the equivalent of about 30 kg of penetrating force and 17 kg of sliding force. The steeper the angle of application, the deeper the penetration into the tissue and the slower the sliding progress through the tissue. It has been stressed already that the technique (after warm up) must be slow to have an optimal effect. One way of putting on the brakes if you are drifting too quickly through the tissue is to bring your weight more directly above the point of application. This makes the vector of entry steeper and thus slows the progress of the stroke while providing more penetration into the tissue. This is much more effective than trying to modulate the pressure through the arm and shoulder muscles alone. The bodyworker can become quite skilled in making subtle trunk movements to vary the depth and direction of their work, rather than using a more muscular effort in the arms and shoulders.

Using gravity

The suggestion to use your weight and gravity alone is an exaggeration. Of course some muscular effort is required because the shoulder girdle needs to be stabilized as you lean into the client. But this work has its martial arts aspect, and one could easily apply to it the basic dictum of judo 'Minimum effort, maximum effect'. This also implies that the practitioner needs a well-developed body awareness. Ida Rolf was known to reject applicants for her training if they were either too cerebral or not very dexterous. The 'judo' of this work is to align your own skeleton such that you require minimal muscular involvement to perform the technique. If you begin to use unnecessary muscular effort then, as in any manual work, you will tire and ultimately damage yourself. The client too will pick up your tremulous energy and will feel less safe, sensing that you are not in control.

Assisting movements

Experience has shown that the MFR technique has a more lasting effect when the client is engaged in appropriate assisting movements in the area being worked. Appropriate lines of stress are thereby placed through the tissue, which is added to the therapist's application of force. Hence there is a compounding of the energy entering the tissue. Giving assisting movements is also an ideal opportunity for incidental proprioceptive learning

to occur; clients can really experience what it is like to lengthen through a particular line.

For areas that are not heavily muscled, any movement seems to help. However, when working over more powerful muscle groups it is important not to work deeply into the tissue *when the underlying muscles are actively shortening*. To do so causes undue discomfort and does not allow useful penetration into the tissue being worked. So in general, try to organize an assisting movement so that underlying muscles are being passively lengthened by their antagonists. This is not always possible or convenient so that at times it is acceptable to work without any assisting movement at all, or just the use of breath. Sometimes the technique works entirely by anchoring tissue with the hands and having the client make all the lengthening movement away from the anchor point. In this way it is possible to introduce tensile vectors into the tissue that can be produced in no other way, through yoga or stretching for instance.

Chapters 16–20 pictorially depict techniques that can be used. They are numbered from T1 to T108. Specific techniques from this point will be referenced by the appropriate number.

Technique T8 exemplifies working into tissue as it is being passively lengthened. The client flexes at the knee by engaging the hamstrings and allowing the quadriceps to be passively lengthened at the same time as you are working into them. Sometimes it is possible for the practitioner to supply the lengthening impulse, rather than the client, as in techniques T31, T78 and T105 for instance. In technique T31 the client is asked to do nothing but allow the practitioner to passively extend the knee, such that the hamstrings are passively lengthening. In this same example it is possible to utilize reciprocal inhibition if the client is simply unable to release – if there is some parasitic co-contraction occurring. Here you can ask the client to actively extend their knee while you gently resist them, allowing them to overcome your resistance. In this way the hamstrings will usually release.

However, these assisting movements need not always be gross. Sometimes micro-movements may be asked for, or sometimes clients may be asked to 'breathe into' an area. This can mean simply to exaggerate the in-breath or out-breath to obtain expansive or contractive movement through specific areas of the thoracic sleeve. It may also mean to visualize the out-breath flowing to a particular area; in this case there may not in fact be any movement except for a subtle release of tonus in the area. This valuable practice originated in yoga, and although superficially it seems like a 'new-age' energetic idea, it has proved in practice to be consistently useful. On the out-breath there is a perceptible reduction in muscular tonus throughout the entire body, so it makes sense to utilize this effect for therapeutic purposes. Breathing into an area can also reduce the discomfort of very deep work.

The use of visualization

Many bodyworkers and movement practitioners have discovered the power of active visualization as a means of achieving some movement quality or some therapeutic benefits for their client. We have already mentioned the practice of having a client 'breathe into' an area. Some of the other 'classic' visualizations are: feeling the body lengthen as if pulled up by puppet strings or a 'skyhook'; sensing the head as floating like a balloon; or even the simple suggestion that you feel the spine lengthening. There is an idiokinetic tradition in dance that uses the power of this idea. This use of visualization has been used by teachers of dance, yoga, Pilates and Trager practitioners, among others, for many years. There is now some research that begins to confirm this intuition. Godard and others have shown that the use of *imaginative directionality* in movement can eliminate unproductive co-contraction of muscles (Godard et al).

The tools of myofascial release

MFR is usually a manual technique; it is the hands and forearms that are most commonly used. The selection of the appropriate tool depends partly on experience and partly on common sense. Experience will show you what will work and where. It is important not to use a gross tool in a delicate area and vice versa. The pressure can be very slight in areas such as the face, scalp and neck, and more forceful where there is a greater underlying muscle mass such as the hamstrings and erector spinae. As with all techniques, you need to individualize them, make them your own, and adapt them to your own body and style of working. So the techniques presented in the next sections are not meant to be definitive in any way; they are merely a starting point. You will need to experiment and discover what works for you. Once the basic principles of the technique are understood you can create an infinite number of variations to suit the precise needs of the moment. In the technical and pictorial sections that follow, different myofascial lines will be described along with specific techniques that address them; from now on, these techniques will be referenced by number: T1, T2 … T100, and so on.

There are great differences between practitioners in their shape, strength, tissue density and dexterity, and a

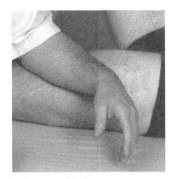

Figure 14.4　The forearm blade.

tool that suits one may not suit another. Practitioners with a tendency to hyperextend at their joints, for instance, should not use their thumbs and perhaps even the 'finger chisel', except sparingly. It is tempting to overuse the fingers because of the rich sensory feedback we receive from them. However, it is possible to use the elbow in most situations where the fingers are used. It can be used with great delicacy and not merely as a blunt instrument.

Forearm blade

The forearm blade (Fig. 14.4) is probably the most versatile tool in the structural bodyworker's toolbox. If you palpate your own forearm right now you can trace the ulna, just beneath the skin's surface, extending continuously from the olecranon to the styloid process at the wrist. The fact that the ulna is such a superficial bone allows it to be used purely as a blade, making broad contact with the tissue in order to 'iron it out'. Then the tip of the olecranon can be used for intense point loading in certain areas of tissue if necessary. It can be used for all variations between these extremes (see Fig. 14.5). The angle of contact can be subtly varied even as you use it, turning it from a blade into a plough. There is even more versatility to this tool, since either side of the ulna you will find relatively dense soft tissue that can be used for a more cushioned contact with the client. This allows the practitioner to rotate the forearm away from the ulna in order to utilize this padding, which can be important for sensitive areas such as the iliotibial tract where bone-to-bone contact could be uncomfortable (your ulna, their femur!).

The finger chisel

The finger chisel (Fig. 14.6) is an effective tool when specificity is required. There are wide individual differences in the relative lengths of our digits, so some experimentation is required to find which disposition of fingers serves best for any practitioner. The chisel can be used singly, as in technique T78, doubled (see Fig. 14.7), or

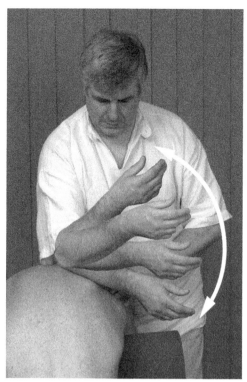

Figure 14.5 Varying the angle of the forearm blade to shift from broad contact to point loading.

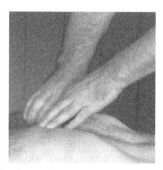

Figure 14.6 The finger chisel.

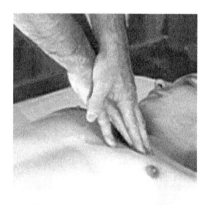

Figure 14.7 The finger chisel doubled.

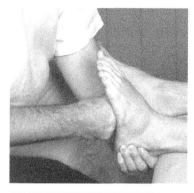

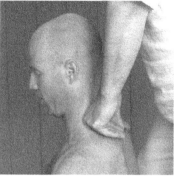

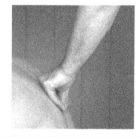

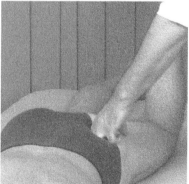

Figure 14.8 The dorsum of the hand, various tools.

overlapped for mutual reinforcement, as in technique T20. In general, the fingers work better if slightly flexed (a natural tendency anyway). Hyperextension of the interphalangeal (IP) joints should be avoided as it will stress them in the longer term.

Dorsum of the hands
There are many ways of using the dorsal side of the hands (Fig. 14.8), with client–practitioner contact

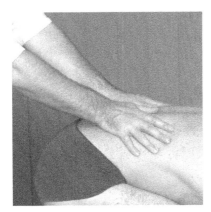

Figure 14.9 The octopus hand.

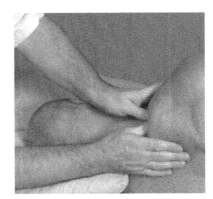

Figure 14.10 Doubled thumbs.

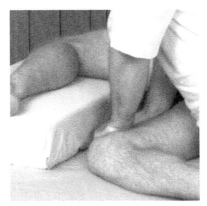

Figure 14.11 The heel of the palm.

coming through the knuckles (metacarpophalangeal joints), the pads of the combined proximal phalanges or middle phalanges. In the full fist the whole hand is flexed, with metacarpals and phalanges at right angles. If the metacarpals and carpals are aligned with the bones of the forearm there is then a direct line of force through the skeleton that requires little muscular effort from the practitioner (see technique T105) and allows the weight to be used more effectively. The same arrangement can be modified to form a 'soft fist', in which the palm is naturally more open and the fingers can shape themselves to more comfortably conform to the shape of the underlying tissue. In technique T58 they are used in this more open and 'moulding' fashion.

For delicate areas such as the neck, pads can be formed from the combined middle or proximal phalanges (see technique T73). In other areas, the saddle-shaped space between the second and third knuckles can be used to slide along spines or crests, for instance along the anterior iliac crest and along the spine of the scapula (see technique T83). Undoubtedly there are other parts of our hands that could also be used.

The octopus hand

The octopus hand is an invaluable tool for palpation, for getting an overall sense of the tissue, for testing the mobility between layers and for evaluating the current tonicity and density of the tissue (see Fig. 14.9). As a technique it relies upon a strong compressive vector into the underlying tissue and then a lateral shearing motion as if to separate the superficial layer from the deep. It is suited to areas in which there is not a great depth of tissues, such as over the ribs and anterior leg, but it can be used almost anywhere to soften or 'warm up' tissue for areas that will require deeper or more detailed work. It is also useful for spreading the effect

of deep work, for 'feathering off' into the surrounding tissue. Traditionally it has been used when you are mostly interested in influencing the superficial fascia. Ida Rolf used a homely image for this kind of work, calling it 'taking out the pins'.

Doubled thumbs

This is a controversial tool (see Fig. 14.10). There is a syndrome colloquially known as 'physiotherapists' thumb', which is an inflammation of the metacarpophalangeal joint of the thumb caused by overuse in the performance of Maitland-style joint mobilization. Shiatsu practitioners may also suffer the same complaint. As with the finger chisel, if you are not loosely ligamented this tool can be used effectively though sparingly, especially when sensitivity is required. Again the pointed elbow can be used in the same way.

Heel of the palm

The heel of the palm (Fig. 14.11) can be used in a bread-kneading fashion in fleshier tissue (see technique T8).

The use of lubricant

This is another controversial area. Ida Rolf herself allowed no use of lubricants at all, except perhaps water. The normal massage practice of applying oil liberally to the client's body does not work for this technique; the surface simply becomes too slippery to allow significant penetration. Sorbolene and other petroleum-based products are also unsuitable since the lighter fractions tend to be quickly absorbed into the skin, leaving the stickier residue coating the surface, which becomes gluey and makes any gliding on the surface impossible. The most workable solution is to use special lubricants created for myofascial release – usually a combination of coconut oil and beeswax, which has the right combination of 'slip' and 'grip'. This lubricant however is never applied directly to the client; it is smeared as a faint film on the actual tool that you will use, your forearm blade or fingertips for instance. Nevertheless, if the client's skin is especially dry then it can be useful to apply a miniscule amount of massage oil to the client: a few drops spread on your palm and dispersed over a wide area of the client's body. This may be particularly useful for clients with very loose superficial fascia where you feel that the MFR technique may just be stretching the skin or causing the sensation of 'Chinese burn'.

Perception of pain

'Pain is an opinion'. This saying is attributed to the famous Gestalt psychologist Fritz Perls after receiving work from Ida Rolf. It is interesting in that it suggests that strong sensations can be reframed in our experience to become less threatening. In any case, people are usually prepared to accept short-lived discomfort if they believe it will help them. The MFR technique is inherently direct and much more robust than traditional massage strokes, yet even at its strongest it causes less discomfort than some of the techniques of approaches such as deep tissue massage, myotherapy, some shiatsu and Chinese massage techniques, trigger-point treatment and some forms of joint mobilization, all of which can at times be excruciating and have been known to bruise the skin. Appropriately applied, MFR should never bruise.

Even now, Rolfing has the lingering reputation of being a painful process. It was once considered to be a tough and painful, though highly effective approach to postural problems, and this perception remains. Although developed from the 1930s it was brought to the world in the 1960s – the era of 'the screaming therapies'. This was a time when psychologists considered it necessary to provoke a deep catharsis in their clients to allow them to discharge their emotional pain. Possibly the early Rolfers got caught up in this historical trend

and believed that part of their unwritten contract with the client was to achieve maximum benefit in the shortest time, and often their work did hurt. However the philosophy has changed; Rolfers realized that painful work was usually counter-productive and so evolved more subtle ways of working. Sensations in the area receiving this deep MFR may range from a pleasant warmth to a type of transient discomfort that bodyworkers usually call 'good pain'. How clients experience this form of MFR depends on sundry factors such as previous injuries, muscular tension caused by chronic stress, or simply a constitutional intolerance to pressure. However, most clients love 'the Rolfing touch'. Any potential challenge or discomfort needs to be negotiated with the client, just as in other approaches such as trigger-point therapy, shiatsu, yoga and physiotherapy in which there is always that delicate balance between 'enough or too much'.

Self care

These techniques can stress the hands and wrists if performed inappropriately. A lot of force is conducted through the bones of the forearm, wrist and hand, which can lead to compaction of the joints, and therefore, in the longer term, a propensity to arthritic changes. The fist tools require sustained flexion in the hands, and some like the 'finger chisel' involve a co-contraction of the wrist–fingers extensors and flexors to stabilize the wrists. Depending on many factors, this can in time lead to repetitive strain injuries, for example compression of the wrist joint and inflammation of the wrist–finger flexor tendons. This does not mean you should not use the fingers in this way, but rather that you should guard against their overuse. It is therefore important to find alternative ways of doing the same thing but with a more robust instrument: particularly the elbow, which with practice can be used with great delicacy. Sometimes, through overuse, the entire forearm may become hypertonic and somewhat ischaemic.

Practitioners can avoid such stress by taking appropriate care of their hands, first by learning to use the minimum necessary muscular effort while working, and secondly by regularly stretching both the flexors and extensors of the finger and hand. Sometimes an alternating hot water/ice water soak can be used to deal with local ischaemia. And of course having the technique applied to oneself is extremely beneficial.

The table

Traditionally a low table is used for structural work, which is half as wide again as the standard massage table and approximately knee height. This allows the practitioner's weight to be easily brought to bear upon the client. It also allows the practitioner to be seated for some work, such as that around the neck. The extra width of the table allows flexed side lying whilst preventing the overhanging of body parts. Massage tables can be used, but if they are too high then exerting any downward pressure becomes difficult and the pressure then comes from muscular strength rather than using your body weight to fullest advantage. A hydraulic table is excellent as it can be set at the exact height required. The best designs go low enough for the client to sit easily for seated work. Many bodyworkers see the hydraulic table as an investment in their own back.

Client care

When preparing to apply the MFR technique in any instance, it is important to apply the necessary force without the client having to accommodate too much to the forces being applied to them; we need to understand in a practical way the simple physics involved in pushing into another body. In seated work (see technique T90 for instance), it can easily be seen that any lateral pressure will tend to unbalance the client, causing them to tense their lateral abdominals to resist the push. This may or may not be appropriate for them at the time. So, when leaning into a client one can sense the vector of pressure and then vary it so they do not have to brace too hard to maintain their position.

Contract–Relax (C–R) stretching

The C–R stretching approach co-evolved within osteopathy and physiotherapy. It is one of a group of related neuromuscular techniques that work by resetting the average resting length of muscles. It has a great advantage over traditional passive stretching in that it is specifically designed to getting under the 'radar' of the stretch reflex. It beguiles the body into allowing tissue to be lengthened beyond what is habitual. The receiver then waits a while in the lengthened position to allow the plastic deformation of the fascia to occur. This technique also has the proprioceptive advantage of enabling clients to focus upon and localize the stretch with pinpoint accuracy, which yoga teachers know can be a difficult task. This is because the muscles to be stretched are activated *immediately prior to stretching*. Like MFR, C–R stretching requires its own time and works partly by directing a controlled stress into the connective tissues. Virtually all traditional stretches have a C–R counterpart; it can be improvized from any existing traditional

passive stretching technique and new forms can always be created once the principles are understood.

The C–R sequence

Having established which area of your client requires stretching, you first test for range of motion (ROM), noting when the lengthening tissue begins to 'put on the brakes'. This is the so-called *first bind* limit of the movement. The first bind is that place in the ROM where the lengthening tissues begin to oppose their lengthening; it is found long before the absolute physiological limit and is discovered when making a passive ROM test for any particular movement. It is a 'stickiness' in the movement which could be pushed through if you chose. Then, starting from that position, use your own body to apply a counterforce to block the return path of that movement. Ask the client to use their own muscular energy to press into you, essentially making an isometric contraction of the muscles to be lengthened, then after relaxing that effort you move to the newly facilitated limit. This process is repeated until a specified limit is reached.

Box 14.3   A general protocol for assisted C–R stretching

For any particular movement restriction:

- Find the first 'bind' or barrier to that movement.
- Block the free return of that movement.
- Ask the client to attempt to press back into you (i.e. away from the limit) while you use your own counterforce to stabilize them in a static position (you are asking for an isometric contraction).
- Remind the client to use no more than 20% of their possible effort (* possibly more for very fibrotic tissue and less for more delicate musculature such as in the neck).
- Hold steadily for 7–12 seconds and ask the client to release (* possible use of breath).
- Move to the newly facilitated limit (* one variation is to use the client's antagonist muscles (CRAC), another is to sensitively assist them to the new limit).
- Repeat until there are no further gains (usually three or four repetitions).
- Remain at this new limit for a while, perhaps asking the client to 'breathe to the area' to allow further lengthening – it is now that the fascia has a chance to 'creep' or lengthen.

* this denotes a point for possible variations in the technique

---

Clients usually experience the technique as safe because they are being asked to apply force *away* from their limitation or point of discomfort, and not into it. Variations of the technique are useful in a wide range of contexts, from the gentlest mobilization of painful tissue to the vigorous challenging of dense or fibrotic tissue. Two forms will be shown in the practical section: a practitioner applied form in which you assist your clients within a sessional framework, and a self-applied version which can be taught to clients for them to use as a resource in their daily homeplay.

C–R stretching works at a relatively low level of neurological organization, even at the level of spinal reflexes. Because of this its effects really need to become integrated into a broader movement repertoire if the results are to be more than just transitory. Clients with a good sensory-motor intelligence may be able to integrate the changes directly; others will need a movement integration approach to maximize the benefits of the technique. At the heart of this technique's efficacy is the fact that muscles are able to lengthen more fully after an isometric exertion, which is a phenomenon known as *post isometric relaxation* (PIR). One variation of the technique, *Contract, Relax, Antagonist Contract* (CRAC), makes use of the client's own antagonists to take them to the new barrier – to the next 'bind'. This variation relies on the muscular reflex known as reciprocal inhibition in which an active agonist muscle will neurologically inhibit its antagonist, thereby allowing it to be passively lengthened. Chaitow (1996) gives an excellent detailed exposition of the many variations of this approach.

Different variants of this technique co-evolved within the osteopathic and the manual medicine traditions. Fred Mitchell Snr. was the osteopath who first called the technique *muscle energy technique*, on the basis that it is the muscles' own energy that is utilized to allow the lengthening to take place. PNF or *proprioceptive neuromuscular facilitation* is actually a highly evolved system of therapeutic exercises that was developed at Kabat-Kaiser Institute in the 1940s. It includes exercises such as maintaining resistance through a range of motion, enhancing postural and righting reflexes, and stretching and exercises to increase muscular endurance (Knott and Voss 1968). It was discovered that the isometric contraction of a muscle facilitated its lengthening, and this technique above all has been absorbed into the full spectrum of manual therapeutic approaches. Many massage therapists are taught one of the isometric techniques, called 'PNF' as if this were the entire PNF system.

The 'contraction' of the C–R technique is an isometric contraction, which strictly speaking is not a contraction in the geometrical sense as the muscle does not actually shorten, it just tries to. Yet, experience has shown that even a strict isometric contraction is not absolutely necessary for this technique to work. An isometric contraction

is perhaps optimal; however, some self-applied techniques will only allow a concentric contraction, although this still allows a subsequent lengthening (see Box 14.3).

The 20% maximum contraction rule means the stretch is taken gently. To invite a client to make an 'all out' effort is to provoke a co-contraction of the musculature on a major scale, which usually results in very undifferentiated muscle action that cannot be useful. It is quite obvious when someone works too hard and mobilizes far too much unnecessary or 'parasitic' co-contraction that this is not the kind of setting in which clients are able to 'listen' more carefully to their bodies – there is too much 'background noise' or neurological static distracting them.

How important is it to have an isometric contraction? Optimal results can be achieved using such contraction. Laughlin (1998) stresses the need to be absolutely immoveable in resisting movement, so that in moving to the next bind there will be a true increase in muscle length. With you and your client as a coupled system it is important that the initial contraction be truly *isometric*, that it does not become *concentric* because you 'give' too much slack. This is an important aspect of technique, again a martial arts aspect, organizing your body to most efficiently resist the impulse from your client. However, as said previously, the technique also seems to work if the contraction is concentric. Hence some of the self-applied stretches can still be useful if a concentric contraction is used (see technique T72 for instance).

Use of the breath

Often, it helps to harness the client's breath in the process. One method is to ask the client to take a deep breath at the beginning of the isometric contraction, and then release the pressure and the breath at the same time. Another is to have them release the isometric contraction first, then take a breath that is released while moving to the next bind. We have already mentioned that research has shown that the average tonus of the body decreases on the out-breath. Therefore, it is always useful when you wish your client to relax.

Developing your verbal 'patter'

It is important to develop your own 'patter' when using C–R stretching. It becomes a standard which your clients begin to understand and can then apply when you use the technique in novel contexts. If the client knows how to respond when you use C–R stretching for their hamstrings, they can very quickly respond appropriately if you are working on their neck since the steps are virtually

---

Box 14.4   The golden rules of assisted C–R stretching

- Avoid the 'arm wrestle' syndrome – some clients will unconsciously believe that this is a contest of strength, you against them!
- Try to organize yourself to be immoveable – if the clients sense that you are unbalanced, or that your energy is tremulous, or that they could push you over if they press too hard, they will not be confident in pushing into you.
- You can use the vector of your own counter pressure to give subtle cues to your client precisely where you wish them to direct their force.
- You can subtly hint to your client that you are about to release the counter pressure (and therefore it is safe for them to release also), either through the verbal 'patter' you establish with them, or by yourself slightly easing off your pressure before saying 'Release'.

---

identical. It will also allow them to learn self-applied techniques more easily. (See the list below and Box 14.4.)

A sample 'patter'

'In a moment I will ask you to … (press into my shoulder, bring your head back to the midline, flex your ankle, etc) … and I want you to use no more than 20% of your strength (effort, oomph, etc).'

'I want you to increase the effort gradually and then hold it steadily for 6 or 7 seconds, until I say "release".'

'Press into me now and maintain that pressure … (1, 2, 3 … 7).'

'And release [here you can cue your client that you are about to release your counter pressure by slightly easing off as you say 'And release'].

'Take a deep breath and on the out-breath we will go a little further … OK, release.'

The partnership of myofascial release and C–R stretching

As a combination of techniques, MFR and C–R stretching complement each other very well. C–R stretching is very useful after an area has been 'opened up' using MFR. The stretching is effective for the overall elongation of an area; however it may not address any microadhesions between muscle layers or fasciculi; the different force vectors at play during the application of the MFR techniques may reduce these microadhesions and anchor tissue in ways that stretching cannot.

Homeplay

Clients can be given stretching and re-patterning exercises as homeplay. Their participation in group-work such as yoga, Pilates or gym work should be encouraged; however in such class situations it is often impossible for the leaders to give individual attention to everyone. Consequently leaders usually 'teach to the middle', to the average person in the group. Often, therefore, the exercises and stretches that people receive may not be particularly appropriate for them. For this kind of structural work it is vital that the homeplay should concentrate on areas that need to be opened or patterns that need to be more deeply felt.

In general, clients do not respond well to home exercise regimens. On the other hand, they will usually agree to find ten minutes a day in which to have 'a sensorial bath': a time just for themselves in which they can try their stretches and re-patterning exercises in a playful way. It can be suggested that they try a new activity for a week in order that it can be learned enough to become part of their repertoire, and then it becomes their resource that can be called upon whenever they need it. In this daily session they should be encouraged to feel what is particularly needed that day and to find sensory enjoyment in it. One has only to look at children and cats to realize that even stretching can be luxuriated!

Passive stretching   If someone stretches forcefully or bounces into stretches they are literally encouraging 'infighting' within the nervous system! The stretch reflex works to prevent tissue from being lengthened to the point of damage; it is the automatic braking system of the musculature. So to use our will (our cortical control) to overrule the wisdom of this lower level response is to encourage strain and a struggle between levels, because the spinal cord is trying to shorten the muscle while the mind is trying to lengthen it. Clients need to be educated into 'gentling' the tissue long. Traditional yoga wisely uses the breath to get 'under the radar' of the stretch reflex. However clients often do not have the luxury of this subtle form of movement education. The self-applied C–R style of stretching can be taught fairly quickly; since the assisted form of this stretching is used within sessions, clients can easily transfer this learning to a self-applied form.

Self-applied C–R stretching   C–R stretching given as homeplay should be taught very carefully. Stretch coaches and yoga teachers know how easy it is for the body to 'cheat' a stretch. Sometimes even with the best intention of stretching any area, the body will subtly find a way of avoiding the stretch – that is what the stretch reflex is there for! So it is important to emphasize aspects of 'form', showing the way to organize the body before even beginning the stretch. Laughlin has developed an extraordinarily comprehensive collection of assisted and self-applied C–R stretches that can fulfil most stretching requirements (Laughlin 1998, 1999).

Occasionally the C–R stretching technique will give rise to a short-lived phenomenon of muscle weakness, usually experienced immediately after a particularly challenging stretch. The muscle has been working outside its customary range and needs a few moments to recover. Simple movement is all that is necessary for functionality to return and the new range to be integrated. This illustrates an important point though, that any technique that actually lengthens tissue changes the body's structure *and therefore needs to be integrated.* After a powerful stretch one always feels a little disorganized. This is obvious for instance if you stretch the hip flexors on one side only and then walk; a lopsided gait cannot be avoided. In his overview of the research into stretching, Tsatsouline (1998) suggests that preperformance stretching has been shown consistently not to enhance performance, despite athletes often believing otherwise. Baseball pitchers who stretch as part of their warm-up routine believe that it improves their pitching, yet their throwing velocities are then actually slightly less. This highlights the importance of integration; a serious stretch changes your structure. You cannot simply stretch and immediately function as effectively as before; therefore, any serious challenge to our structure, whether through stretching or MFR, will need to be integrated.

Integration work – embodiment

Ideally integration work should be woven into the fabric of the whole session, but it is especially important at the end. Clients often fall into a light alpha state during the early stages of this work. Often are signs (borborygmus, muscular twitching, deep sighing breaths, and so on) that the autonomic nervous system is shifting towards the parasympathetic. Clients do need to be brought back into the real world gently, to re-adjust to gravity and to allow the changes to ripple through the whole system. Traditional massage often does not take this into account and sends its clients into the world in a vague, pleasant and relaxed, but nonetheless disorganized, state. Driving in such a state can be highly dangerous so some grounding work at the end of a session is absolutely necessary.

Here it can be useful to use Alexander or Feldenkrais style hands-on work to suggest new postural or movement possibilities, to track and encourage a new range of movement, or to explore a new pattern of coordination. At the very minimum clients should be encouraged to walk around and try to feel any changes that might have occurred and to explore new options for movement with them. This is also an ideal time to ask the client to use some of the visualizations that have been mentioned or to give time for new sensory impressions to sink in.

Clients often 'feel strange' when shown new postural or movement options because a different proprioceptive experience can sometimes feel rather alien. For instance, the client with military squared shoulders who felt 'like a gorilla' when at last he was able to accept his shoulders in a more neutral position. Similarly, when clients with an anterior shift in the pelvis are brought back to 'the Line', they often feel unbalanced, and it seems strange although not necessarily unpleasant. Clients need time to get over the strangeness of new options. Relearning, integration is always needed when ancient, deeply learned patterns are challenged.

The integration walk

A good general suggestion is to ask clients to take an 'integration walk' after the session. Immediately afterwards is best, but definitely before bedtime; unintegrated work has been known to affect sleeping patterns and emotional balance. Generally a ten-minute walk is ample, provided it is done with the attention directed inwardly to the sensations of walking. Clients can be asked to observe and enjoy their walking as if they were watching themselves on TV. The Feldenkrais approach suggests that this kind of attention to our sensorial life is the most potent means of allowing our sensory motor intelligence to adjust to the differences induced by somatic work, and to integrate new patterns.

REFERENCES

Barnes J 1990 Myofascial release: the search for excellence. Rehabilitation Services Inc., Paoli, Pennsylvania

Chaitow L 1996 Muscle energy techniques. Churchill Livingstone, New York

Cottingham J 1987 Healing through touch. Rolf Institute, Boulder, pp 147–162

Flury H 1987 Structural levels at the pelvis. In H Flury (ed.) Notes on Structural Integration, 1: 25–34

Flury H, Harder W 1988 The tilt of the pelvis. In H Flury (ed) Notes on Structural Integration 1: 6–15

Godard H et al Neurophysiological study of the emotion. Unpublished study. Online. Available: http://*www.somatics.de*

Godard H 2000 Notes from Bodywisdom conference. Coromandel, New Zealand

Greenman P 1996 Principles of manual medicine. Lippincott, Williams & Wilkins, Baltimore

Knott M, Voss D 1968 Proprioceptive neuromuscular facilitation: patterns and techniques. Harper and Rowe, New York

Laughlin K 1998 Overcome neck and back pain. Simon and Schuster, New York

Laughlin K 1999 Stretching and flexibility. Simon and Schuster, Sydney

Stanborough M 2004 Direct release myofascial technique. Churchill Livingstone, Edinburgh

Tsatsouline P 1998 Beyond stretching: Russian flexibility breakthroughs. Dragon Door Publications, St. Paul, Minnesota

CHAPTER 15

A FIRST APPROXIMATION TO BALANCING STRUCTURE

In the next chapters we will look at the practical application of the techniques covered in Chapter 14 and how they can be used to address the following five fundamental structural themes:

- working in the sagittal plane – balancing the front and the back
- working in the frontal plane – balancing left and right
- working in the transverse plane – unwinding longitudinal rotations
- working with shoulder girdle displacements
- working with externally rotated legs.

Addressing these themes alone is an ideal approach to achieving a 'first approximation' to balancing structure.

In Chapter 14 a two-pronged approach was suggested for making an initial assessment of our clients: observing their standing organization and observing their gait. For the assessment of standing organization, in the frontal plane we looked at left–right symmetry, in the sagittal plane the organization of the spine, ribs, pelvis and legs, and in the transverse plane rotations of the vertically stacked segments: legs, pelvic and thoracic segments and the head. In assessing gait patterns we looked for the following undulatory patterns that are inherent in efficient walking:

- the lateral sway of the pelvis in the frontal plane
- a rocking of the pelvis in the sagittal plane
- the counter-rotation of the shoulder and pelvic girdles in the transverse plane – a slight twisting and untwisting around the longitudinal axis of the body.

There is an obvious correlation between the fascial continuities in these three planes and the potential for movement through them during gait; soft-tissue restrictions in standing organization will relate to restricted gait patterns, and therefore freeing up these soft-tissue restrictions is an excellent means of approaching more efficient walking. Looking at how our clients walk is one of the most effective methods of seeing where both structural and functional restrictions exist. Very occasionally the restriction may be purely functional, owing to the fact that there may simply be motor concepts that the client has never fully learned. In this case, perhaps movement work alone may be called for; however, such restrictions must in time become reflected in the structural body, so that it is usual to find that some relieving structural work may be called for, even if only minor.

For each of the above five structural themes we will examine the key 'lines' or fascial continuities that will become the focus of that work. Much of the myofascial work will then consist of progressively releasing areas of shortness within those lines. In the sagittal organization we will look at *the back line* and *the front line*; in the frontal organization we will look at *the lateral line* and the *inner-leg line*, and in the transverse organization we will cover just a few releases to help differentiate the thoracic and pelvic segments. Myers, in his masterly analysis of these longitudinal fascial continuities (Myers 2001), proposes what he calls the *superficial front lines* and *superficial back lines*. The lines examined here are similar to but not identical with those. He also expands upon what he calls *spiral lines*, which obviously relate to our transverse organization; however, working with spiral and oblique lines calls for a more advanced understanding of structure and cannot be explored in detail in an introductory book such as this. More in-depth information about the spiral lines may be found in Myers' *Anatomy Trains* (Myers 2001).

OPENING THE GAIT

Detailed mathematical modelling of the human spine suggests that efficient gait is driven by the action of the spine rather than the legs (Gracovetsky 1988). Gracovetsky notes that in many animals it is undulation through the spine that supplies the entire energy of locomotion; we see this still in fish and to a lesser extent in reptiles and amphibians. He believes that this is still the case in mammals, and one only has to look at the slow-motion picture of a cheetah in full flight to see the extraordinary power of locomotion that comes from the vigorous flexion and extension of the animal's spine. He suggests that this 'spinal engine' forms the motive power for locomotion even in human beings; it is the complex motion of frontal and sagittal undulation combined with the counter-rotation of the spine about its own axis that drives our gait. Gracovetsky (1988) gives a dramatic account of a man born with no legs who is able to 'walk' with a spinal motion that is only a slightly exaggerated form of our own. The legs amplify the action of the spinal engine but are not essential for locomotion.

In order to clarify the three components of pelvic undulation we can perhaps illustrate them with their more exaggerated forms, which are caricatures of the movements. The frontal undulation is a side-to-side translation of the pelvis that is also accompanied by a tendency for the hips to alternately lift and drop; it has been called the 'Marilyn Monroe' walk, but is also seen in competitive walking and so-called 'power walking'. The sagittal rocking of the pelvis and spine in walking and dance is very evident in some traditional African cultures, but is also seen in the relaxed rocking pelvis of trained dancers. In Rolfing circles it is sometimes referred to as 'the psoas walk', however it could also be called the 'Jar Jar Binks' walk in reference to the Star Wars character who walks in this way. The transverse undulation of the pelvis is the counter-rotation of the shoulder and pelvic girdles around the longitudinal axis of the body, which is most apparent in an exaggerated form as the 'cat-walk' of trained models. Our gait contains all three components but in very different degrees; the mixture is often a reflection of our cultural milieu: for instance, one sees more movement of the hips in the streets of Rio de Janeiro than in London. Aspects of these component undulations are intrinsic to our structure. As an example, the typical female pelvis is wider proportionally than the male pelvis and therefore has a proportionally greater distance between the femoral heads. During the 'swing' phase of gait, the swinging leg is therefore suspended from a longer lever, making the dropping of the

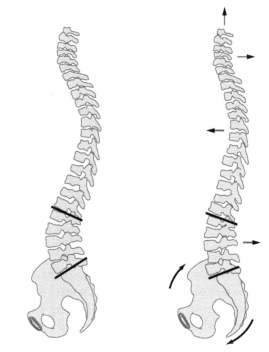

Figure 15.1 Sagittal undulation (after Gorman).

ungrounded hip a natural adaptation. So the Marilyn Monroe walk is not necessarily a 'put on' but is a natural consequence of having wider hips!

All three components of efficient gait demand differentiated movement of the head and the thoracic and pelvic segments, which means that these vertically stacked segments of the body can move somewhat independently of each other. For instance, the thoracic and pelvic segments can counter-rotate against each other to the degree that spiral fascial lines will permit, and in the frontal plane these same segments can move laterally, in opposite directions. This kind of differentiated movement requires a free spine and for abdominal muscles (particularly the obliques) to work in a subtle and complex way, otherwise these segments simply move together as an undifferentiated block. Differentiated motion will be inhibited if there is a generalized tightening of the abdominal muscles as this can form a muscular 'corset', suppressing natural gait. We will now look at these three undulations in more detail.

Sagittal lines, sagittal undulation

The sagittal undulation of the spine and pelvis is a fundamental and distinguishing movement of mammals (see Figs 15.1 & 15.2). It consists of a subtle wave-like rippling, like a skipping rope gently wriggled from one end. In humans in upright stance the pelvic segment

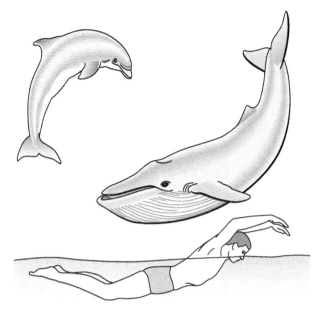

Figure 15.2 Sagittal undulation.

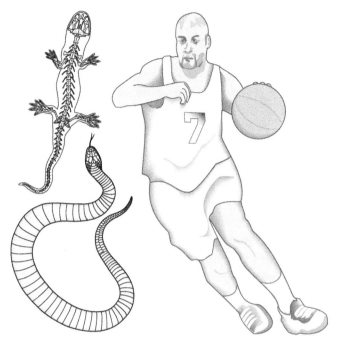

Figure 15.3 Lateral undulation throughout the world of vertebrates.

rocks anterior–posterior through the axis that passes through the acetabula, and this is coupled with a sinusoidal wave that passes up the spine and is combined with a periodic shortening and lengthening of the entire spine. The same kind of motion can be seen very clearly in the powerful locomotory movements of dolphins and whales, and can be seen dramatically in human beings performing the butterfly stroke in swimming. Mammals are capable of utilizing this sagittal undulation in combination with the lateral undulation that is more characteristic of fish and reptiles.

Lateral lines, lateral undulation

Lateral movement within the frontal plane is a distinguishing movement in all vertebrates (Fig. 15.3). It can be expressed as simple side-flexion, or as a lateral undulatory wave that progresses longitudinally through the length of the animal. In fish this wave becomes their principal means of locomotion. Humans, as vertebrates, have the same potential for a 'wavy spine' through this plane. If we look at the main structural segments in their frontal aspect, we see the three main skeletal masses of the head, the thorax and the pelvis connected respectively by the cervical and lumbar spines (Fig. 15.4). It also shows the main ways that lateral movement can be expressed – as lateral flexion and lateral undulation. But we are also bipedal, which means that, in standing, our spine and legs have the same longitudinal orientation as the trunk, so this longitudinal wave can continue

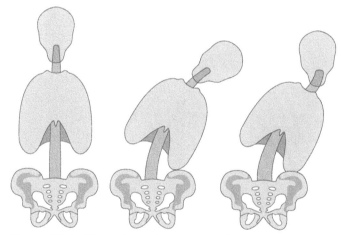

Figure 15.4 The main trunk segments in frontal organization showing lateral flexion and lateral undulation.

through the hip, bypassing the knees (because of the collateral ligaments) before reaching the ankles and feet. The hip joints are designed to abduct and adduct freely, and thus have the potential to translate laterally within the frontal plane (Fig. 15.5). In walking, this becomes the rhythmic swaying of the hips that accompanies the weight shift from one supporting leg to the other.

Transverse lines, transverse undulation

Movement in the transverse plane is possible because our major axial segments – the head, and the thoracic and pelvic segments – are stacked vertically above each

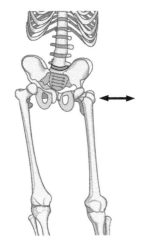

Figure 15.5 Lateral translation of the hips in the frontal plane (after Versalius).

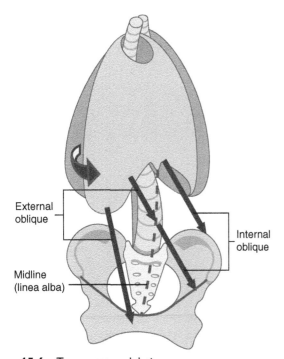

External oblique

Internal oblique

Midline (linea alba)

Figure 15.6 Transverse undulation.

of the matador to rotate around his own axis, the matador will usually win out (Feldenkrais 1949). Many of the Eastern forms of martial art capitalize on the power of helical and rotatory movements, whereas in the West we seem to focus on orthogonal planes of movement in our exercise regimens and in the design of exercise equipment, paying less heed to rotatory patterns.

KEEPING A LEVEL HEAD

A perfectly functioning spine–pelvis complex has the potential for all three kinds of undulation in movement, particularly in gait. Yet on top of this whole mobile arrangement is a head that needs to be relatively stable in movement.

This presents the interesting scenario of a pelvic segment with the potential to undulate in a highly complex fashion, and a swaying sacral base connected to a spine on top of which is a head that ideally should *not* sway in movement too much. Our vertebrae are designed to allow flexion–extension and side-flexion–extension throughout the entire length of the spine, and rotation through the thoracic and cervical regions, and this would suggest that with good co-ordination it should be possible to have a moving sacral base, a complex undulation of the spine and a head that is able both to remain vertical and to track forward in space during walking without too much lateral displacement. And this kind of gait is quite evident in many traditional cultures, and is seen in its most beautiful expression in the flowing gait of some African cultures, particularly when it is normal practice to carry heavy loads on top of the head. However, this elegant way of moving is seen much less in the West, where cultural constraints often will not allow the full and natural expression of movement.

What we so often find are hips that move very little and a head–thorax–pelvis complex that virtually moves as one piece; there is very little differentiated movement between the segments, and the thorax–abdomen–pelvis becomes *the trunk* (with an obvious semantic relation to tree trunk!). And we know that if any constraint is placed on the full expression of our movement potentiality then eventually that constraint will become consolidated in the flesh; it will manifest first as a fascial restriction, and later as joint stiffness and immobility.

But why does the head need to be stable in movement? As was outlined in Chapter 12, the head is the repository of our main orienting senses of sight, hearing and sense of smell, and also of the semi-circular canals or vestibular complex that informs us of our orientation in

other and able to rotate relative to each other around a longitudinal axis, to the degree that the spiral lines and the facet joints at each spinal segment permit (see Fig. 15.6). These rotatory movements are driven by the spiralling orientation of the muscle fibres, which suggests that the human body is designed to support spiral or helical movement patterns.

Feldenkrais suggests that a rotation around our longitudinal axis is an extremely efficient kind of movement in humans. He notes that when the enormous linear momentum of a bull is pitted against the ability space. Our senses will generally work better atop a stable platform. The perceptual processing involved in vision, for instance, is a much simpler process in a non-swaying universe. And anyone who has visited an amusement park knows the effect of too much movement of the semi-circular canals! So what is necessary to accommodate the ideal poise of the head when everything below is in complex movement? What are the options open to the body? And how is this affected by the extremely common pattern of an undifferentiated head–thorax–pelvis complex?

We have spoken a lot about the sensory-motor intelligence of the body. Let us imagine that this intelligence could articulate its reasons for choosing to move in a certain way. How would it try to solve the following movement problem?

How can I help this body maintain a stable platform for the head given that the thorax and the pelvis move as one piece?

Its 'reasoning' might proceed as follows:

a. If a lateral swaying of the hips is permitted then the head can only remain stable in space if the lateral movement at the hip is counter-balanced by a contrary (and possibly excessive) side-flexion of the neck.
b. Another solution might be to dispense with the swaying of the hips entirely, or at least to inhibit their lateral sway as much as possible. This will not only stabilize the head, but the whole trunk as well! (This could be called the 'brick on legs' syndrome, a pattern very common in the West.)
c. The only other alternative is to accept that the head will displace from side-to-side in walking, and this will result in a swaggering gait like the motion of an inverted pendulum.

Each of these 'solutions' has its associated problems. In solution a., by minimizing movement in one place we encourage excess movement elsewhere, and all the repetitive stresses that this entails. In solution b., we are employing large-scale co-contraction of muscle groups to inhibit the expression of natural movement. This is inefficient mechanically and ultimately very destructive of joints. Or in solution c., the inverted pendulum syndrome, the centre of gravity of the head and chest is being systematically displaced from the midline. Apart from the fact that the head is not stable in walking, the movement is mechanically inefficient because energy is expended in bringing the upper centre of gravity back to the midline twice each gait cycle. All such inefficient gait patterns will leave their imprint in the structural body.

FIVE STRUCTURAL THEMES

In the following technical chapters we will address five structural themes – three axial and two appendicular:

- working in the sagittal plane
- working in the frontal plane
- working in the transverse plane
- addressing shoulder girdle displacements
- addressing the external rotation of the legs.

For each theme we will first examine the relevant myofascial lines and structures that may need to be addressed. This will be followed by a pictorial section outlining a series of techniques that can be used to address these myofascial lines. The three axial themes will also include some simple Feldenkrais-style integrative work that can be used following structural work.

The integrative work will be shown firstly as a Feldenkrais *Awareness Through Movement* (*ATM*) script, followed by a pictorial exposition of the kind of 'hands-on' movement work that is typically used by Alexander or Feldenkrais practitioners. In Feldenkrais circles this is known as *Functional Integration.*

The Feldenkrais ATM scripts consist of a series of verbal directions that guide the client through a carefully structured movement exploration. These ATMs are typically conducted with the client lying down on the floor or on your table; this eliminates much of the 'anti-gravity' processing required of the nervous system in standing and gives the client more 'space' in which to attend closely to new sensory information. ATMs typically begin with a process of sensorial focussing: an attempt to bring the client's awareness to their inner world of sensory and kinaesthetic impressions, and to 'awaken' areas of their body that will be engaged in the exploration. Verbal directions are then used to guide the client towards some specific movement patterns or coordinations that usually start simply and build in complexity. These movements must never try to challenge the client's structure; they are usually performed slowly, with small amplitude and with eyes closed, so they can be more deeply sensed. ATMs will often then take the movement pattern into other bodily orientations. You will notice also that 'rests' are given fairly often. These are not a rest from physical exertion but a space to allow the nervous system to integrate the new impressions. It is suggested that you experience the lesson yourself before using it with your clients. In the ATM scripts that follow, a certain amount of anatomical language has been used; this may not be appropriate for your clients and you may need to find a more colloquial language that is appropriate for them.

Following each ATM script you will find a pictorial section that shows how you can use your hands to direct or enhance aspects of the clients' movements. They can be used by themselves or as a means of enhancing the ATM work.

REFERENCES

Feldenkrais M 1949 Body and mature behaviour: a study of anxiety, sex, gravitation and learning. International Universities Press, New York

Gracovetsky S 1988 The spinal engine. Springer, Vienna

Myers T 2001 Anatomy trains: myofascial meridians for manual and movement therapists. Churchill Livingstone, Edinburgh

CHAPTER 16

WORKING IN THE SAGITTAL PLANE

Work in the sagittal plane means addressing the spinal curves, dealing with dysfunctional patterns of rib organization, finding an appropriate tilt of the pelvic segment and finally 'getting the head on top'. Working with the spinal curves means directing attention to exaggerated or diminished primary and secondary curves and finding a more balanced relationship between the pelvic segment and the spine. This necessarily also entails working with the anterior and posterior aspects of the lower limbs as these are major myofascial determiners of the tilt of the pelvic segment.

FASCIAL LINES THAT AFFECT MOVEMENT IN THE SAGITTAL PLANE

Figure 16.1 shows the fascial continuities that run through the dorsal and ventral aspects of the whole body that, here, will be called *the front line* and *the back line*.

The front line runs through the anterior aspects of both the legs and the trunk. It consists of the connected fascial continuity that flows from the dorsum of the feet, through the anterior aspect of the crural fascia, the anterior aspect of the fascia lata overlying the rectus femoris, reaching to the anterior superior iliac spine (ASIS). In the trunk there is a primary line running from pubic bone up to and including the sternal fascia and thence flowing into the anterior fasciae of the neck. There are also key areas more lateral to this line that 'feather off' laterally: the more anterior attachments of the obliques, the costal arch and the more anterior fascia overlying the ribs.

The back line consists of the fascial continuity running from the plantar fascia, the posterior aspect of the crural

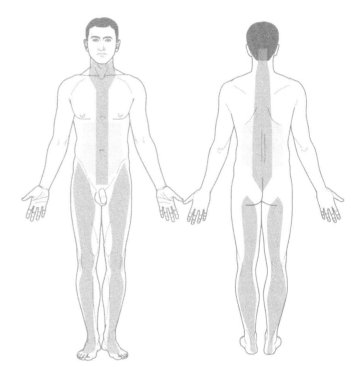

Figure 16.1   The front and back lines.

fascia that invests the calcaneus, calcaneal tendon and the gastrocnemius, and the posterior aspect of the fascia lata that invests the hamstrings and the fascial environment of the sacrotuberous ligament. In the trunk there is a primary line consisting of the multiple fascial layers that overlie the multifidus and erector spinae group, connecting the multifidus triangle over the sacrum into the galea (epicranial aponeurosis) of the scalp. There are also key areas lateral to this primary line: the thoracolumbar fascia and the fasciae overlying the posterior aspect of the ribs.

THE FRONT LINE (SEE TECHNIQUES T1–T23)

In the technical section that follows, a series of techniques will be outlined for addressing the following areas:

- the antero-lateral compartment of the leg (tibialis anterior and the more anterior of the peroneal group) and the fascia overlying the flat, anterior surface of the tibia (T1, T2)
- the anterior aspect of the fascia lata, in a line connecting the patella and the ASIS, and more laterally to the tensor fasciae latae and the sartorius attachments, then more medially to the short adductors (T3–T16)
- the ASIS and the superior–anterior aspect of the iliac crest (T17)
- the costal arch (T18)
- the anterior belly wall (T19)
- the sternal fascia and the more medial aspects of the pectoral fascia (T20)
- the ventral aspect of the trunk generally (T21)
- the anterior fasciae of the neck, and the deeper layers that invest the longus collis (T22, T23 and also T73, T74 and T75).

THE BACK LINE (SEE TECHNIQUES T24–T55)

These areas will be addressed in the technical section that follows:

- the plantar aponeuroses (T24)
- the posterior aspect of crural fascia, calcaneal tendon, the heads of the gastrocnemius, and more laterally to the edges of the soleus (T25, T26 and also T78)
- the hamstrings (T27–T35)
- the multifidus triangle, the thoracolumbar fascia, the erector spinae from mid-sacrum to the nuchal ligament and occiput (T36–T55).

We will also look at the internal ligamentous structure of the spine, especially the anterior and posterior longitudinal ligament.

SOME GENERAL PROTOCOLS FOR ADDRESSING IMBALANCES IN THE SAGITTAL PLANE

What follows is a summary of some common features of the front and back lines in which one would normally consider some lengthening work (see Fig. 16.2). However these 'point form' suggestions should not be taken as a simple formula that can be applied without considering the organization as a whole. It is again emphasized that the order in which any of these areas are opened up depends on coming from a broader strategic perspective, for instance by applying the 'rules of thumb' for strategizing sessions that were outlined in Chapter 14 (see Box 14.1, p. 133).

Excessive cervical lordosis
Lengthen the local erector fascia, open the suboccipital area and perhaps also the sternocleidomastoid and scalenes (T48–T55, T73–T75).

Diminished cervical lordosis
Lengthen the anterior cervical compartment including the infrahyoids (T22, T23, T73–T75).

Excessive kyphosis
Generally lengthen the entire ventral aspect of the trunk. Give counter-curve stretches to the thoracic spine, aiming to influence the anterior longitudinal ligament. Strongly lengthen any ventral area that is found to be tight during a counter-curve stretch (T17–T21).

Diminished kyphosis (flat thoracics)
Lengthen the thoracic erectors and the posterior aspect of the ribs after positioning the client in a flexed, even foetal position (T39–T41, T86).

Excessive lumbar lordosis
Lengthen the lumbar erector fascia, then more broadly into the thoracolumbar fascia. Lengthen the psoas (T36–T39, T42–T44, T12, T13).

Diminished (or flat) lumbar lordosis
Lengthen the hamstrings, the anterior belly wall and the superior attachments of the ASIS. Perhaps also give lumbar extension stretches or exercises (T27–T35, T17–T19).

Forward lean (from ankle to hip)
Lengthen the plantar fascia, the fascia investing the calcaneus and around the calcaneal tendon (to decompact the calcaneus and give 'more heel'). Broadly lengthen the antero-lateral compartment and the superficial fascia investing the tibia (T24, T25, T1, T2).

Excessive anterior pelvic tilt
Lengthen the thoracolumbar fascia, the lumbar erectors, the rectus femoris, the vasti group, the anterior aspect of the short adductors and the iliopsoas (T36–T39, T42–T44, T3–T16).

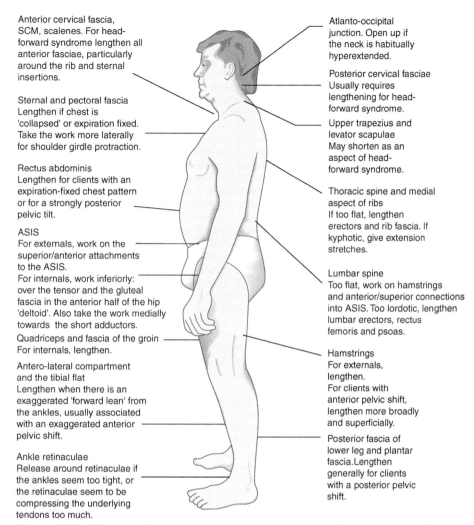

Anterior cervical fascia, SCM, scalenes. For head-forward syndrome lengthen all anterior fasciae, particularly around the rib and sternal insertions.

Sternal and pectoral fascia Lengthen if chest is 'collapsed' or expiration fixed. Take the work more laterally for shoulder girdle protraction.

Rectus abdominis Lengthen for clients with an expiration-fixed chest pattern or for a strongly posterior pelvic tilt.

ASIS For externals, work on the superior/anterior attachments to the ASIS. For internals, work inferiorly: over the tensor and the gluteal fascia in the anterior half of the hip 'deltoid'. Also take the work medially towards the short adductors.

Quadriceps and fascia of the groin For internals, lengthen.

Antero-lateral compartment and the tibial flat Lengthen when there is an exaggerated 'forward lean' from the ankles, usually associated with an exaggerated anterior pelvic shift.

Ankle retinaculae Release around retinaculae if the ankles seem too tight, or the retinaculae seem to be compressing the underlying tendons too much.

Atlanto-occipital junction. Open up if the neck is habitually hyperextended.

Posterior cervical fasciae Usually requires lengthening for head-forward syndrome.

Upper trapezius and levator scapulae May shorten as an aspect of head-forward syndrome.

Thoracic spine and medial aspect of ribs If too flat, lengthen erectors and rib fascia. If kyphotic, give extension stretches.

Lumbar spine Too flat, work on hamstrings and anterior/superior connections into ASIS. Too lordotic, lengthen lumbar erectors, rectus femoris and psoas.

Hamstrings For externals, lengthen. For clients with anterior pelvic shift, lengthen more broadly and superficially.

Posterior fascia of lower leg and plantar fascia. Lengthen generally for clients with a posterior pelvic shift.

Figure 16.2 The sagittal organization showing key areas that often need to be addressed.

Excessive posterior pelvic tilt
Lengthen the hamstrings, the lower abdominals and the more anterior oblique attachments superior to the ASIS. At a ligamentous level, lengthen the anterior longitudinal ligament in the lumbar spine through lumbar extension stretching (T27–T35, T17, T19).

Excessive anterior shift – shortened back line
Broadly lengthen the back line: the plantar fascia, fasciae of the calcaneus, the calcaneal tendon, the gastrocnemius, the hamstrings, the fascia investing the sacrotuberus ligament, the thoracolumbar fascia, the erector spinae group, the nuchal ligament, the suboccipitals, the occipital fascia and the fascia of the scalp and brow. Most effect will come from broad work on the hamstrings and along the full length of the back (T28, T39).

Excessive posterior shift – shortened front line
Broadly lengthen the front line: the dorsal fascia of the foot, the antero-lateral compartment of the leg, the fascia overlying the flat of the tibia, the rectus femoris, rectus

abdominis, and the pectoral–sternal fascia (T4–T7, T17–T21).

Expiration fix
Lengthen the sleeve of the thorax generally. Work between the ribs, under the costal arch and the length of the tendinous borders of the rectus abdominis. Use stretches to influence the internal fascial connections between the costal arch–xyphoid process and the crural attachments of the lumbar spine (T18–T20, T39–T47, T70–T72).

Inspiration fix
Lengthen the dorsal aspect of the thorax. If the shoulder girdle is retracted, lengthen the fasciae investing the mid-trapezius, rhomboids and superficial scapular musculature (T39–T41, T86).

The forward head syndrome
This is a large scale pattern and is thus a longer-term project that includes lifting the ribs, lengthening the

pectoral and clavipectoral fasciae, opening the sub-occipital region, lengthening the upper trapezius, the levator scapulae, the sternocleidomastoid and scalenes. Broadly lengthen the entire ventral aspect of the trunk especially the upper abdominals and the costal arch (T18–T23, T45–T55, T73–T75, T83–T93, T96–T100).

Thoracic inlet syndrome
Lengthen the pectoralis minor and the scalenes. Broadly work all the connections into the axilla. Consider giving a neuro-stretch for the brachial plexus if you are confident there is no nerve inflammation (T96, T23, T73–T77, T94–T100).

SAGITTAL ORGANIZATION

Front line

T1

MFR technique – shin
Use the 'octopus grip' for a broad contact since it is only the superficial fascia that needs to be engaged. Slide superiorly. You can work specifically on the flat of the tibia, then use fingertip contact to work on the borders of the tibia.

Assisting movements
Ask for a slow flexion–extension of the ankle.

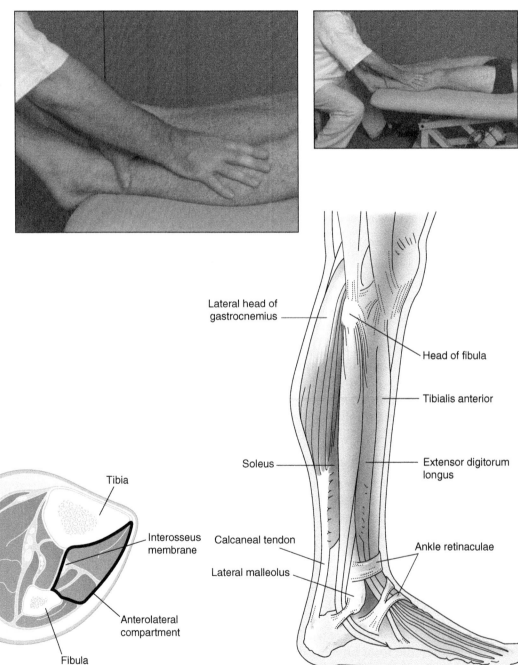

T2

MFR technique – antero-lateral compartment
Slide superiorly using the forearm blade but avoiding any hard contact with the tibial border. The client can be placed in a side-lying position if you require specific access to the peroneals.

Assisting movements
Ask for a slow flexion–extension of the ankle.

Alternative
Use doubled thumbs along lateral tibial border.

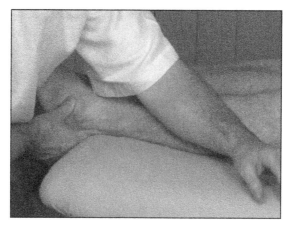

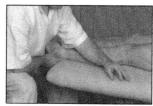

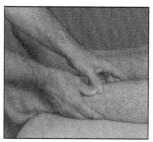

The quadriceps
It should be borne in mind when working with the quadriceps that the four muscles in the group have two kinds of action. The rectus femoris is a two joint muscle, spanning the knee and the hip, and acts as a hip flexor as well as a knee extensor. The vasti only extend the knee, yet they are packaged in the same fascial compartment of the anterior thigh (see Fig. 9.4, p. 61). Hence a generalized lengthening of the quadriceps, including the vasti, will assist hip extension.

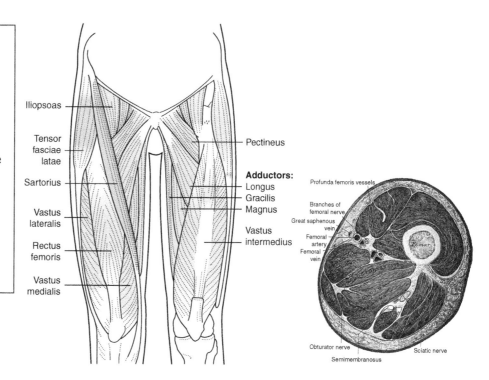

T3

Test for hip flexors
The client lays supine and hugs one knee to the chest in order to flatten and stabilize the lumbars. If the hip of the suspended knee remains slightly flexed then the psoas is short. If the knee lifts as it is passively flexed (as in this photo), then the rectus is short.

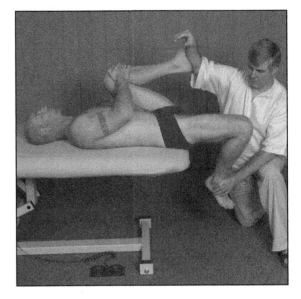

T4

MFR technique – quadriceps
Work along the rectus to the ASIS. Repeat with more lateral and more medial strokes taking in the vasti. Work along the 'valley' of the sartorius, which separates the adductor mass from the quadriceps.

Assisting movements
Ask for a gentle pelvic rock, assisted if necessary by having the opposite leg flexed with the foot flat on the table.

Alternative
Use the 'octopus hand' to spread the work.

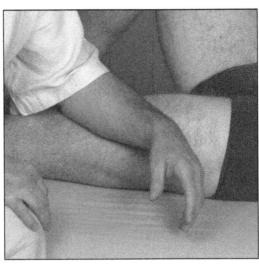
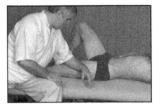
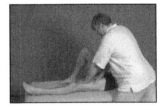

T5

MFR technique – insertion of sartorius
Gently settle on the sartorius tendon close to the ASIS. Gradually lean and increase the pressure while sliding laterally very slowly.

Assisting movements
Ask for a gentle pelvic rock, assisted if necessary by having the opposite leg flexed with the foot flat on the table.

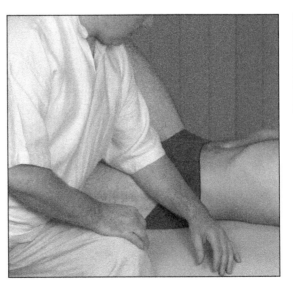
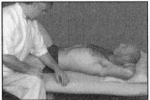

T6

MFR technique – quadriceps, lateral aspect

This area can be tender and full of trigger points and is close to the femur, so this work should be relatively superficial and using the 'fleshy' part of the forearm blade to avoid sharp contact.

Gather the superficial fascia and work medially or laterally.

Assisting movements

Ask the client to breathe into the area or to perform a small pelvic rock.

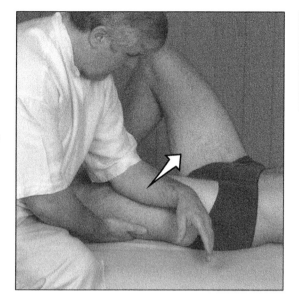
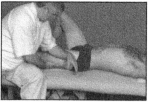

T7

MFR technique – quadriceps, medial aspect

Using the full length of the forearm blade, settle in the valley of the sartorius, gather the mass of superficial fascia and work laterally.

Assisting movements

Ask the client to breathe into the area or to perform a small pelvic rock.

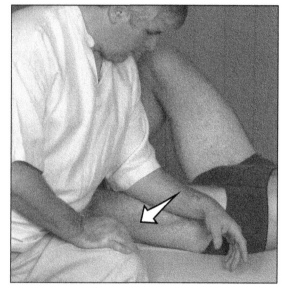

T8

MFR technique – quadriceps, medial aspect

Grip the quadriceps with both hands and lean your body weight into the tissue under the 'heel' of the palms.

Assisting movements

Knee flexion. 'Slowly draw your heel towards me.'

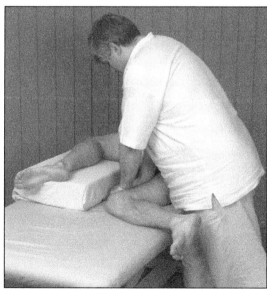
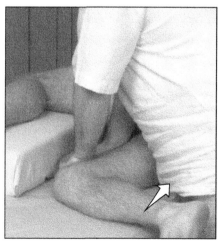

T9

MFR technique – inner thigh, adductors

Place the client's leg on an angled roller or Torson bolster. Using the 'forearm blade' and the softer surrounding tissue as the tool, sink into the tissue of the inner thigh. (If you do not have a bolster use a pillow for support and work without the client's assisting movement.)

Assisting movements

Leg abduction. 'Slowly draw your knee towards me.'

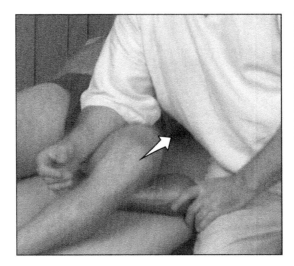

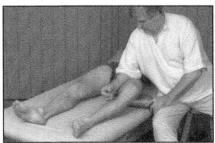

T10

C–R stretch – quadriceps

Passively flex the knee to the first bind.

Isometric contraction

Knee extension. 'Press your foot into my shoulder.'

Next position

Knee flexion. 'On the out-breath let me bring your heel towards you.' For clients with a strong lumbar lordosis, place a pillow under the abdomen to stabilize and flatten the lumbars.

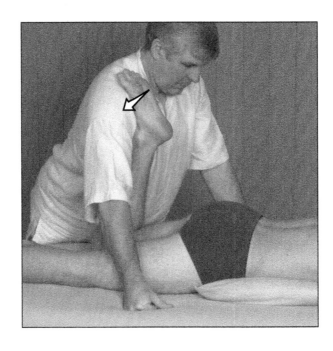

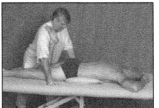

T11

Self-applied C–R stretch – quadriceps

This stretch is similar to the traditional sports stretch for the quadriceps, but without the need to maintain balance on one leg. Clients can use a table or desk with the edge padded with a towel.

Isometric contraction

Knee extension. 'Press your foot down into the table.'

Next position

This is an important and versatile stretch with various ways of increasing the stretch:

- hip extension, 'Drop your knee.'
- knee flexion, 'Lean back, using your hands for support.'
- flexion of the lumbar spine, 'Tuck your tail under.'

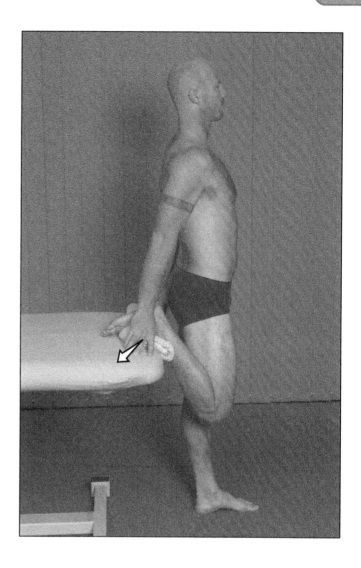

T12

C–R stretch – groin area and psoas

Have client sit on the edge of the table with sit-bones sliding off the table. Ask them to hold one knee and roll back leaving the other leg behind. The client can stabilize the lumbars by drawing the held knee closer to their chest and resting their foot against your hip.

Isometric contraction

Hip flexion. 'Lift your knee towards the ceiling.'

Next position

Hip extension. 'On the out-breath drop your knee towards the floor.' Some gentle assistance may be necessary.

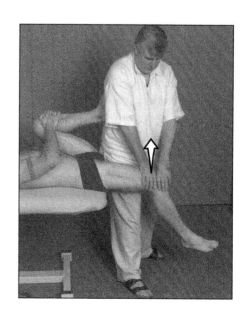

T13

Passive stretch – fascia of groin and psoas
This is a passive form of the above stretch – allowing gravity to do the work.

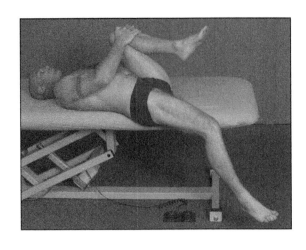

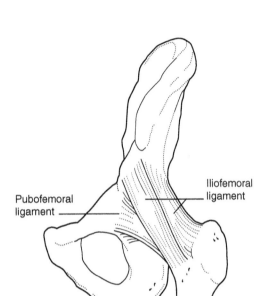

Pubofemoral ligament

Iliofemoral ligament

T14

Ligamentous challenge
Sometimes the iliofemoral ligament is the chief limiting factor that prevents a fuller extension of the hip. In this ligament stretch you lift the client's knee while leaning with the other hand into the femur. Repeat in a bouncing fashion.

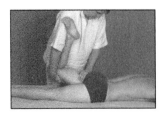

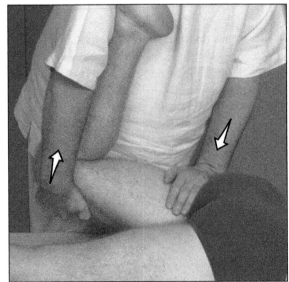

T15

Self-applied C–R stretch – fascia of groin and psoas

For this 'lunge' stretch to be effective, it is often necessary first to teach the 'pelvic rock' so that clients know how to stabilize the lumbars while doing this stretch.

Isometric contraction

Hip flexion. 'Attempt to slide your kneeling knee forward.'

Next position

Keeping the spine upright, the tail 'tucked under' and, with a sense of lengthening upwards through the trunk, gently lunge forward extending at the hip. If the distance travelled in this lunge is large then probably some points of form were missed. Usually only small increments are possible.

    When comfortably balanced, it is possible to introduce a slight twist away from the extended hip to reach more lateral fibres.

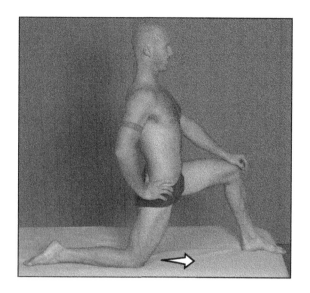

T16

Self-applied C–R stretch – hip flexors and knee extensors

This is an extreme stretch that works on both the hip flexors and the knee extensors. As for other hip flexor stretches the lumbars need to be stabilized with a 'tail tuck'.

Isometric contraction

Knee extension. 'Press your foot down into the chair.'

Next position

Knee flexion, hip extension. 'Lean back and bring your buttocks closer to your heels.'

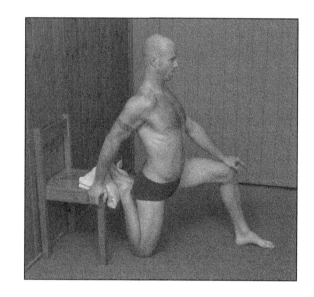

T17

MFR technique – superior to the ASIS

Make initial contact with the lateral–superior aspect of the iliac crest and slowly slide anteriorly towards the ASIS while maintaining contact with the crest.

Assisting movements

Hip extension–adduction. Starting with both hips flexed: 'Slowly straighten your leg and reach back with your heel till your foot slides off the table.'

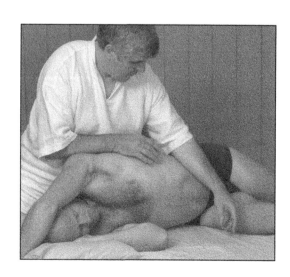

T18

MFR technique – costal arch

Starting close to the xiphoid process (but avoid pressing into it), slide laterally while maintaining contact with the inferior surface of the ribs. If the rectus is very tight use the free hand to take up the slack in the superficial fascia of the ribs.

Assisting movements

Ask for breathing in the upper chest.

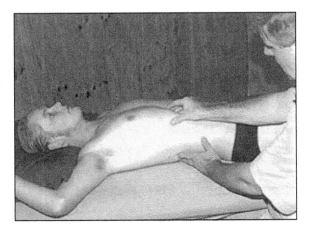

T19

MFR technique – rectus abdominis

Work bilaterally on the fascial borders of the rectus and the obliques. The direction is medial, as if trying to reach beneath the rectus, then slide either superiorly or inferiorly.

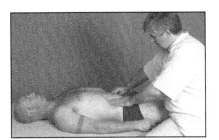

Assisting movements

Ask the client to exaggerate breath to the upper chest, or even to slightly raise and lower their head.

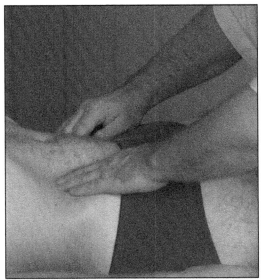

T20

MFR technique – rectus tendons and sternal fascia

Anchor in the tissue of the rectus tendons, then continue along the sternum and work over the sternal origin of the pectoralis major.

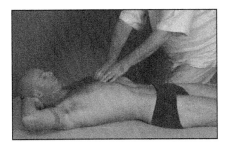

Assisting movements

Neck flexion. 'Gently raise your head a little, as if to look to your feet.' Suggest they support their head with both hands.

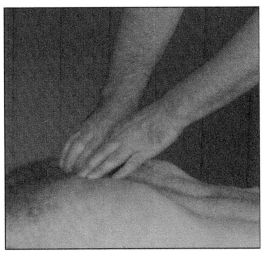

The thoracic visceral fasciae

Ultimately, lengthening through the front line needs to be matched with an internal lengthening of the thoracic visceral fasciae. The thoracic cavity is densely networked with visceral fasciae: prevertebral and pretracheal fasciae, the mediastinal ligaments, the pericardium and the fascia of the diaphragm. These fasciae are inevitably linked together forming a network from the base of the skull, through the thoracic outlet, and connecting to the crura of the diaphragm. We can perhaps only influence these fasciae indirectly, by stretches such as the following.

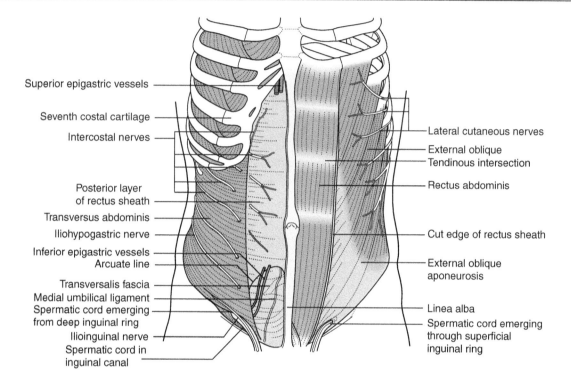

Superior epigastric vessels

Seventh costal cartilage

Intercostal nerves

Posterior layer of rectus sheath

Transversus abdominis

Iliohypogastric nerve

Inferior epigastric vessels

Arcuate line

Transversalis fascia

Medial umbilical ligament

Spermatic cord emerging from deep inguinal ring

Ilioinguinal nerve

Spermatic cord in inguinal canal

Lateral cutaneous nerves

External oblique

Tendinous intersection

Rectus abdominis

Cut edge of rectus sheath

External oblique aponeurosis

Linea alba

Spermatic cord emerging through superficial inguinal ring

T21

C–R stretch – ventral aspect of trunk

A good stretch for unifying previous MFR work on the trunk, generally opening up the front line. When constructing the pillow mound, try to make the apex coincide with the maximum point of curvature in the kyphosis. Clients with a strong lordosis should be asked to bend their knees and flex their lumbar spine to prevent the stretch affecting the lumbars.

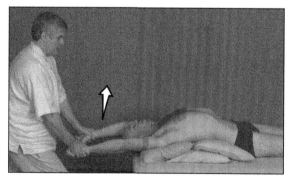

Isometric contraction

Shoulder extension. 'Try to lift me.'

Next position

Shoulder flexion. Gently traction the arms while taking them further into shoulder flexion and trunk extension.

Alternative

Lever from the elbows if the previous technique is too stressful for the shoulders.

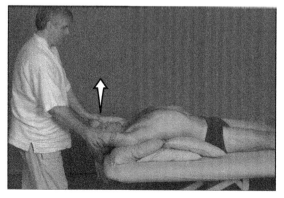

T22

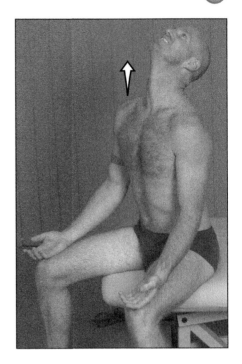

Passive stretch – infrahyoid area
This stretch actually lengthens the infrahyoids but also seems to reach into the chest and affect the thoracic viscera. For this stretch, the client needs to sense the difference between cervical and capital extension, and may need to be tutored in this, then:

● open the jaw wide
● drop the head backwards (more cervical extension than capital extension). Clients can be told 'Think of lengthening up through the front rather than folding at the back'.
● close the mouth bringing the teeth together gently
● reach up towards the ceiling with the chin. 'Feel yourself lengthening through the front including the ribs.'
● relax the jaw
● repeat.

T23

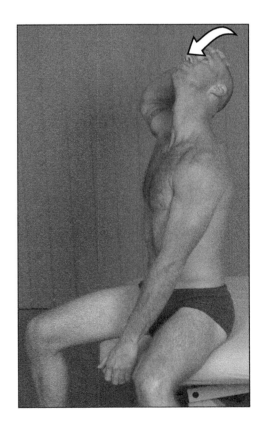

Self-applied C–R stretch – scalenes and sternocleidomastoid
This is one of the most difficult stretches to get right, but it is one of the most important for mitigating the effects of the forward head syndrome. Clients need to sense exactly where the stretch is acting, and if necessary modify the vectors of the stretch to place the stretch directly into the scalenes.
Caution: It is important not to jam the facet joints on the side opposite the stretch, so an emphasis on lengthening in the front of the neck while performing this stretch needs to be conveyed to the client.

Isometric contraction
Neck flexion. 'Press your forehead into the hand using about a 10% effort.'

Next position
Neck extension. 'Take the head a little further back at a diagonal while maintaining a general sense of lengthening in the neck.'

Back line

T24

MFR technique – plantar fascia

Using the phalangeal surface of the fist and with the elbow stabilized against your own knee, work slowly toward the heel.

Assisting movements

Toe and ankle flexion– extension. 'Curl your toes up, now your foot.'

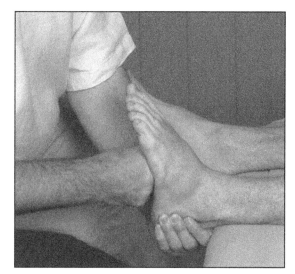

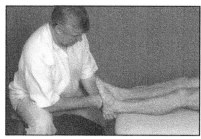

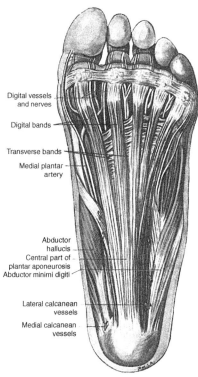

Digital vessels and nerves

Digital bands

Transverse bands

Medial plantar artery

Abductor hallucis

Central part of plantar aponeurosis

Abductor minimi digiti

Lateral calcanean vessels

Medial calcanean vessels

T25

MFR technique – calcaneal tendon

Using the forearm blade work superiorly. Take care when approaching the heads of the gastrocnemius as this area can be quite sensitive and often has active trigger points. Use a broad technique like the octopus hand over the heads to the gastrocnemius.

Assisting movements

Ankle flexion and extension. 'Slowly flex and extend your ankle.'

Alternatives

Use the 'octopus grip' to broadly lengthen the crural fascia. Use the finger chisel bilaterally starting from the calcaneus and working superiorly along the tendon.

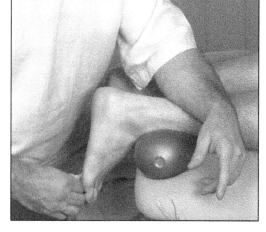

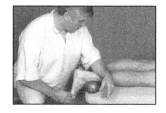

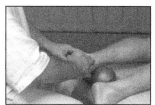

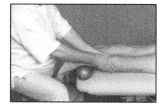

T26

Self-applied C–R stretch – gastrocnemius and soleus
Using a straight leg to stretch the gastrocnemius or a flexed knee to stretch the soleus.

Isometric contraction
Plantar flexion. 'Press the balls of your foot into the floor.'

Next position
Hip extension, dorsiflexion. 'Translate your pelvis toward the wall.'

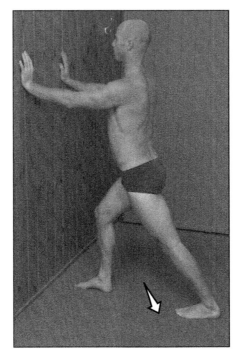

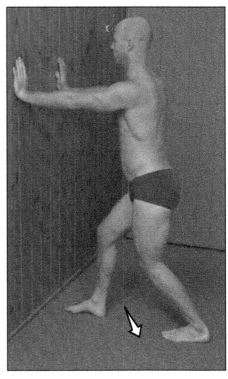

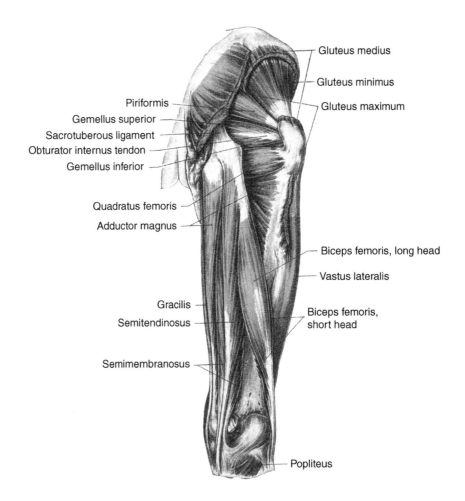

Piriformis

Gemellus superior

Sacrotuberous ligament

Obturator internus tendon

Gemellus inferior

Quadratus femoris

Adductor magnus

Gracilis

Semitendinosus

Semimembranosus

Gluteus medius

Gluteus minimus

Gluteus maximus

Biceps femoris, long head

Vastus lateralis

Biceps femoris, short head

Popliteus

T27

Straight leg raise test – to check hamstring length

When first lifting the heel allow the whole leg to be suspended *loosely* in a relaxed hand. This will encourage the client to relax the quadriceps before doing the test.

Then elevate the foot to the place where the hamstrings begin to 'put on the brakes', at which point the knee will tend to flex slightly.

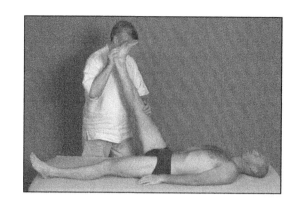

T28

MFR technique – the hamstrings

First perform a broad stroke with the forearm blade from distal to proximal to 'warm up' the tissue.

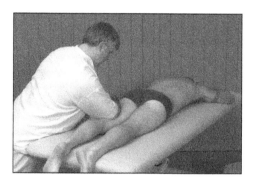

Then, with more point loading, follow the lines of the medial and lateral hamstrings. On meeting the ischial tuberosity, work around the common tendon of the hamstrings.

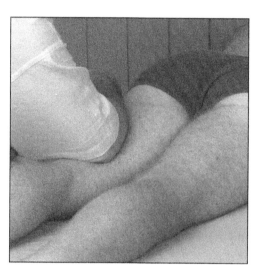

Assisting movements

Slight hip flexion. 'Gently and rhythmically, press your knee into the table.'

T29

MFR technique – medial hamstrings

Using the forearm blade, work medially with short transverse strokes, gradually working inferiorly.

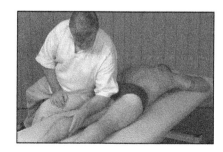

Assisting movements

Slight hip flexion. 'Gently and rhythmically, press your knee into the table.'

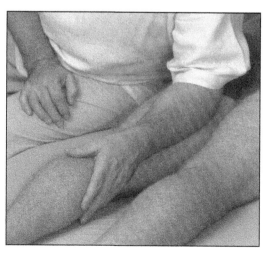

T30

MFR technique – lateral hamstrings

Using the forearm blade and starting from the fascia-rich area behind the trochanter, work towards the knee.

Assisting movements

Slight hip flexion. 'Gently and rhythmically, press your knee into the table.'

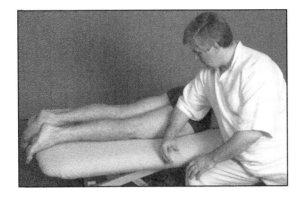

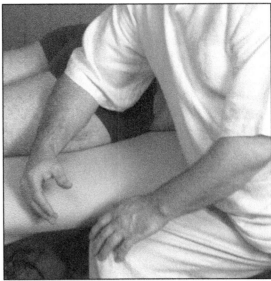

T31

MFR technique – hamstrings, distal aspect

Using a soft fist, work in turn the medial and lateral tendon areas.

Assisting movements

Use the free hand to lower the leg to the table. If the client cannot relax the hamstrings, have them extend the knee gently while you resist. 'Gently press your foot into my hand. I will resist a little.'

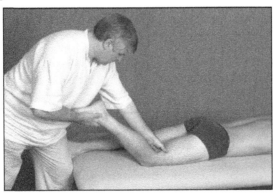

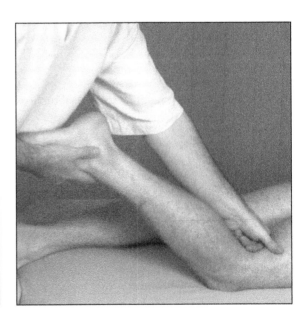

Using reciprocal inhibition

This technique makes use of reciprocal inhibition. If the client is unable to 'give' you their leg, oblige them to use the hamstring antagonists, the quadriceps, to enable the hamstrings to release.

T32

MFR technique – inner line of the medial hamstrings

Begin with the knee as flexed as possible, and then using soft fists bring your weight to bear on the hamstring. Use the knuckles as if to separate the hamstrings from the adductor mass.

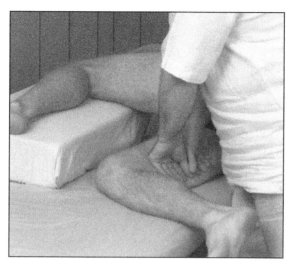
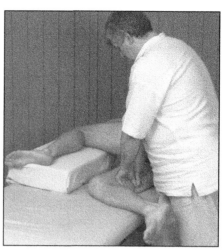

Assisting movements

Knee extension. 'Slowly straighten your leg.'

T33

C–R stretch – hamstrings

Test for the first bind by doing a straight leg raise, and begin the stretch at the first bind. For clients with a tendency to hyperextend at the knee, apply the counter-force as close as possible to the knee to avoid stressing the posterior ligaments.

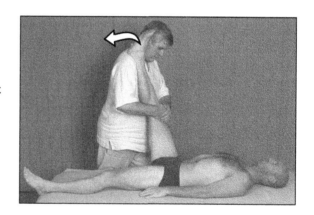

Isometric contraction

Hip extension. 'Keeping a straight leg, push into my shoulder.'

Next position

Hip flexion. On the out-breath take the hip further into flexion until you feel the next bind. Alternately use the CRAC method and ask the client to actively move to the next position (using their hip flexors).

General comment on hamstring stretches

Any major flexion at the hip (as for instance in the 'dog pose' of yoga) will impart a lengthening tendency throughout the entire back line, from the scalp to the toes. However, where the stretch 'goes' depends on which sections of the back line are shortest. For instance, external clients typically have very shortened hamstrings and a loosened posterior longitudinal ligament in the lumbar spine. Therefore, when they flex at the hip the stretch inevitably goes to the lower back (which will flex too easily) instead of to the hamstrings. Hence, points of

form are vital in hamstring stretches otherwise the stretch will not go where it needs to go. When giving hamstring stretches to external clients it is important to show them how to flex at the hip without flexing in the lumbar spine. Ask them to visualize an axis through the trochanters. Have them take their chest forward, maintaining the straight relationship in everything above the hip. They will not go far. Language is important so ask them to 'hinge' rather than 'curl' forward. You can even ask them to maintain a slight lumbar lordosis.

T34

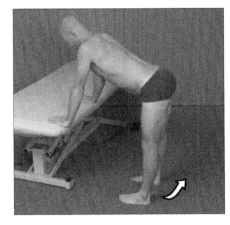
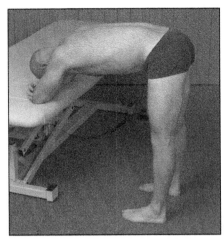

Self-applied C–R stretch – hamstrings

This stretch is unusual in that each hamstring is contracted successively prior to moving to the next position. Using a chair or table for support, hinge forward from the hips (taking care not to flex the lumbar spine).

Isometric contraction

Knee flexion. 'Draw your heel backwards as if trying to bring your heel to your backside.' Then repeat for the other leg.

Next position

Hip flexion. 'Pivot from your hips, taking your chest forward and keeping a straight back.'

T35

Passive stretch – hamstrings

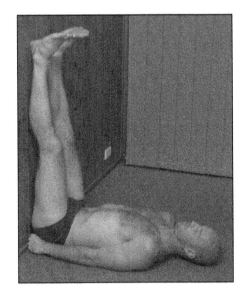

A stretch from the Iyengar tradition. Try to keep the sacrum on the floor and the sit-bones in contact with the wall. The knees need to be straight and the feet need to be in as neutral position as possible, neither in plantarflexion nor lateral rotation as these will decrease the effectiveness of the stretch.

For clients with an external pelvis, placing a roll under the lumbars can increase the stretch. This also tends to encourage more of a lumbar curve. However, extreme externals may not be able to do this stretch straight away as their entire sacrum will be lifted from the floor. They may need to use a C–R approach first.

T36

MFR technique – multifidus triangle and inferior erectors

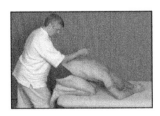
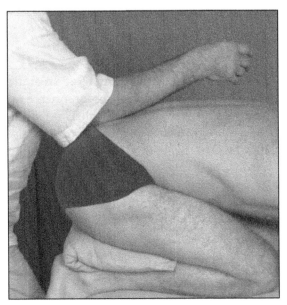

Similar to 'the pose of the child' of yoga, this working position allows good access to the most inferior erectors and less directly to the iliolumbar ligaments. Ask the client to use their elbows and head to form a triangle of support in order to resist being pushed forward. A pillow placed between the heels and the buttocks can prevent excessive compression of the patella.

Assisting movements

Ask the client to breathe into the lower back.

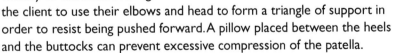
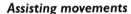

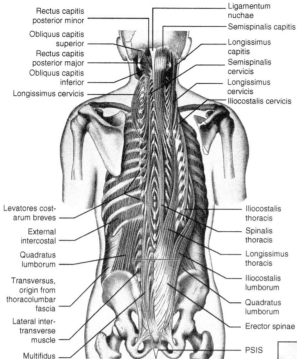

Rectus capitis posterior minor
Obliquus capitis superior
Rectus capitis posterior major
Obliquus capitis inferior
Longissimus cervicis

Ligamentum nuchae
Semispinalis capitis
Longissimus capitis
Semispinalis cervicis
Longissimus cervicis
Iliocostalis cervicis

Levatores cost-arum breves
External intercostal
Quadratus lumborum
Transversus, origin from thoracolumbar fascia
Lateral inter-transverse muscle
Multifidus

Iliocostalis thoracis
Spinalis thoracis
Longissimus thoracis
Iliocostalis lumborum
Quadratus lumborum
Erector spinae
PSIS

T37

MFR technique – thoracolumbar fascia

This working position allows good access to the thoracolumbar fascia as it meets the iliac crest. It also allows broad access to the fascia overlying the floating ribs. Use the octopus hand or soft forearm blade.

Assisting movements

Ask the client to breathe into the lower back.

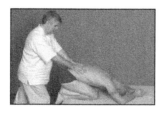

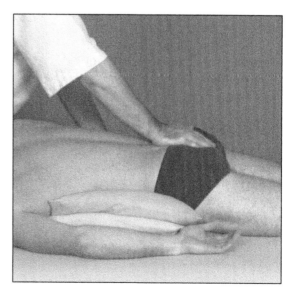

T38

C–R stretch – lumbar erectors

This technique follows naturally from the previous one. Place several pillows on the table and ask the client to lie face down. Take care to align the edge of the pillows with the ASIS. Place the heel of your palm at about S2 or S3, depending on which gives the better purchase.

Isometric contraction

Lumbar extension. 'Arch your lower back and stick your backside out.'

Next position

Lumbar flexion. 'Tuck the tail under and allow your lower back to lengthen.'

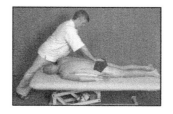

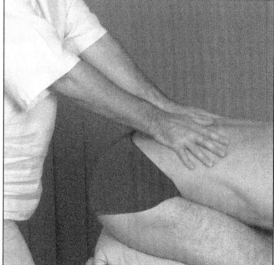

T39

MFR technique – erector fasciae

Ask the client to place the feet slightly in advance of their knees. This allows them greater control during the folding forward. Starting at around C7, make broad contact with the tissue either side of the spinous processes and gradually glide inferiorly. This can be taken right to the apex of the sacrum. Ask the client to allow their arms to hang to reduce tonus in the rhomboids.

Proprioceptively, this technique can give a strong unified impression of the whole back and, incidentally, provides the practitioner with an ideal opportunity to check on any scoliotic tendency.

Assisting movements

Spinal flexion. 'Allow your chin to drop to your chest then slowly roll forward, allowing your arms to hang down like old ropes.'

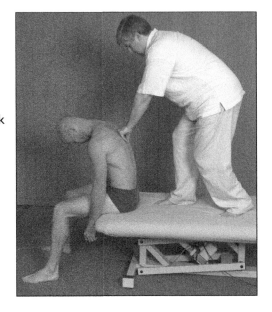

T40

MFR technique – upper thoracic area

The support beneath the chest removes the need for stabilizing tonus in the erector group. It gives good access to the thoracic erectors, the rhomboids and central trapezius, and to the more lateral fascia of the ribcage.

Assisting movements

Ask the client to exaggerate the in-breath and allow the ribs to expand backwards.

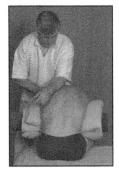

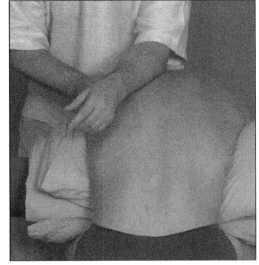

T41

MFR technique – upper thoracic area, whilst side-lying

This is an ideal position to work on the upper trapezius, rhomboids and the more superficial rotator cuff muscles. Use a bolster or rolled pillow to pack the chest of the client and allow a supported and rotated position of the thorax. The support minimizes the need for resisting tonus in the trunk when pressure is applied. Bring the knees up towards a foetal position.

Assisting movements

Ask the client to breathe into the area.

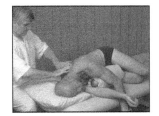

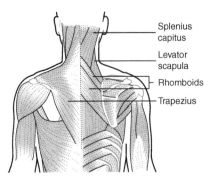

Splenius capitus

Levator scapula

Rhomboids

Trapezius

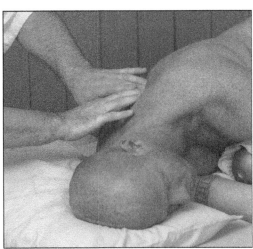

T42

MFR technique – erectors

This is a general technique that can be used anywhere along the spine, wherever more detailed work is required. Position the client with a supporting roll as in the previous technique. Using the point of the elbow, make longitudinal strokes along the erectors or in short lateral strokes from the laminar groove.

Assisting movements

Ask the client to breathe into the area, or minimally flex the spine into you.

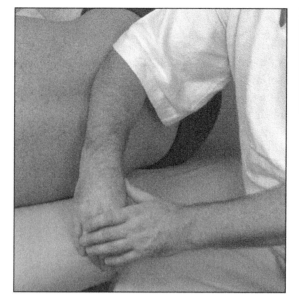
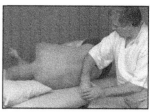

T43

MFR technique – erectors, laminar groove

Using either a reinforced finger chisel or the point of the elbow. Apply successive transverse strokes laterally from the laminar groove.

Assisting movements

Ask the client to breathe into the area.

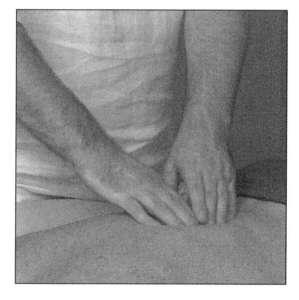
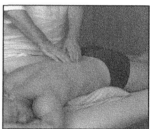

T44

MFR technique – erectors, working medially

Use reinforced double thumbs to make several transverse strokes towards the spine.

Assisting movements

Ask the client to breathe into the area.

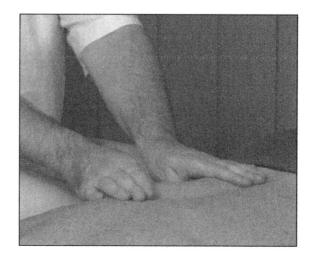
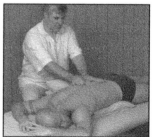

T45

Passive stretch – thoracic spine, ALL

This is a counter-curve stretch of the thoracic spine. It is one of the few means of lengthening the ventral surface of the trunk while directly influencing excessive kyphosis.

The hands should be clasped behind the head to prevent neck hyperextension and to lengthen the pectoral fascia at the same time.

This is also a good working position for myofascial work on a shortened front line. All of the myofascial techniques for lengthening the ventral aspect of the trunk can be used with the client in this position. Clients can be asked to sense the specific areas of tightness in the chest, which may then be released.

Clients with a gym ball can be encouraged to use this stretch as homeplay.

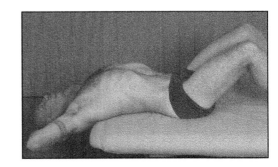
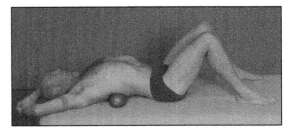

T46

C–R stretch – thoracic spine and ALL

NB: This is identical with T21, which is used for lengthening the anterior thorax.

Construct a mound out of pillows, rollers etc, ensuring that when the client lies back the neck does not hyperextend.

Isometric contraction

Shoulder flexion. 'Gently try to lift me.'

Next position

While maintaining a slight traction through the arms, assist the client further into spinal extension.

Alternative

Use flexed arms if the shoulders are stressed.

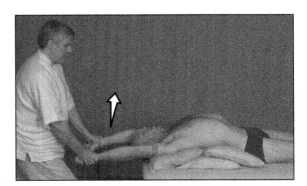

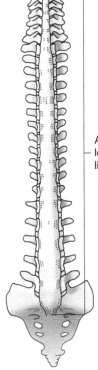

Anterior longitudinal ligament

The anterior longitudinal ligament (ALL)

For clients with a pronounced kyphosis, it is often the shortened anterior longitudinal ligament of the spine that is the chief factor maintaining the curve. Possibly the only way of influencing this ligament directly is with a counter-curve stretch. A rolled towel, Torson bolster or several pillows can be used (in Iyengar yoga a wooden block is sometimes used), using graded thicknesses to avoid strain.

T47

C–R stretch – pectoral fascia
This stretch follows naturally from the previous one. Ask the client to interlace their fingers behind the head.

Isometric contraction
Arm adduction. 'Raise your elbows to the ceiling.'

Next position
Arm abduction.

Caution: Any pain felt deep in the shoulder on either side should be a contraindication as there could be some dysfunction in the rotator cuff.

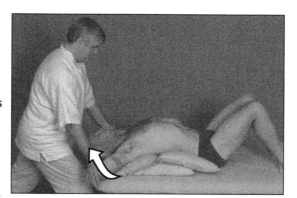

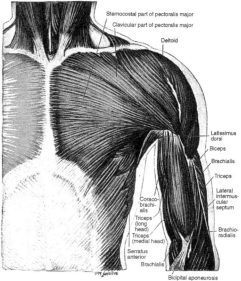

T48

MFR technique – posterior cervical fascia
Starting around T2, press up into the laminar grooves. Work bilaterally with finger chisels, using the back of the hands on the table to obtain leverage. Work superiorly each side of the nuchal line to the occiput and then into the galea aponeurosis.

Assisting movements
None, or perhaps a very slight capital flexion. 'Draw in your chin.'

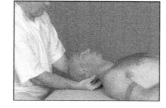

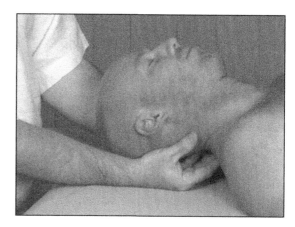

T49

MFR technique – occipital ridge
This technique looks severe but the contact can be firm, yet gentle. The first and second knuckles contact the mastoid process, while the third and fourth contact the cervical fascia. The head is compressed slightly into the pillow. Slide medially whilst maintaining a vector of force towards the centre of the cranium (i.e. try to avoid making the client tense up to stabilize the head).

Assisting movements
Eye rotation. 'Look towards the pillow.'

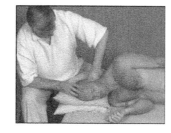

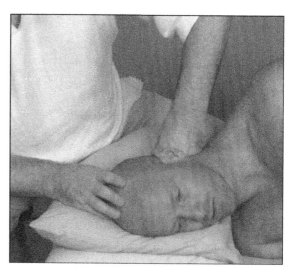

T50

MFR technique – occipital ridge

An alternate method is to reach under the neck and work on the opposite side of the occipital ridge. Using finger-pad pressure, slowly slide along the occipital ridge from the mastoid process to the nuchal line.

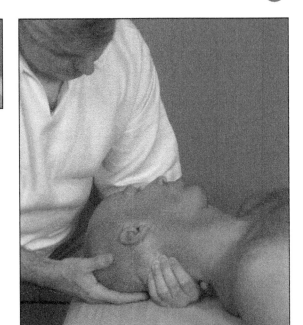

Assisting movements
None.

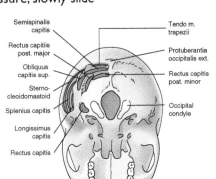

Semispinalis capitis

Rectus capitiis post. major

Obliquus capitis sup.

Sterno-cleoidomastoid

Splenius capitis

Longissimus capitis

Rectus capitis

Tendo m. trapezii

Protuberantia occipitalis ext.

Rectus capitis post. minor

Occipital condyle

T51

Movement education – the chin tuck

Few clients are able to flex their neck while keeping the head parallel with their mid-line. This technique is a first approximation to discovering this movement.

Using a roller or flattened Torson bolster, show the client how to flex their neck in a way that opens the junction of the neck with the occiput. The roller takes away the friction of the head with the table and allows a free exploration of this movement.

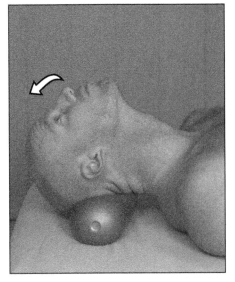
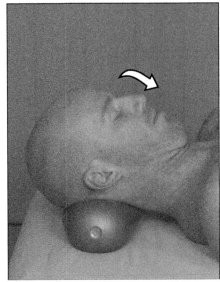

T52

Passive stretch – atlanto-occipital junction

This neck retraction is the 'chin tuck' of yoga.

Initially ask the client to stand with heels and buttocks touching the wall. Ask them to draw in or tuck in the chin, while at the same time lengthening through the back of the neck. The aim is to keep the face parallel with the wall. Once this unusual neck flexion is sensed, it can be performed without using the wall.

This stretch is very useful for dealing with the consolidated results of the head forward syndrome.

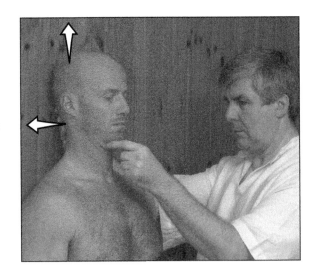

T53

C–R stretch – atlanto-occipital junction

Flex the neck to the first bind. If you feel insufficient weight then the client is trying to 'assist' by tensing the abdominals and is not resting back into your hands. If so, ask them to relax the abdomen.

Isometric contraction

Cervical extension, capital flexion. 'Press gently back into my hands, at the same time taking the tip of your nose towards your chest.'

Next position

Cervical flexion. Ask client to maintain the pressure while taking a big breath and then release. At the same time take the head to the next barrier.

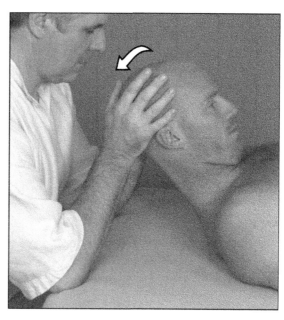

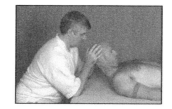

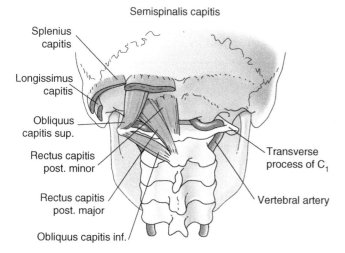

Semispinalis capitis

Splenius capitis

Longissimus capitis

Obliquus capitis sup.

Rectus capitis post. minor

Rectus capitis post. major

Obliquus capitis inf.

Transverse process of C$_1$

Vertebral artery

T54

Self-applied C–R stretch – occiput and posterior fasciae of neck

This stretch can lengthen the entire posterior fascia of the neck, including the occipital region. It flows naturally into the following technique, which then concentrates the stretch at the atlanto-occipital junction. By performing a pelvic rock in this position, the point of the stretch can be localized in different parts of the upper back and neck. If the stretch is being felt more in the mid to lower thoracic region then try lifting the sternum more.

Isometric contraction

Cervical extension. 'Press your head *gently* back into your hands.'

Next position

Cervical flexion. 'Draw your chin to your chest.'

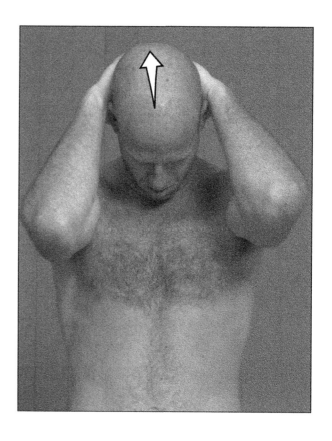

T55

Self-applied C–R stretch – sub-occipitals
Maintain the final position of the previous technique. This technique can also be repeated with a slight rotation to reach the oblique sub-occipital muscles.

Isometric contraction
Capital extension. 'Try to tip your head back, using your eyes to look up through your forehead.'

Next position
Capital flexion. 'On the out-breath tip your head forward, using the eyes to look down.'

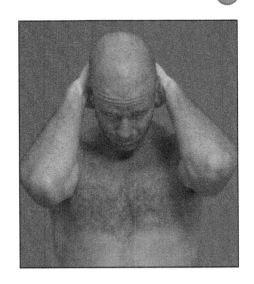

This vital stretch is unusual in that it works best as a self-applied technique. The hand position of the doer is ideally placed to resist the powerful forces of capital flexion and extension. A practitioner's help does not easily duplicate this.

The use of the eyes is very important. Research has shown that looking up will induce generalized spinal extension, and looking down: generalized spinal flexion.

MOVEMENT WORK FOR SAGITTAL UNDULATION

A key movement exploration will now be shown that can give the client a kinesthetic feel for sagittal undulation. First there is an ATM script and then a section on tactile guidance. It begins with a supine exploration of a sagittal rocking motion that in Feldenkrais circles is known as 'the pelvic rock'. This will be generalized into different orientations of the body and will finally be taken into walking.

Feldenkrais Awareness Through Movement (ATM) exploration – the 'Pelvic Rock'

Sensorial focusing

Lie on your back with your arms and legs long. Sense your contact with the floor. Which parts of you are in contact with the floor? Which parts are not? Sense the shape of the spaces behind you. Sense the cervical lordosis – how far from the ground is the highest point of that curve? Move your attention further down your spine. At what point does the spine re-contact the ground? Sense the ribs that contact the floor each side of the thoracic vertebrae. Where does the lumbar lordosis begin? How far from the ground is its highest point? Sense the contact of your pelvis with the floor. Rest.

Flattening the lumbar lordosis, with legs long

Remain lying with legs long. Rhythmically and gently press your lumbar area towards the floor. Use your own hands to gently cradle your ASIS. What is happening to your pelvis? How is it moving? Note the tendency for the tailbone to 'tuck under' and move towards the ceiling as you press your lumbar region towards the floor. Rest. Again rhythmically press your lumbars towards the floor. This time palpate your abdominal region and notice which muscles become active.

Feet in standing, posterior pelvic tilt, lumbar flexion

Lie long and sense the areas of contact with the floor. Notice the pattern of curvature of the entire spine: the extent of the cervical and lumbar lordoses and the thoracic kyphosis. Flex at the hip, bringing your feet up into a standing position. Notice how the whole shape of the spine changes to accommodate this new position. From this neutral position, gently press your feet into the floor and release. Repeat in a slow rhythmical way. Sense what is happening to the pelvis. Note the rocking motion of the sacrum as the tailbone 'tucks under'. Rest. Continue, but palpating the abdominals to better sense their activity. See if you can allow the abdominals to do less work. Rest.

Feet in standing, anterior pelvic tilt, lumbar extension

From the neutral position, gently rock your pelvis in the reverse direction, as it were, by pressing your tailbone towards the floor while at the same time gently arching your lumbar area away from the floor. Release and relax back into the neutral position. Repeat a number of times sensing how your abdomen swells towards your knees. Sense how this movement translates through the spine and evokes a gentle rocking of your head. Rest.

Combining posterior and anterior tilt

Now alternate these two opposite rocking motions to create one coordinated movement. Repeat many times while sensing the rolling contact of the sacrum with the floor. See if there are any points in this movement where there is a sense of jerkiness, and try to smooth it out. Try to reduce the effort and bring a lazy, cat-like quality into the pelvic rock. Rest.

Expanding the focus of the attention to include the breath

Check in with the rhythm of your breathing. Sense what areas are moving most. Least. On the in-breath sense how the expanding ribs gently press against the floor. When the rhythm of your breath is clear, begin to synchronise your pelvic rock with the rhythm of the breath, so that for every breath cycle there is a cycle of the pelvic rocking

motion. Repeat many times. Notice whether you inhale while flattening the lumbars, or the opposite. What does it feel like when you do the reverse? Rest.

Including a full-length flexion of the spine

Bring your feet to standing. Interlace your fingers and place them behind your head. Find a way of comfortably cradling the back of your skull. Begin to raise the elbows from the floor and towards each other. When your elbows are at their highest point, raise your head as if to examine your feet. After your head returns to the floor, allow the elbows to drop back to the floor like wings. Do this a few times, noticing how the cervical and thoracic spine responds. Rest. Repeat, but gradually introduce a pelvic rock so that the lumbars flatten as the head is raised. Repeat many times, using minimal effort. Briefly try to do the opposite!

This basic 'pelvic rock' exploration can be undertaken in other orientations:

- Sit on the floor, resting back with your hands behind you, soles of your feet together and knees dropped wide. Begin a slow pelvic rock in this position. Add in head and neck flexion and extension, i.e. as the lumbars curve back towards the floor, allow your head to drop to your chest. As the lumbars arch forward and the abdomen swells towards your knees, allow your head to look up to the ceiling and have a sense of a general lengthening throughout the entire front of your chest and neck. Sense how the chest can slide back and forth between the scapulae.
- Explore the same movement but change the previous position so that you are resting back on your elbows instead of your hands.
- Explore the same movement seated upright in a chair.

'Hands-on' movement exploration – the pelvic rock

Pelvic rock – neutral position, sensorial focussing

The client lies supine with standing legs. Have the client sense their contact with the table. You could use some aspects of the sensorial focussing that were suggested in the preceding ATM script. Ask the client to press their feet into the table, noticing how their pelvis and lumbar spine respond.

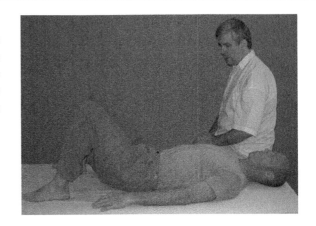

Pelvic rock – lumbar flexion phase, posterior pelvic tilt

With your hands gently moulded around the anterior pelvic crests, thumbs contacting the ASIS, use your hands to *suggest* a posterior tilt, and then allow a relaxed return to neutral. It is important not to use your hands forcefully here: the client provides the necessary muscular force, you just indicate the trajectory.

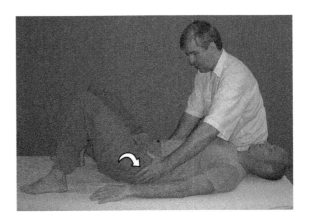

Pelvic rock – lumbar extension, anterior pelvic tilt

In the same way, use your hands to suggest an anterior tilt, then relaxing back to neutral.

Ask the client to combine the flexion and extension phases into one coordinated movement. You could then draw the client's attention to how this movement 'ripples' through the system – how it demands a coordinated response from the rest of the spine, the chest and the head.

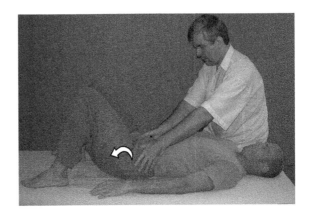

Pelvic rock – in sitting, full spine extension and flexion

Bring the client to sitting then recapitulate the pelvic movements just rehearsed in the supine position, positioning your hands over the ASIS as in that work. When the slow pelvic rocking is established, reposition your hands as in these photos to encourage full spine flexion and extension. Have the client use their eyes to assist – looking up during spinal extension and down during spinal flexion. Use your hands as a guide wherever you see there is more potential for movement in the pelvis, the ribs or the spine.

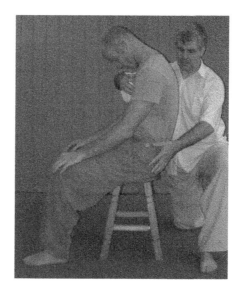

Now the client is sensitized to this undulatory pattern, have them walk around while noticing what is happening to the pelvis and lumbar spine. You can then ask them to exaggerate the rocking motion into a 'Jar Jar Binks' walk.

They can then drop the exaggerated pattern to find a natural degree of sagittal undulation might be right for them.

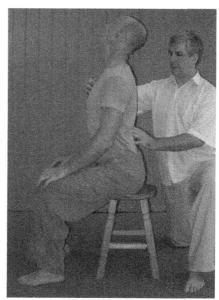

WORKING IN THE FRONTAL PLANE

When working in the frontal plane in any particular session there will inevitably arise the question of whether to work symmetrically or asymmetrically. For compressed structures a general lengthening each side of the mid-sagittal plane is required. A generalized shortness in both iliotibial tracts, for instance, will inhibit the lateral sway of the hips, while shortness in the lateral abdominal and thoracic fasciae will restrict side flexion and lateral undulation of the spine, and in both of these cases symmetrical work will be called for. For structures in which a left–right imbalance predominates, it may be necessary to work asymmetrically, addressing a different pattern of shortness either side of the mid-sagittal plane. Such imbalances may arise from asymmetrical usage or from skeletal asymmetries such as leg length discrepancy (LLD). It will be recalled from the 'rules of thumb' suggestions for strategizing a series of sessions (see Box 14.1) that generalized lengthening work usually precedes work on left–right imbalances, so in most cases in which significant such balancing is required, the asymmetrical work would be taken up later in the series following initial work to decompress the structure. Let us now look at the key fascial continuities that will affect movement in the frontal plane.

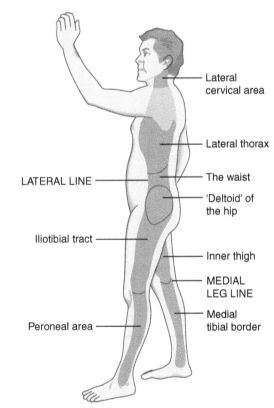

Figure 17.1 The lateral line and medial leg line.

THE FASCIAL LINES THAT EFFECT LATERAL MOVEMENT

If we consider the gross myofascial lines that influence lateral movement, we have *the lateral lines*, running from the lateral malleolus to the mastoid process each side, and *the medial leg lines*, running from the medial malleolus to the ischio-pubic ramus and pelvic floor (Fig. 17.1).

The lateral line

The crural fascia wraps the lower leg. On the lateral side it is anchored to the malleolus and the head of the fibula. It hugs the knee very tightly and is continuous with the fascia lata above. The lateral line in the upper leg is defined by the iliotibial tract (which is nothing else than a localized thickening of the fascia lata), and it runs from the head of the fibula and lateral tibial condyle to the greater trochanter and thence to the crest of the ilium, blending with the lateral gluteal fascia.

Immediately above the iliac crest arise the aponeuroses of the transversalis and obliques, which become the several layers of the lateral abdominal fasciae that span the space between the crest and the lower ribs, the transversalis fascia being the deepest. More posterior is the lateral edge of the thoracolumbar fascia, and deep to that the fascia of the quadratus lumborum.

The fasciae on the lateral seam of the thorax are not continuous but span the intercostal spaces, and in effect span the lateral seam up to the axilla and thence beneath the shoulder girdle to the base of the neck. More posteriorly is the lateral margin of the latissimus. From the base of the neck several layers of cervical fascia reach up to the mastoid process.

In practical terms, the following are the key areas in the lateral line that can be addressed:

1. The peroneal area, which extends from the peroneal retinaculae at the lateral malleolus to the head of the fibula (T56).
2. The distal aspect of the iliotibial tract, extending from the head of the fibula to the trochanter (T57, T58).
3. The 'deltoid of the hip', which includes a broad fan of fascia that radiates from somewhat below the trochanter up to the full arc of the iliac crest, and includes the gluteals and tensor fasciae latae (T59–T65).
4. The waist, which spans the iliac crest and lower ribs, and the quadratus (T66–T69).
5. The lateral seam of the thorax (T70–T72).
6. The superficial laminae of the lateral cervical fascia (T73–T77).

Like the front and back lines, these are not sharply defined areas and are best seen as 'feathering off' the more we move anterior or posterior from them.

The medial leg line

This line starts at the medial malleolus and follows the medial border of the tibia to the pes anserinus at the medial tibial condyle. From here it continues into the medial aspect of the fascia lata to the ischio-pubic ramus and blends with the obturator fascia of the pelvic floor.

In practical terms there are two key areas that can be addressed:

1. The medial border of the tibia as it blends with the crural fasciae of the soleus and gastrocnemius (T78).
2. The inner thigh line (T79, T80).

WORKING WITH ASYMMETRIES IN THE FRONTAL PLANE

In Chapter 4 we spoke of two kinds of working strategies – *decompressing* and *balancing*. Sometimes we find a 'balance' in the frontal plane in which there is overall shortness in both lateral lines. Decompression means lengthening both sides equally, thereby giving more potential for lateral sway in gait. Sometimes there is asymmetry between the left and right lateral lines. Balancing in this case means deliberately working asymmetrically, trying to 'equalize' or at least bring more congruence to the fascial continuities either side of the midline. Working in this asymmetrical fashion somehow needs more integration than work to achieve front–back balance, and usually requires definite preparatory work. Some of the main themes for working with frontal organization can be found in Figure 17.2.

Working with scoliosis

After the general work of decompressing and lengthening, it is possible to take some of the strain out of the scoliotic system by lengthening work on the concavities of the curves. It may seem as if the erectors are hypertoned on the convex side of the curve; however, this is actually more likely to be the erector tissue being pushed out by the transverse processes on that side since vertebrae tend to rotate in side bending.

If the scoliosis has been induced by a LLD then the following adaptations typically occur:

- The hips will displace laterally towards the side of the longer leg, giving it a fuller appearance on that side.
- The sacral base will slope towards the shorter leg, initiating a scoliotic adaptation that initially curves towards the side of the shorter leg.
- The following fascial planes will shorten: on the side of the shorter leg – the iliotibial tract (ITB), the more lateral aspect of the gluteal fascia superior to the trochanter; on the side of the longer leg – the fascia of the inner thigh and adductors.
- There will be a torsion set up within the pelvis which will cause one ilium to rotate forward and the other back.
- The pelvic torsion will set up an asymmetry in the associated soft tissues: the external rotators, the hip flexors (including the iliopsoas) and hip extensors, the abductors and adductors, the sacrotuberous, sacrospinous, sacro-iliac, iliolumbar and lumbosacral ligaments.
- There will probably be asymmetry in the quadrati.

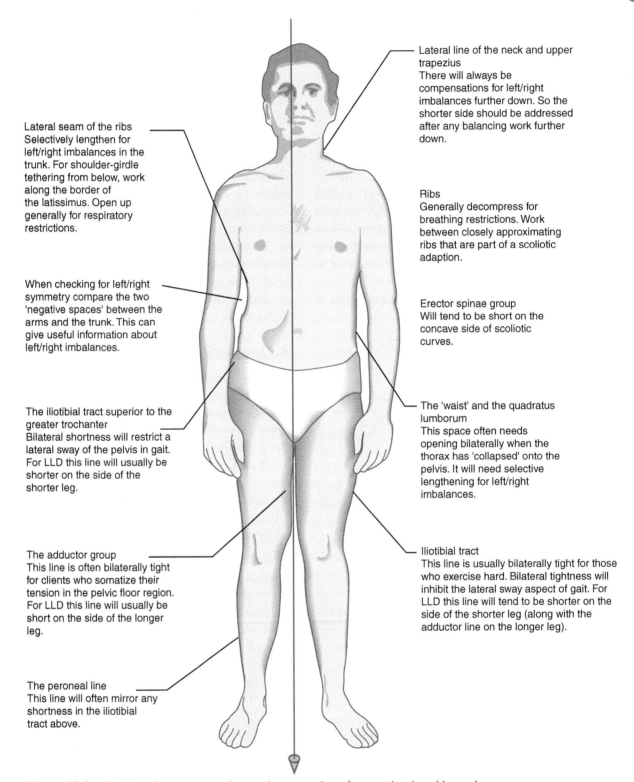

Lateral line of the neck and upper trapezius
There will always be compensations for left/right imbalances further down. So the shorter side should be addressed after any balancing work further down.

Ribs
Generally decompress for breathing restrictions. Work between closely approximating ribs that are part of a scoliotic adaption.

Erector spinae group
Will tend to be short on the concave side of scoliotic curves.

The 'waist' and the quadratus lumborum
This space often needs opening bilaterally when the thorax has 'collapsed' onto the pelvis. It will need selective lengthening for left/right imbalances.

Iliotibial tract
This line is usually bilaterally tight for those who exercise hard. Bilateral tightness will inhibit the lateral sway aspect of gait. For LLD this line will tend to be shorter on the side of the shorter leg (along with the adductor line on the longer leg).

Lateral seam of the ribs
Selectively lengthen for left/right imbalances in the trunk. For shoulder-girdle tethering from below, work along the border of the latissimus. Open up generally for respiratory restrictions.

When checking for left/right symmetry compare the two 'negative spaces' between the arms and the trunk. This can give useful information about left/right imbalances.

The iliotibial tract superior to the greater trochanter
Bilateral shortness will restrict a lateral sway of the pelvis in gait. For LLD this line will usually be shorter on the side of the shorter leg.

The adductor group
This line is often bilaterally tight for clients who somatize their tension in the pelvic floor region. For LLD this line will usually be short on the side of the longer leg.

The peroneal line
This line will often mirror any shortness in the iliotibial tract above.

Figure 17.2 The frontal organization showing key areas that often need to be addressed.

Scoliotic patterns will inevitably induce adaptations in the rib cage, so the lengthening work should be taken wider into the surrounding ribs. Ribs will have compressed on the concave side and expanded on the convex. If X-rays are not available then the areas of the ribs that need to be opened can be found by careful palpation. Laughlin outlines some excellent protocols for examining and treating LLD (Laughlin 1998).

FRONTAL ORGANIZATION

Lateral line

The peroneal area

The fascia of the peroneal area is continuous with the iliotibial tract (ITB). Therefore, it may usefully be lengthened along with the ITB to address hip asymmetries in the frontal plane. It also marks the functional separation of the front and back of the leg, so work in this area can help to functionally differentiate the anterior and posterior compartments and free up the ankle.

T56

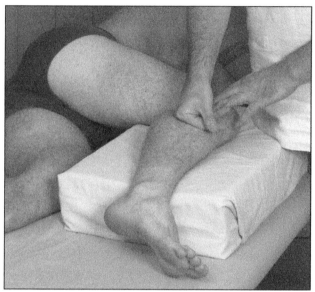

MFR technique – peroneals

First work the area broadly, then use more point loading to separate the underlying muscular compartments.

Assisting movements

Ankle flexion–extension. 'Slowly flex and extend your ankle.'

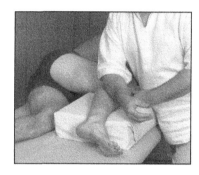

T57

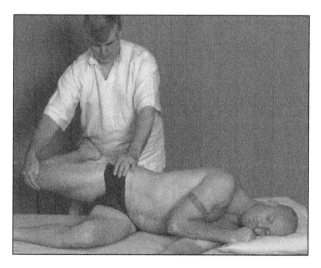

Ober test – test for shortness in the iliotibial tract

With the hip in a neutral position and the knee flexed at right angles, support the knee with one hand to inhibit any medial or lateral rotation of the thigh while stabilizing the pelvis with the other.

Allow the knee to drop to the table, sensing the tension in the ITB. A drop to just below horizontal is considered to be a normal length.

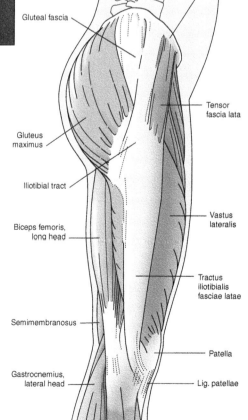

Iliac crest

Gluteal fascia

Tensor fascia lata

Gluteus maximus

Iliotibial tract

Vastus lateralis

Biceps femoris, long head

Tractus iliotibialis fasciae latae

Semimembranosus

Patella

Gastrocnemius, lateral head

Lig. patellae

The iliotibial tract

The ITB is often a sensitive area to work, particularly for athletic clients. The underlying vastus lateralis is easily compressed onto the femur. Trigger points are commonly present about two-thirds of the way down to the knee. So check with the client as you approach the spot and ease the pressure as necessary.

T58

MFR technique – ITB

Starting on and around the trochanter work towards the fibular head. Either use double soft fists to contour to the shape of the thigh, or use the forearm blade to 'iron out' the ITB. You can use various transverse strokes to 'feather out' from the midline of the ITB.

Assisting movements

If the ITB is particularly sensitive you can ask the client to 'breathe into' the area.

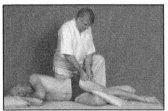
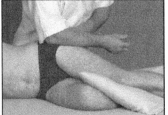
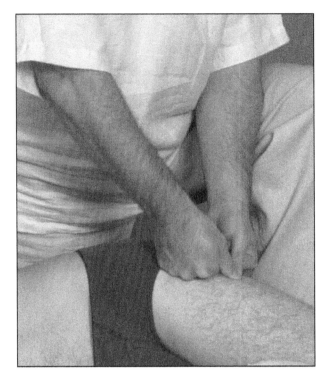

T59

MFR technique – hip deltoid

Start with the hip and leg flexed. Using the forearm blade, sink into the gluteal fascia at the trochanter and work towards the crest. The successive strokes can progress anteriorly or posteriorly, depending on the area that needs most release. You can work over the trochanter itself with soft fists.

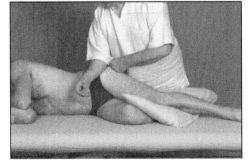
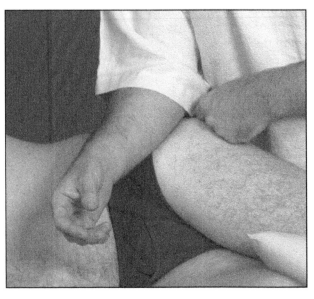

Assisting movements

Hip flexion–extension. 'Slowly lengthen the leg, reaching through the heel, then draw your knee forward again.'

T60

MFR technique – iliotibial tract, above the trochanter
This deeper technique can be used following the broader work of the previous techniques. Using doubled thumbs or elbow, work in short strokes across the ITB.

Assisting movements
Ask the client to breathe into the area.

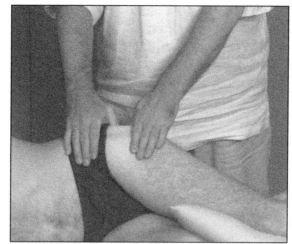

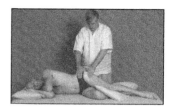

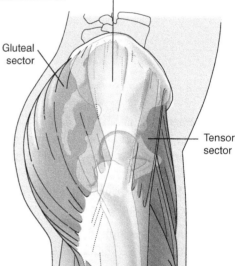

Central sector

Gluteal sector

Tensor sector

Deltoid of the hip
Fibres radiate in a broad fan from a point below the trochanter towards the arc of the iliac crest, not unlike the shoulder deltoid. Work in this area can allow freer lateral translation of the hips and can also influence pelvic tilt.

To encourage freer lateral translation of the hips concentrate on the central sector. To encourage anterior tilt work more in the gluteal sector. To encourage posterior tilt work more in the tensor sector.

T61

MFR technique – tensor fasciae lata
Start with the hip and leg flexed. Use the forearm blade or finger chisel to work from the trochanter towards the anterior superior iliac spine (ASIS).

Assisting movements
Hip extension. 'Slowly reach back through your heel. Straighten the leg till it hangs off the table.' Encourage the client to slide the leg, not elevate it, so as to minimize the tonus in the abductors.

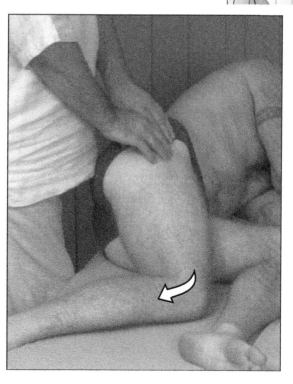

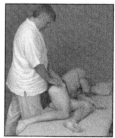

T62

MFR technique – gluteal fascia in side-lying
Use double fists to hook into the tissue behind the trochanter and work medially towards the sacrum.

Assisting movements
Hip flexion and internal rotation. 'Draw your knee towards your chest. Then allow it to drop to the table.'

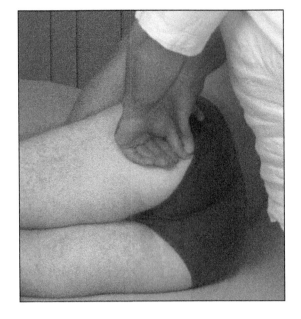

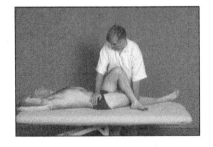

T63

C–R stretch – ITB and hip deltoid
This stretch focuses on the full length of the ITB, from the crest to the fibular head. The operator stabilizes the hip with one hand on the ASIS while the other is near the knee. The operator can avoid wrist-strain by leaning onto the fist.

Isometric contraction
Leg abduction. 'Press your leg back towards the midline.'

Next position
Assist the client to adduct the leg to the next position.

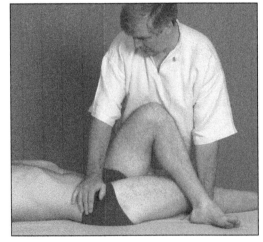

T64

C–R stretch – ITB, hip deltoid and quadratus
This stretch is less specific than the previous one and, depending on where the client has shortened, may include the lateral abdominal fascia and quadratus. It is important to position the client precisely side-on to the table. This prevents them from rolling back and engaging the hip flexors in the isometric contraction, instead of their hip abductors.

Isometric contraction
Leg abduction. 'Draw your leg towards the ceiling.'

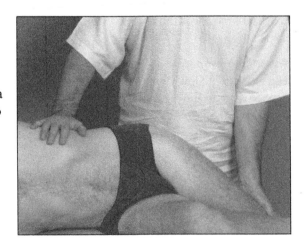

Next position
Stabilize the client at the ribs and ask them to drop the leg to the floor on the out-breath.

T65

Self-applied C–R stretch – the entire lateral line
Instruct the client to maintain a straight arm, allow the head to hang sideways and keep most weight on the outside leg.

Isometric contraction
Abduction of the supporting leg. 'As if you are trying to slide your foot sideways.'

Next position
On the out-breath, drop further into the hip. After 3 or 4 repetitions, stay there, breathing into the hip and allowing the stretch to work.

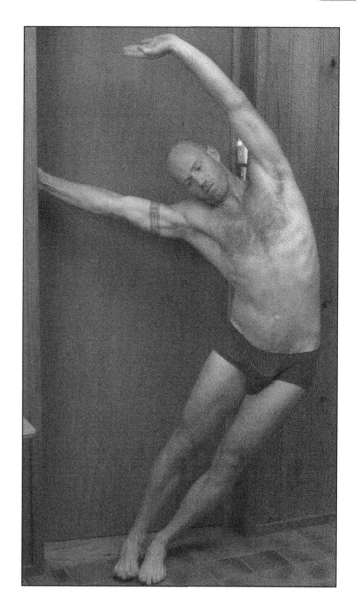

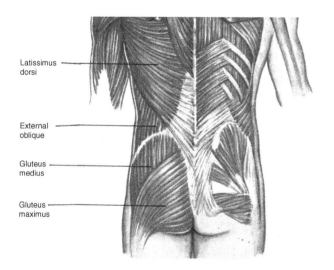

Latissimus dorsi

External oblique

Gluteus medius

Gluteus maximus

The waist
When you palpate the crest you often find what seems like a large investing fibrous pad. This is actually the collective thicknesses of all the aponeuroses that attach there, making this is an effective area to work.

As for the hip deltoid, a different emphasis in the work here can produce different outcomes:

● Working the most lateral line will influence lateral translation of the hip.
● Working more posteriorly will encourage posterior tilt.
● Working more anteriorly will encourage anterior tilt.

T66

MFR technique – waist

This working position allows good access to all the fasciae that connect into the iliac crest: the lateral abdominal fasciae and the most lateral aspect of the thoracolumbar fascia. It also allows broad access to the quadratus and the fascia overlying the floating ribs.

Assisting movements

There are several possibilities: a slow pelvic rock, a rhythmic reaching through the heel of the upper leg, or a reaching of the arm combined with the breath.

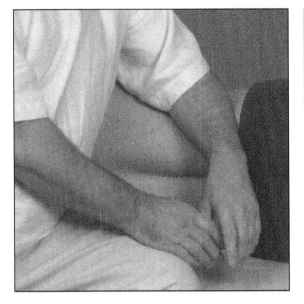
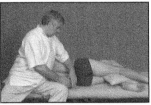

T67

MFR technique – anterior aponeuroses of the abdominals

You can ask the client to drop the upper leg off the table to further open the line you are working on. The client may feel more stable using a hand to grip the edge of the table.

Assisting movements

'Reach through the heel then relax back.'

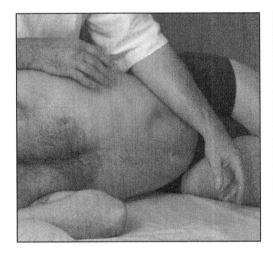
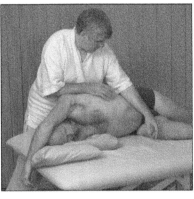

T68

MFR technique – quadratus

This detailed work can follow the more generalized freeing work of the previous techniques. Use doubled thumbs to reach the lateral border of the quadratus. Entry can be from the 12th rib end, or from the crest end by following the line of the crest medially until you meet the fibres of the quadratus. Work very slowly.

Assisting movements

Ask for deep breathing into the region or a slow pelvic rock.

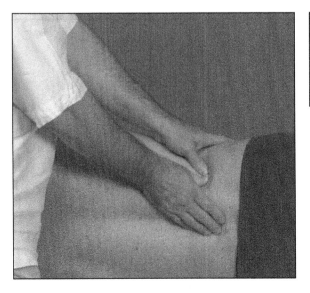
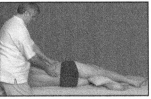

T69

C–R stretch – lateral abdominals and the quadratus lumborum

This stretch has two phases. In order to reach the quadratus, the lateral abdominals must first release, so the direction of this stretch is first lateral and then with a slight anterior rotation to allow the stretch to reach the quadratus.

Isometric contraction

Side extension. The client laterally extends into your hand, which is placed at the axilla. Repeat. Then to reach the quadratus, the vector needs to be slightly more posterior, so as the operator you will need to reposition yourself further behind your client.

Next position

Ask the client to drop further into side-flexion on the out-breath.

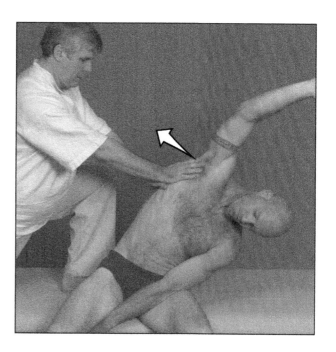

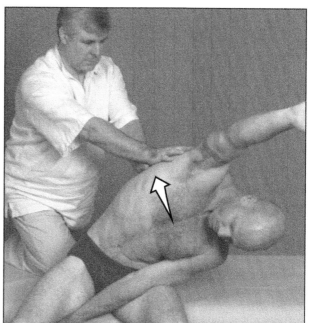

T70

MFR technique – lateral seam

Using an octopus handgrip, mould your hands to the shape of the ribcage using some compression. Try to engage the whole underlying superficial fascia and shear the tissue superiorly. A bolster beneath the client can assist in opening up the ribs you are working.

Assisting movements

Ask for deep breathing into the ribs coordinated with reaching through the arm.

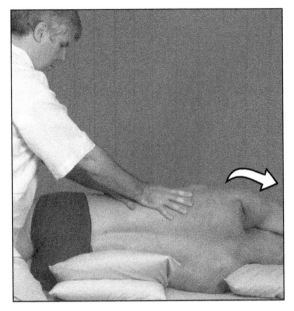

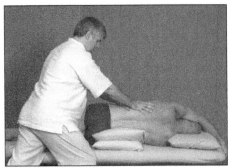

T71

MFR technique – intercostal spaces

This technique can be used to ease respiration generally, or to encourage opening in specific areas of the ribs, as in scoliosis. Using the finger chisel, work between the ribs that need to open more.

Assisting movements

Ask for deep breathing.

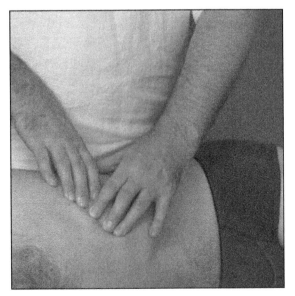

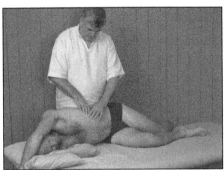

The lateral seam of the thorax

Using MFR in the lateral seam we can influence the more superficial layers: the superficial thoracic fascia and the deeper investing fasciae of the obliques and serratus. The deepest layers can probably only be affected by stretching – particularly the transversalis fascia, which is continuous with the endothoracic fascia beneath the ribs.

Work in the lateral seam can affect respiration as well as postural organization in the frontal plane. For clients with respiratory restrictions this work should be supplemented with more pointed MFR into the intercostal spaces.

T72

Passive stretch – lateral seam
There are many possible variations for this stretch, using a gym ball, a bed, piles of cushions and so on. It can be turned into a C–R stretch by using the upper arm to reach alternately to the ceiling and the floor. If using a table it is important to pad the edge for comfort.

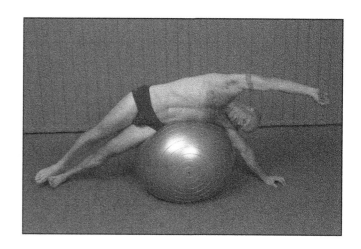

The superficial cervical fasciae – a word of caution
In this general area there are sensitive structures such as the brachial plexus, the jugular vein and carotid artery, so it is essential to get to know the area by gentle exploratory palpation. Explore your own neck first before moving on to other people's necks. The techniques described below are soft, and although it is possible to work more directly and more deeply in this area, it is best to wait and learn in a supervised context from someone experienced in handling necks.

T73

MFR technique – superficial cervical fasciae
Start with the client facing ahead. You can use the finger pads as if to reach beneath the clavicle towards the scalene insertions, or broadly contact the 'scalene triangle' using either the finger pads or the dorsal surface of the middle phalanges, using the 'soft fist' to anchor the superficial tissue. Sink in until you begin to sense the underlying

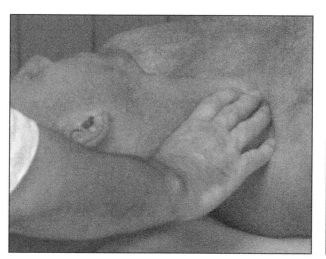

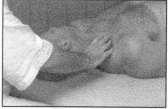

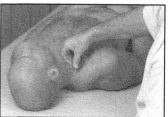

transverse processes, and then ask for movement. Maintain a firm smearing pressure as you work posteriorly, successively working the sternocleidomastoid (SCM), scalenes and the upper trapezius.

Assisting movements
Cervical rotation. 'Slowly rotate your head away.'

T74

MFR technique – sternocleidomastoid (SCM)

With one hand contacting the jugular notch and the other lateral to the SCM, scoop beneath the SCM and slide the fingers in opposite directions, placing a shearing force through the fascia that invests the SCM.

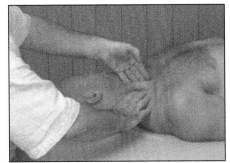

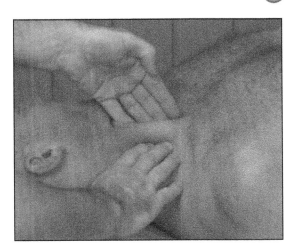

Assisting movements

Ask the client to make micro-movements of rotation or flexion–extension.

T75

MFR technique – SCM bilaterally

Keeping the back of your hands resting on the table, contact the dorsal aspect of the SCMs bilaterally. In a slow scooping motion slide ventrally while maintaining contact with the mastoid process.

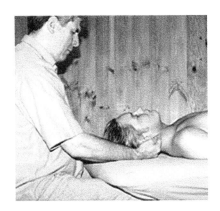

Assisting movements

Ask the client to have a spatial awareness of their 'overhead' region. Such a simple perceptual shift can assist the neck to relax and lengthen.

T76

C–R stretch – lateral cervical fasciae

When working with neck stretches it is important to impart the sense of a *general* lengthening of the neck even while stretching one side. Note the operator's hand positions here and how one arm is used as a brace.

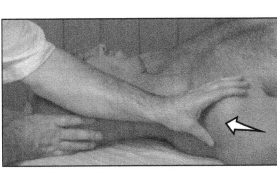

Isometric contraction

Lateral extension of the neck. 'Gently draw your head towards the midline. At the same time be aware of a general lengthening of your whole neck.' With neck stretches it is important always to remind the client to use a 5–10% effort in the isometric contraction.

Next position

Side flexion of the neck. You can apply a slight traction to the head as you assist the client to the next position.

T77

Self-applied C–R stretch – lateral cervical fasciae
First stabilize the shoulder girdle by grasping the edge of the seat
and leaning away until the shoulder girdle is felt to sit firmly on the
upper ribs. Bring the fingers close to the ear, using finger pad pressure
alone. Without forcing, allow the head to drop sideways.

Isometric contraction
Side extension of the neck. 'Press the head into your fingertips
using no more than a 10% effort.'

Next position
Side flexion. 'On the out-breath let gravity take your head to
a new position.'

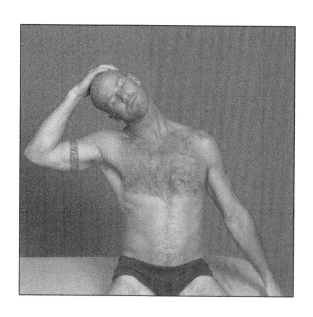

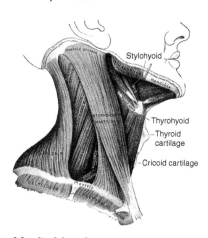

Medial leg line

Medial tibial border
This area should be worked in conjunction with the inner
thigh line, particularly when there is a side-shift
asymmetry in the frontal organization of the pelvis. Like
work in the peroneal area, work in this line can help
establish a functional differentiation between the back and
front of the leg.

T78

MFR technique – medial tibial border
Stabilize the foot in a
plantarflexed, inverted
position to obtain
maximum slackness in the
tissue. Using the finger
chisel, work slowly along
the tibial border, reaching
successively for flexor
digitorum longus, soleus
and gastrocnemius.

Assisting movements
With your free hand,
passively evert–invert the foot.

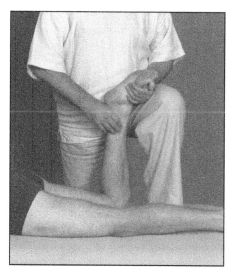

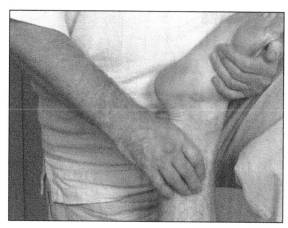

Inner thigh
Different structural results can be obtained by emphasizing either the anterior or posterior aspects of the inner thigh line:

● Working the most medial line will influence lateral translation of the hips.
● Working the hamstring side will encourage anterior tilt.
● Working the quads side will encourage posterior tilt.

T79

MFR technique – adductor group
Slide superiorly using a broad forearm blade. Repeat if necessary with more point loading. Then work in transverse strokes. You can work separately over the pes anserinus using a finger chisel.

Assisting movements
Ask for a slow pelvic rock. You can ask clients to emphasize different phases of the pelvic rock – extending the lumbar spine to encourage anterior tilt; flexing the lumbar spine to encourage posterior tilt.

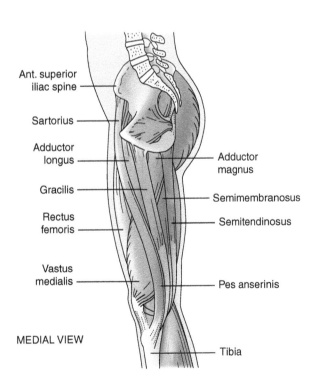

Ant. superior iliac spine
Sartorius
Adductor longus
Gracilis
Rectus femoris
Vastus medialis
Adductor magnus
Semimembranosus
Semitendinosus
Pes anserinis
Tibia
MEDIAL VIEW

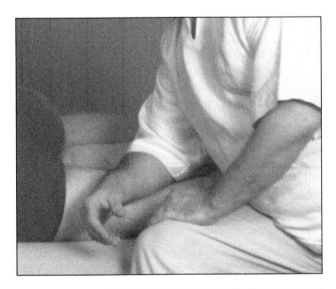

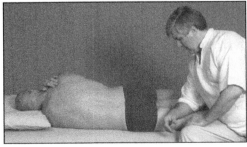

T80

C–R stretch – anterior adductors

This is one of a group of techniques in which it is useful to employ some compressible material as a support. Here the use of pillows removes the need for the client to engage the adductors protectively. Clients find it easier to release into a supporting surface. Stabilize the contralateral ASIS.

Isometric contraction

Hip adduction and internal rotation. 'Lift your knee towards the ceiling.'

Next position

Hip abduction and external rotation. Press the knee into the pillow taking it to a more abducted position.

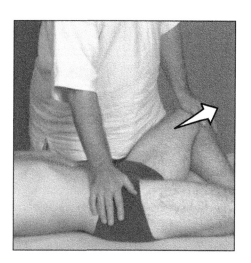

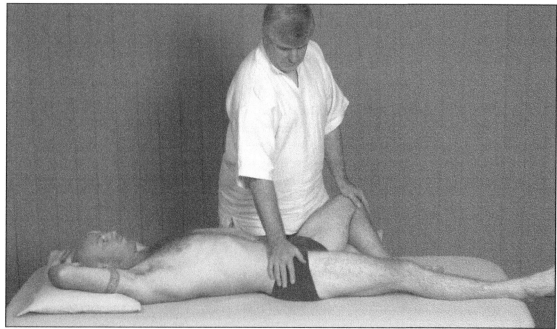

MOVEMENT WORK FOR FRONTAL UNDULATION

A key movement exploration will now be shown that can give the client a kinesthetic feel for frontal undulation, again, first as an ATM script and then using tactile guidance. It looks at two closely related movements in the frontal plane: 1) the pure lateral translation of the pelvis each side of the midline, and 2) the alternating 'hitching' of the hips around a sagittal–transverse axis. Generally they appear together in gait patterns, both involving contralateral abduction and adduction at the hip joints. The photos that follow show how this movement pattern can then be generalized into standing and walking.

Feldenkrais Awareness Through Movement (ATM) exploration – frontal undulation

Sensorial focusing, the mid-sagittal plane
Lie on your back with your arms and legs long. Sense your contact with the floor. Which parts of you are in contact with the floor? Which parts are not? With your eyes closed visualize that someone is tracing your own midline; starting from your crown then moving through the midline of your scalp and forehead, between the eyebrows, the bridge of the nose, the septum of the nostrils, the cleft of

the upper lip, the cleft of the chin, the sternal notch, the middle of the chest to the xiphoid process, the umbilicus, the pubis and around the line of the perineum. Continue along the cleft of the buttocks to the tailbone, through the middle of the sacrum and gradually trace over the spinous processes for the full length of the spine – the lumbar area, the thorax, the central ligament of the neck, the occipital bump and returning once more to the crown. Have you drawn a straight line down the front of your body? Do any of the body's segments feel displaced from the midline or non-symmetrical? Compare the left and right halves of the body: do they feel the same? How are they different?

1. Lateral translation of the pelvis

A pelvic rock, lifting the spine 'like a chain' to forming a 'bridge'

Bring your feet into a standing position. Begin a slow pelvic rock: alternately flattening and then arching the lumbar spine. Rest. Continue with the pelvic rocking but each time you flatten the lumbar area go just a little further and, eventually, the pelvis will lift from the ground. Continue, but with each pelvic rocking motion allow the spine to 'peel' a little further from the floor, vertebra by vertebra, like a chain being lifted link by link from the floor. Gradually you will approach a 'bridge' position. As you return to the floor try to reverse the movement precisely, vertebra by vertebra until your pelvis reaches the floor. Rest.

Forming a 'bridge', lateral translation

Bring your feet to standing about hip-width apart. Press though your feet, tucking the tail under, lifting the pelvis, and successively peeling your vertebra from the ground until finally you reach the shoulders (the thoracic–cervical junction in anatomical terms). You are now bridging from your feet to your shoulders. From this position begin to take your pelvis just a short distance left and right of your midline, trying to keep the pelvis parallel to the ground. Rest. Again come up into the previous bridge position. Again take the pelvis left and right of your midline but now go just a little further each time, still keeping the pelvis level with the ground. Only go as far as you can without strain. Rest.

Forming successively smaller bridges (isolating the movement further down the spine)

Form a bridge resting on your shoulders and resume the movement left and right of your midline. Rest. Next time you roll up your spine to form the bridge do not go so far up the spine – stop before you reach the shoulders, making a smaller bridge. In this new position, take your pelvis to the

left and right of the midline, keeping it parallel with the floor. Now the displacement left and right is achieved over a smaller length of spine. Only displace as far from the midline as is comfortable and without strain. Rest. Try a few more times, each time forming a smaller, lower bridge. Rest.

2. Hip-hiking

Reaching through the heel

Lie down with your arms and legs long. Reach through your right heel, trying to slide it away from you along the floor; relax back to a neutral position. Repeat in a rhythmical way reaching through the heel and noticing the response further up your body. Keep the movement small, just a few centimetres. What are the left and right hips doing? Allow the hips to participate more. What is happening in the lumbar spine? Rest. Continue reaching through the right heel in this rhythmical fashion but use your hands to gently palpate your ribcage, noticing how the ribs respond to this reaching movement. How is the head responding? Rest.

Hitching the opposite hip

Lying with arms and legs long, keep your left leg straight as you draw your left heel towards you, hitching your left hip. Repeat in a slow rhythm noticing once more how the rest of the body responds: the lumbar spine, the ribs, the shoulders and the head. Rest.

Combining the reaching and the hitching

Now combine both of these movements: as you reach through the right heel, draw your left heel in towards you. Repeat in a slow rhythm trying to make the coordinated movement as smooth and effortless as possible. Notice now the partial undulation of the spine. Rest.

Repeat on the opposite side

Recall the sequence for the right side: reaching through the right heel, hitching the left hip and then combining both. Now recapitulate this sequence of movements on the opposite side, starting with reaching through the left heel. Take a few minutes then rest.

Contralateral movement including the shoulder girdle

Lying with legs long and arms lying long beside you, reach alternately through the right and left heels. Gradually make the movement larger. Sense the undulatory pattern throughout the entire spine. Rest. Continue with this movement but now slide your hands alternately down towards the hip that is hitching. Notice how this movement enhances the undulatory pattern through the spine. Rest.

'Hands-on' movement exploration – lateral undulation

Lateral translation of the pelvis – neutral position

Guide the client through a series of pelvic rocking movements. Gradually allow the lumbar flexion to increase until the pelvis leaves the table; each time moving further up the spine till this 'bridge' position is reached.

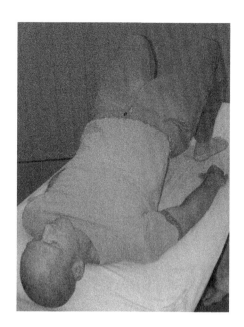

Lateral translation of the pelvis – displacement from the midline

Ask the client to shift the pelvis left and right of the midline. Initially keep the shift small – a few centimetres perhaps. Use your hands to suggest a movement *absolutely* in the frontal plane as there may be a strong tendency for the pelvis to rotate through a transverse plane; you could suggest the client aims to keep both buttocks an equal distance from the table.

Allow the amplitude of the movement to increase gradually but stop well short of a position of strain. As in the preceding ATM script, ask the client to repeat the movement with successively smaller 'bridges'.

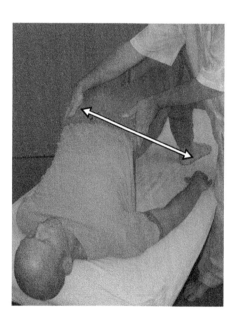

Rotation of the pelvis through the frontal plane – hip-hitching

Follow a sequence of movements as in the preceding ATM script.

Ask the client to reach through one leg; use your hand beneath the client's heel to reinforce the sense of lengthening from that hip. Next, ask the client to hitch the opposite hip. Then combine the 'reaching' of one leg and the 'hitching' of the opposite hip into one coordinated movement.

Repeat for the other side.

Ask for alternate reaching through the heels.

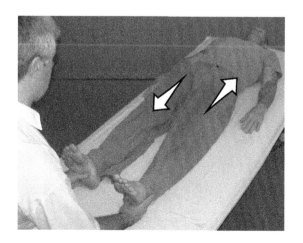

Have the client continue this movement on their own. Use your hands now to amplify any complementary movements of the ribs and head that you find, as well as the undulatory response of the entire spine. Then bring the client to standing.

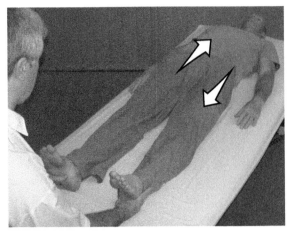

Frontal undulation in standing – stabilize head

Position yourself behind the client and use your hands to track the lateral displacement of the hips from the midline. Note the overall response to this movement. Is the amplitude of movement limited in this plane? Is the head stable in space or does it tend to displace left and right with the trunk?

When the movement is established use your hands softly to stabilize the head in space. Then progress through the following series of constraints that are designed to elicit differentiated movement between the pelvis, thorax and head.

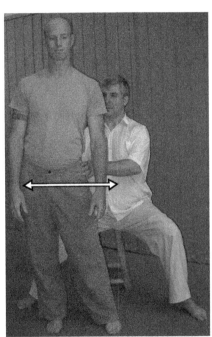

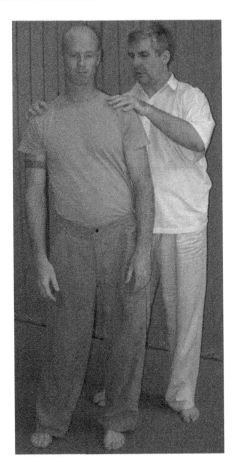

Frontal undulation in standing – stabilize shoulders

Now have the client continue the side-to-side movement of the pelvis but position your hands lightly on the shoulders and ask the client to maintain their position in space while the pelvis and spine continue their swaying movement below. It is important not to restrain the shoulders forcefully; merely use your hands as sources of proprioceptive feedback for the client. Ask the client to maintain their shoulders relatively immobile.

Frontal undulation in standing – stabilize ribs

Shift your hands to softly palpate the client's ribs. They should continue the lateral undulation but limited more to the lower spine. You could indicate that this is the kind of differentiation required in much of Latin-American dance.

Then ask the client to walk and notice any difference in their gait.

Ask them to exaggerate the lateral sway of the pelvis. You can evoke images of the 'Marilyn Monroe' walk (or the 'power' walk for male clients!).

Then ask the client to drop the exaggerated pattern and find what is an appropriate degree of lateral sway in walking.

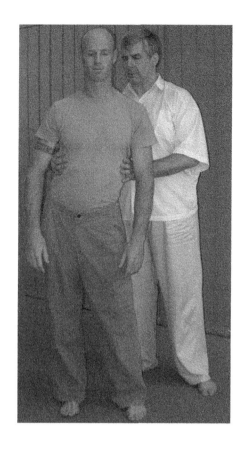

REFERENCE

Laughlin K 1998 Overcome neck and back pain. Simon and Schuster, New York

WORKING IN THE TRANSVERSE PLANE

For 'first approximation' structural bodywork it is sufficient to release all around the abdominal attachments before using the C–R stretches and then performing the functional work required to give the client a sense of differentiated movement of the chest and pelvis.

Release all connections between the thorax and pelvis: the pubic bone, the iliac crests from posterior to anterior superior iliac spine (PSIS to ASIS). The oblique attachments on the lower ribs, the rectus attachment around the sternum, the thoracolumbar fascia, the lateral and posterior ribs, the latissimus dorsi, quadratus lumborum and psoas (T17, T18, T20, T37, T66, T67, T68, shown in Chapters 16 & 17).

The C–R stretches should be used after assessing the longitudinal rotational tendencies, taking careful note of the *winding direction* of the rotation (from standing on a stool behind the client, see Fig. 14.1, p. 132), and performing the stretch contrary to the winding direction of the existing rotational pattern. There should then be more emphasis on engaging the obliques in movement explorations that differentiate the pelvis and thorax (T81, T82).

TRANSVERSE ORGANIZATION

The following two techniques are excellent means of addressing the soft-tissue adaptations to rotatory patterns around the longitudinal midline. The first technique addresses rotations at the lumbo-sacral end of the spine, and the second addresses rotations in the thoracic region. There are ways of working spiral adaptations of tissue using MFR techniques but these require a sure geometric vision of patterns of shortness.

T81

C–R stretch – lumbo-sacral region
Use this technique as part of the general alleviation of a rotoscoliotic pattern, or use bilaterally to promote more rotational ease of the pelvis in walking. Have the client look to the outstretched hand. Apply counter force at the PSIS.

Isometric contraction
Ask the client to unwind the trunk by pressing back into your hand.

Next position
Ask the client to go further into rotation by reaching through the upper knee. After 3 or 4 repetitions ask the client to breathe deeply into the lower back.

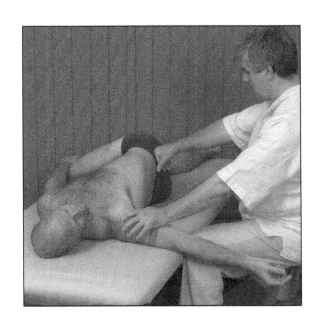

T82

C–R stretch – thoracolumbar region
In this seated position, have the client grip the back of the chair and pull into a rotated position of first bind. Stabilize the shoulder girdle.

Isometric contraction
Ask the client to unwind the upper torso into you.

Next position
Ask the client to pull further into rotation.

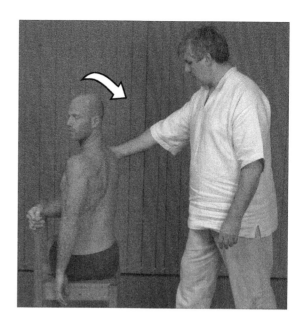

MOVEMENT WORK FOR TRANSVERSE UNDULATION

A key movement exploration will now be shown that can give the client a kinesthetic feel for transverse undulation – first as an ATM script and then using tactile guidance. Using the classic Feldenkrais 'knees to the side' exploration, it shows how the movements of the pelvic and thoracic segments can be differentiated, that is, allowed to rotate somewhat independently of each other around a longitudinal axis; then the head is added in a counter-rotatory pattern. Efficient gait requires that the head should track forward in space in a relatively straight line. This means that, with the pelvis and chest counter-rotating against each other, the neck must constantly adjust the orientation of the head so that it remains facing forward. This ATM is conducted in a supine position, and the photos that follow show how this movement can then be explored in standing and in walking.

Feldenkrais Awareness Through Movement (ATM) exploration – 'knees to the side'

Sensorial focusing
Lie on your back with your arms and legs long. Sense your contact with the floor. Which parts of you are in contact with the floor? Which parts are not? Sense the weight of your different segments as they rest on the floor: the head, the thorax, the pelvic segment, the arms and the legs. Sense the shape of the imprint of the soft tissues of the pelvic segment on the floor. Can you visualize this imprint? Is it symmetrical? Does one side seem to rest more firmly on the floor? Can you sense where the bones of the sacrum and ilia press through the soft tissues to the floor? Rest.

imprint changed? Maintaining a constant distance between the knees, begin to take them to the left a little, just a few centimetres, then bring them back to the midline. Repeat in a rhythmical way sensing how the pelvis responds. Rest. Continue now taking the knees to the left but each time going a little further. Note how at a certain point the pelvis begins to follow the knees in rotating to the left. Sense how the weight of the entire pelvic segment shifts to the left then returns to the midline. Rest. Repeat, this time explore the sensation of taking the knees to the right. Rest.

Knees to one side
Bring your feet up into a standing position, about hip-width apart and the knees apart. Again sense the contact of the pelvic segment with the floor. Has the shape of its

Taking the knees to both sides
Bring your feet to standing and begin taking the knees to the left and the right. Make it a small movement at first but increasing the amplitude by degrees. Sense how the

pelvis rolls from side to side and how different parts of the pelvis come into contact with the floor. As you increase the size of the movement note how the trunk responds – how, after a short delay, the ribs follow the pelvis in rotation. Note how this 'twisting' movement progresses up the spine until one shoulder begins to leave the ground. Use your hands to gently mould to your own ribs and 'urge' them into further involvement. Rest.

Counter-rotating the head

Bring your feet to standing and begin taking the knees to the left and the right, very gradually increasing the size of the movement. This time allow the head to rotate in the opposite direction to the pelvis, which leads in time to a twisting motion through the full length of the spine. Coordinate the movement so that both the head and the knees reach their comfortable end limit at the same time, and so that on their return they pass through the midline together. Try to bring a lazy, luxurious quality to the movement. Rest.

Neck–eye coordination

Lie with legs and arms long. Sense the weight of your head on the floor. Roll your head to the left and right; allow it to roll (rather than rotate around the midline) so that the chin moves towards the shoulders alternately. Pause. Notice some detail on the ceiling above, a speck or a detail of the surface texture, and fix your eyes on that point as you now rotate your head to the left and right. Pause. Continue rolling the head but now allow your eyes to rotate opposite to the head's movement. You can imagine you are following the movement of a train on the horizon. Rest.

Include eye fixation into the pattern

Bring the feet to standing and begin taking the knees to the left and right. Now introduce a counter-rotation of the head while, at the same time, keeping the eyes fixed on that point on the ceiling. Continue now but try to bring an even and relaxed quality to the movement. Try to luxuriate the movement. Rest.

'Hands-on' movement exploration – transverse undulation

Transverse undulation – knees to the side

The client lies supine with standing legs, and with feet and knees about hip width apart. Ask the client to begin a small movement, taking the knees to the left and right, and maintaining an even distance between the knees.

Have the client slowly increase the amplitude of the movement and use your hands successively to encourage a rotation of the pelvis, ribs and shoulders (as in these photos).

Then, ask for a contrary movement of the head; this requires a transverse rotation through the full length of the spine.

Bring the client to standing.

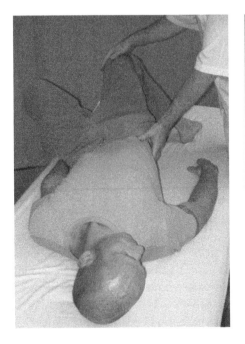
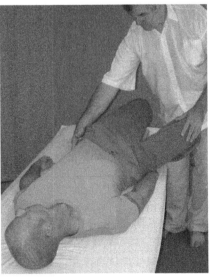

**Transverse undulation in
standing – stabilize
the hips**

Whilst gently stabilizing the hips,
ask the client to rotate the chest to
the left and right as if scanning the
horizon with the chest. Allow
the head to follow the rotation of
the trunk so that they move as
one. Again use your hands only to
provide proprioceptive feedback,
not to actually restrain the movement of the hips as that is the
client's job.

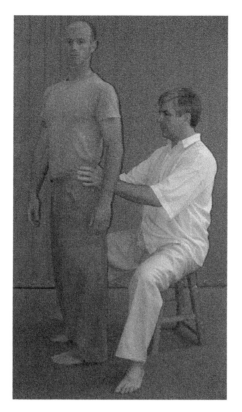
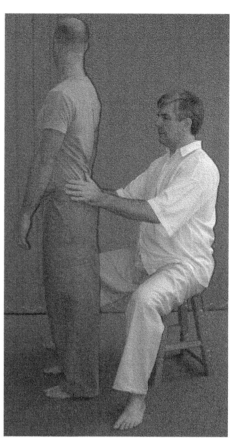

**Transverse undulation in standing – stabilize
the hips, counter-rotate the head**

Ask the client to continue rotating the trunk whilst
keeping the hips still. Then ask for a contrary movement of the head. You can ask them to turn their head as
if to look over the shoulder that is moving forward.

This coordination is vital if the client is to be able
to counter-rotate the shoulders against the hips in
walking while at the same time maintaining the head
oriented straight ahead.

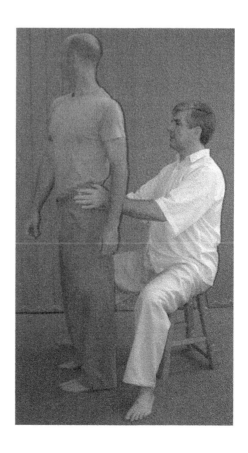

Transverse undulation in standing – stabilize the shoulders, counter-rotate the hips

Ask the client to rotate the hips – taking one hip forward while the other moves back, and then the other side. You could ask them to recall the 'Twist'. Rest your hands gently on the shoulders to assist the client in tracking the tendency for the shoulders to rotate with the hips.

For completeness, you could also extend this exploration to include a counter-rotation of the head, first against the hips then against the chest.

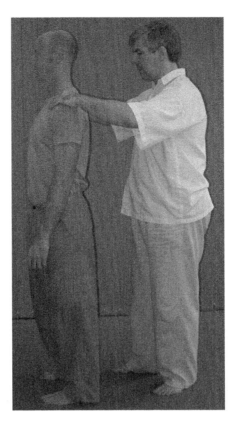
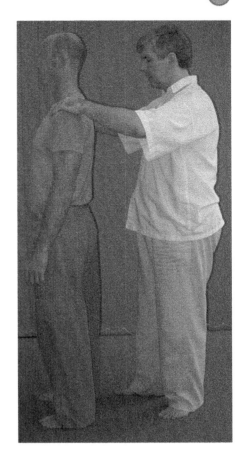

Transverse undulation in walking – counter-rotating hips and chest

Ask the client to combine all of the above rotatory movements into walking. You can walk behind the client using your hands to suggest the counter-rotation of the axis of the shoulder girdle against the pelvic girdle. When that is established, use your hands to stabilize the client's head such that it tracks directly forward in space. Then ask that the arms be completely relaxed, that their swing is determined solely by the fact that they are suspended from a moving shoulder girdle.

Ask the client to exaggerate the pattern into the 'cat-walk' of trained models.

Next, ask the client to drop the exaggerated form and find an amount of counter-rotation that feels appropriate.

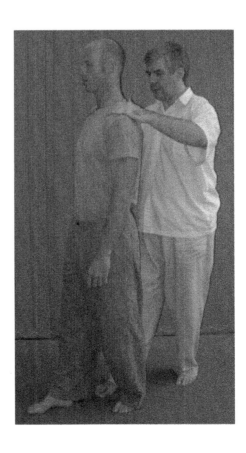

CHAPTER 19

WORKING WITH THE SHOULDER GIRDLES

What follows is a summary of the chief kinds of shoulder girdle displacement and the areas that one would normally consider for lengthening work. Once again these 'point form' suggestions need to be considered in the context of working with the organization of the body as a whole. It is emphasized once more that the order in which any of these areas are opened up depends on coming from a broader strategic perspective.

Elevated shoulder girdle
Lengthen the upper trapezius, the levator scapulae, especially its insertion onto the superior angle of the scapula. If the arms are abducted then work on the mid-deltoids too (T83–T93).

Depressed shoulder girdle
Lengthen the pectoralis minor and the lateral border of the latissimus dorsi (T94–T97).

Protracted shoulder girdle
Lengthen the pectoral fascia and the superficial fascia of the clavicles. Work deeply into the delto-pectoral groove (T97–T100).

Retracted shoulder girdle
Lengthen the posterior aspect of the shoulder girdle including the mid-trapezius, the rhomboids, the infraspinatus and teres minor. If the arms are habitually held hyperextended at the shoulder then lengthen the triceps (T40, T41, T86).

The elevated/protracted pattern
This is due to the synergistic operation of the shoulder girdle elevators and the pectoralis minor and is usually an aspect of the forward head syndrome.

SHOULDER GIRDLE DISPLACEMENTS

Elevated

Shoulder girdle – in elevation
The shoulder girdle elevation is an aspect of 'the body pattern of anxiety' and is one of the most common structural dysfunctions found today. The upper trapezius and the levator scapulae are mostly implicated, but this pattern is often combined with the depressive action of the pectoralis minor. Working synergistically, these muscles act to bring the scapulae 'up and over' the upper ribs into the common round-shouldered pattern.

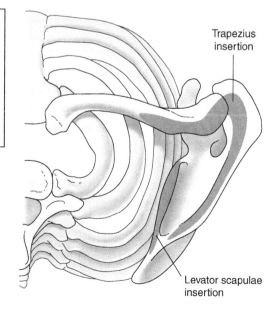

Trapezius insertion

Levator scapulae insertion

T83

MFR technique – spine of scapula

The fibres of the upper trapezius insert onto the spine of the scapula, making this an effective place to work. The space between the first and second knuckles fits nicely over the ridge of the spine. Starting at the acromion, follow the spine of the scapula medially.

Assisting movements

Ask the client to breathe into the area.

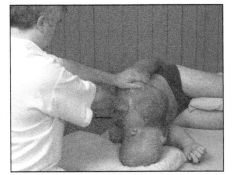
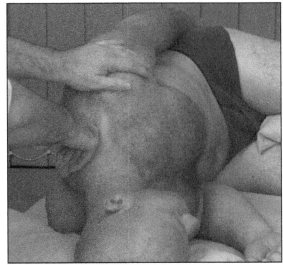

T84

MFR technique – upper trapezius

Use one hand to stabilize the shoulder girdle so that it sits firmly on the upper ribs, and then starting at the acromion work medially following the border of the upper trapezius.

Assisting movements

Ask the client to breathe into the area.

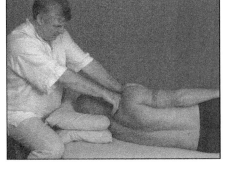
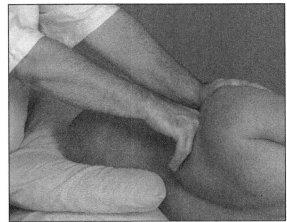

T85

C–R stretch – upper trapezius

Stabilize the shoulder girdle. You can vary the direction of your counter force to engage different muscles or different groups of fibres. As a subtle cue not to side-flex the neck you can gently rest an elbow on the side of the client's head.

Isometric contraction

Shoulder elevation. 'Lift your shoulder into my hands.'

Next position

Shoulder depression. 'Gently reach towards your feet.'

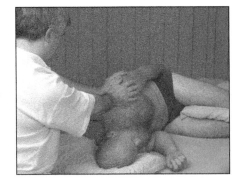
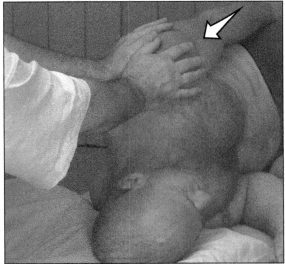

T86

MFR technique – upper trapezius, rhomboids, serratus posterior superior or levator scapulae insertion
This is an alternative position for working into

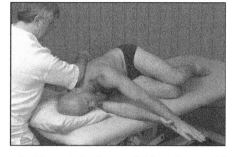

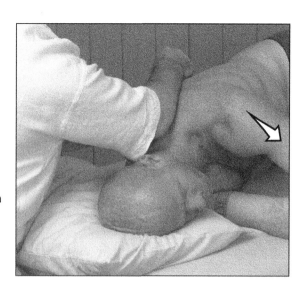

the upper trapezius or the rhomboids, so it is also useful for clients with habitually retracted scapulae – the 'military squared' shoulder girdle. It can be used very specifically to work on the levator scapulae insertion by maintaining strong contact with the superior angle of the scapula.

Ask the client to place their palms together in front of them. Gently depress the shoulder girdle (it will elevate when relaxed in this orientation), and then using the forearm blade contact the upper trapezius and work medially and inferiorly.

Assisting movements
Shoulder protraction. 'Reach slowly through your upper arm, sliding over the lower palm.'
It is important that the upper arm be supported on the lower arm in order to minimize the eccentric tonus in the rhomboids.

T87

MFR technique – upper trapezius, lateral
This technique blends naturally with the next.

Keeping fists at right angles to the upper line of the trapezius, slowly work laterally to the acromia.

Assisting movements
Neck retraction. 'Draw in your chin and lengthen through the crown.'

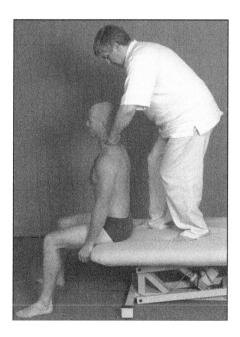

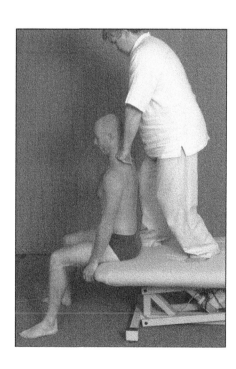

T88

MFR technique – the upper trapezius, posterior

Use your knees to support the upper back. This reduces the need for the client to engage the trunk flexors in performing the assisting movement. Gather the mass of tissue in the mid-trapezius region as if to bring over and back.

Assisting movements

Neck flexion. 'Slowly drop your chin to your chest and have a sense of lengthening through the crown.'

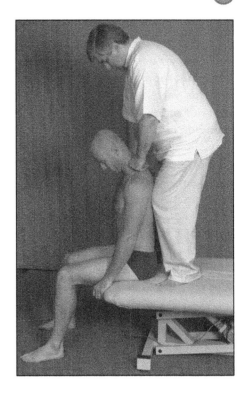

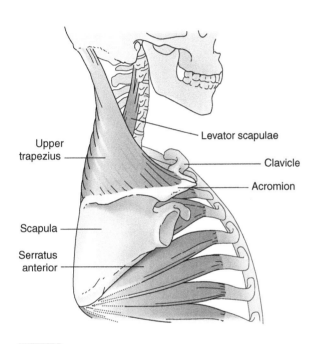

Upper trapezius

Levator scapulae

Clavicle

Acromion

Scapula

Serratus anterior

T89

C–R stretch – upper trapezius

Using your body weight through locked arms bear down upon the shoulders.

Alternatively, place a pillow in the lumbar region of the client and ask them to slump back into your legs 'like into an old armchair'. This lessens the need to mobilize the trunk muscles to resist the downward vector from the shoulders and allows the client to concentrate on the shoulders rather than in maintaining an upright posture.

Isometric contraction

Shoulder elevation. 'With no more than a 20% effort shrug your shoulders into my hands.'

Next position

Shoulder girdle depression. 'On the out-breath allow your elbows to drop towards the floor.'

This is a very strong stretch and should be performed gently if the client seems soft-bodied or loosely ligamented (it is possible to stress the sternoclavicular joint).

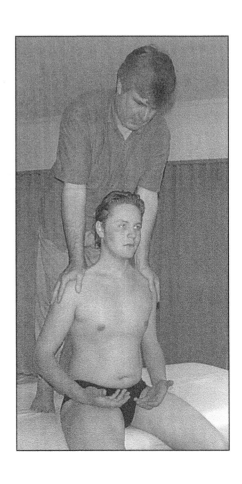

T90

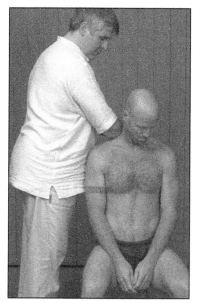
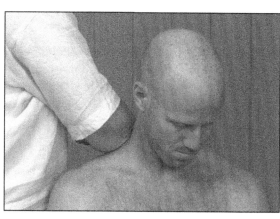

MFR technique – upper trapezius, seated position
Sink into the upper trapezius tissue and work medially and inferiorly.

Assisting movements
Cervical rotation and flexion. 'Slowly rotate your head away and then drop it forward and diagonally to your chest.'

T91

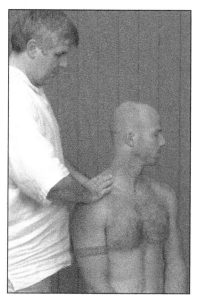
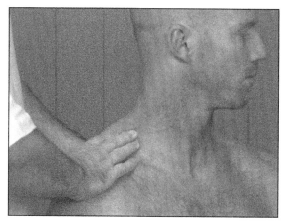

MFR technique – upper trapezius, seated position
Stabilize the thumb close to the shoulder joint. Direct the fingers as if trying to reach beneath the layer of the upper trapezius. During the application of this technique it is useful to keep asking the client to retract the neck, the chin-tuck position.

Assisting movements
Cervical rotation. 'Slowly rotate your head away from me.' It is common to get trigger point referral to above the eyebrow.

T92

MFR technique – levator scapulae insertion
Work superiorly along the vertebral border of the scapula towards the superior angle. You can use the forearm blade or reinforced thumbs. This area is usually rich in trigger points.

Assisting movements
Ask the client to breathe into the area.

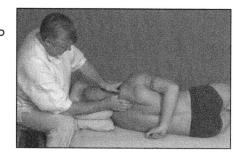
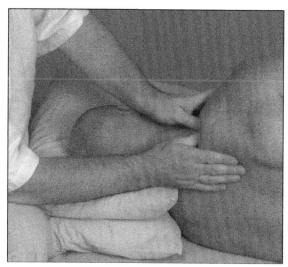

T93

Self-applied C–R stretch – levator scapulae
Rotate the head 45°. Bring the hand overhead and grasp near the nuchal line. The eyes should be looking at the crook of the elbow. Grasp the chair behind and lean forward to stabilize the shoulder girdle.

Isometric contraction
Cervical extension. 'While lengthening through your crown, press back gently into your hand.'

Next position
Cervical flexion. 'Drop your chin to your chest.'

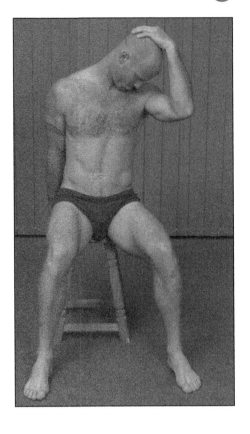

Depressed

Shoulder girdle – in depression
As a singular dysfunction, a shoulder girdle in depression is relatively rare and is found mostly in soft-tissue types. Paradoxically, however, it is often found in combination with an elevating tendency, which brings the shoulder girdle into the common, round shouldered 'up and over' pattern.

T94

MFR technique – latissimus
Using a 'soft' forearm blade, follow the lateral edge of the latissimus.

Assisting movements
Arm abduction, shoulder girdle elevation. 'Reach overhead through your elbow.'

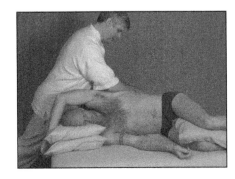

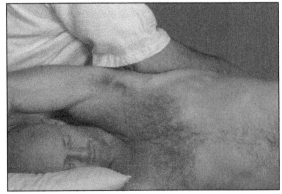

T95

C–R stretch – latissimus
Reach through the extended arm keeping the thumb uppermost while supporting the body weight on the other forearm.

Isometric contraction
Arm extension. 'Press the side of your hand into the floor.'

Next position
Arm flexion. 'Drop the shoulder towards the floor and reach though the arm.'

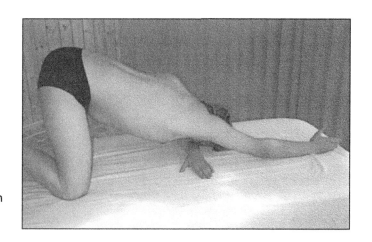

T96

MFR technique – pectoralis minor
Using doubled thumbs, reach under the pectoralis major to the origins of the pectoralis minor. Work superiorly with successive transverse strokes.
NB: this is a sensitive area!

Assisting movements
Arm abduction. Ask client to breathe into the area, or slowly reach overhead.

Alternative
Use finger chisel to reach for pectoralis minor.

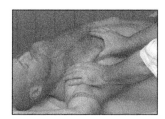

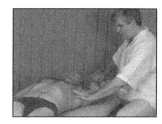

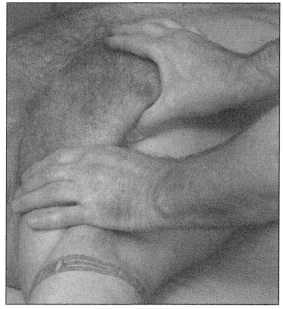

T97

MFR technique – latissimus tendon
Find the latissimus tendon between the biceps and triceps and anchor with finger pressure.

Assisting movements
Arm abduction. 'Slowly reach overhead, straightening the arm at the same time. Bring the arm as close as possible to your head.'

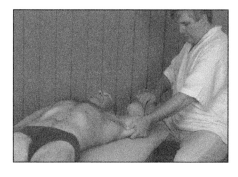

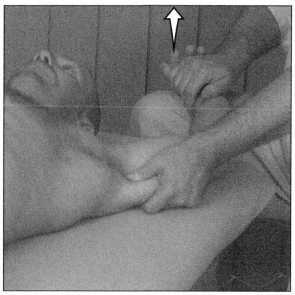

Protracted

Shoulder girdle – in protraction

The protracted shoulder girdle is associated with various emotional patterns. It is an aspect of 'the body pattern of anxiety'. It is also seen as a gesture of withdrawal, protectiveness or emotional hiding.

T98

MFR technique – superficial pectoral fascia

For shoulder girdle protraction or depression.

Starting mid-sternum, work laterally towards the coracoid process. Use several parallel strokes. Take care when working through the top of the breast tissue of women.

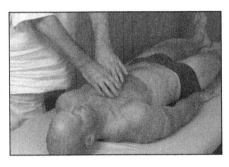
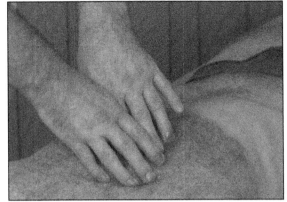

Assisting movements

Ask for deep upper-chest breathing.

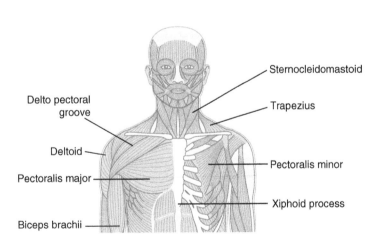
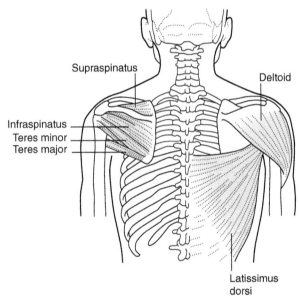

T99

MFR technique – deltopectoral groove
Gently place fist in the deltopectoral groove. Gradually increase the pressure by bringing your weight more vertically over the client. Tend to slide inferiorly.

Assisting movements
Cervical rotation. 'Slowly turn you head away from me and sense the stretch beneath your collar-bone.'

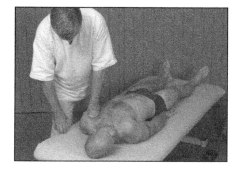

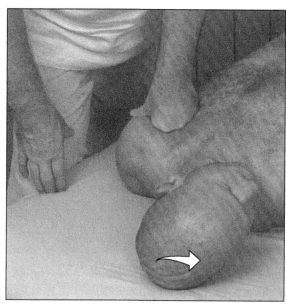

T100

MFR technique – pectoral fascia, pectoralis major tendon and deltopectoral groove
This is an alternative to the previous technique. Starting midway along the clavicle, work in slow strokes at right angles to the fibres of the pectoralis major muscle, ending up in the deltopectoral groove.

Assisting movements
Cervical rotation. 'Slowly turn your head away from me and sense the stretch beneath your collar-bone.'

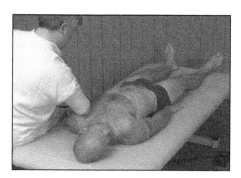

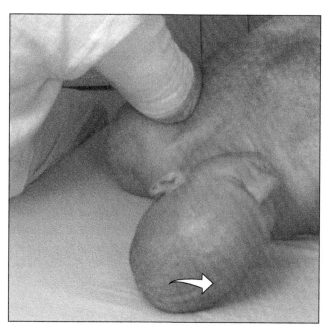

Retracted

Shoulder girdle – in retraction
The 'military squared' organization of the shoulder girdle is often a habit arising from the common postural 'advice' – 'Shoulders back'. It leads to a chronic holding pattern in the rhomboids and mid-trapezius. The techniques that address this pattern have been covered previously and are those that address the posterior aspect of the thorax (T40, T41 and T86).

WORKING WITH THE EXTERNAL ROTATION OF THE LEG

The 'toe out' pattern is usually associated with the external organization, or flat-backed tendency. Some typical myofascial adaptations to it are: a shortening of the external rotators, the gluteus maximus, the medial hamstrings, the medial aspect of the gastrocnemius–soleus complex, the tibialis anterior and the fascia of the lateral arch of the feet. It should be remembered, however, that a certain asymmetry between the legs is expected from segmental standard rotation.

The following areas can be worked:

- The posterior aspect of the gluteal fascia (T59, T62, T103).
- The medial insertion of the gluteus maximus, from coccyx to PSIS and beyond on the iliac crest (T101).
- The soft tissue overlying the linea aspera up to the greater trochanter (T102).
- The deep rotators, especially the piriformis (T104–T106, T108).
- The medial and inferior aspect of the calcaneal tendon and soleus (T78).
- The lateral arches of the feet (T24).

DE-ROTATE LEGS

The following techniques can be applied when there is marked external rotation of the feet when walking or standing, and when the external rotation comes from the hip rather than from a segmental rotation of the lower leg. Marked external rotation of the feet will produce an inefficient waddling gait and will tend to stress the medial arch of the foot, stretching the ligaments and encouraging pronation, and bunion formation in the longer term.

Note that it is common for the right foot to be more externally rotated than the left (segmental standard rotation), so it is not necessary to work for exact symmetry of the feet.

T101

MFR technique – medial gluteus maximus insertion
Initially contact the sacrotuberous ligament then slide superiorly in a slow arc, maintaining pressure against the gluteal insertions.

Assisting movements
Internal rotation of the femur. 'Slowly rotate your leg inwards, then relax back to a neutral position.'

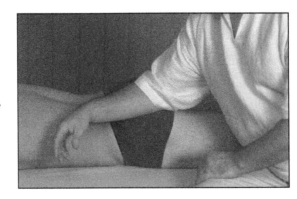

T102

MFR technique – lateral rotator insertions, gluteal insertions
Using the point of the olecranon sink down as if to reach the lineae asperae and slide superiorly. If there is too much resistance in the tissue, re-enter in a series of applications working superiorly. Work as if reaching for the lesser trochanter, then work around the greater trochanter.

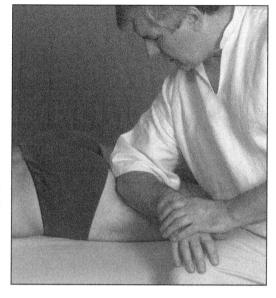
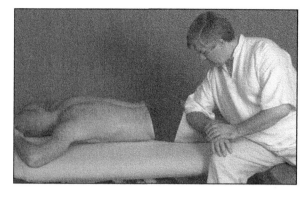
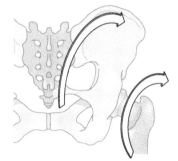

Assisting movements
Internal rotation of the femur. 'Slowly rotate your leg inwards, then relax back to a neutral position.'

T103

MFR technique – gluteal region
Gently contact the PSIS and edge of the sacrum. Increase the pressure by bringing your weight more vertically over the client. Slide towards the greater trochanter, or else make several applications moving laterally.

Assisting movements
Internal rotation of the femur. 'Slowly rotate your leg inwards, then relax back to a neutral position.'

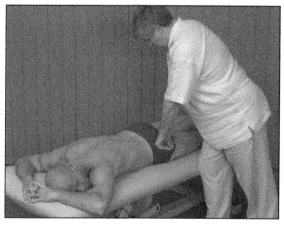

T104

C–R stretch – external rotation of leg from hip
While holding the leg in traction, rotate the foot internally.

Isometric contraction
External rotation of the femur. 'Rotate your leg outwards.'

Next position
Internal rotation of the femur. Check with the client that the knee ligaments are not being stressed.

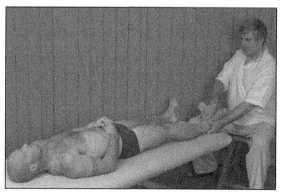

T105

MFR technique – piriformis, broad

Holding the heel of the flexed leg, locate the approximate position of the piriformis (on the line connecting the mid-sacrum to the tip of the greater trochanter). Gently sink through the gluteal layer with the free hand.

Assisting movements

Passively rotate the leg internally–externally.

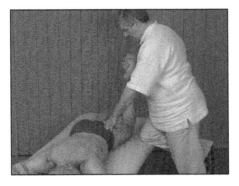

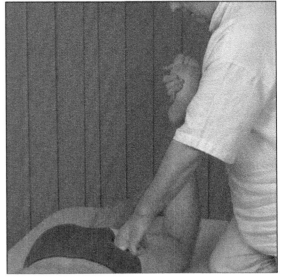

T106

MFR technique – piriformis, specific

Use doubled thumbs to first locate the posterior aspect of the greater trochanter. Slowly work medially.

Assisting movements

Internal rotation of the femur. 'Roll your foot inwards then release.'

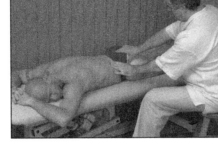

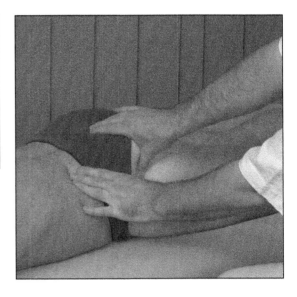

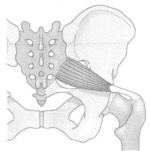

T107

Tracking

Rolfing tracking techniques are used to gently challenge ligamentous restrictions, or perhaps they work more by 'educating' joints proprioceptively into feeling different possible planes of movement.

For this technique ask the client to bring the inside of the feet unnaturally parallel (they will probably feel pigeon-toed). Ask them to perform slow knee bends. Use your hands to guide the knees forward over the big toe. The knees will want to track inwards. Clients may report feeling ligamentous challenge in the collateral knee ligaments and around the ankle joint. Persist if it is not experienced as stressful.

Then ask the client to take this into walking, consciously increasing the internal rotation of the leg say 10°. The preceding soft-tissue releases should make this quite easy.

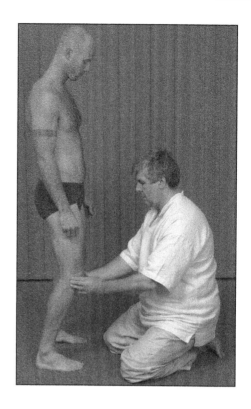

T108

Self-applied C–R stretch – piriformis

Sit on a table or massage table with the knee flexed at a right angle. On the breath lean forward from the hip (avoid flexing the spine). Take the chest towards the foot (not the knee).

Isometric contraction

Press the heel down into the table.

Next position

Take the chest forward and down to the next limit.

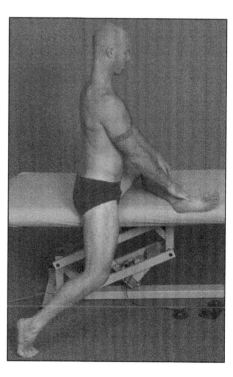

STRUCTURAL AND FUNCTIONAL BODYWORK TRAINING

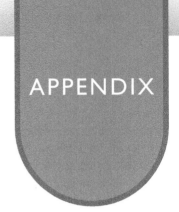

STRUCTURAL APPROACHES-TRAINING AND MEMBERSHIP ORGANIZATIONS

Rolfing

Rolf Institute
5055 Chaparral Ct. Ste. 103,
Boulder, CO 80301, USA
Ph: 303-449-5903
Fax: 303-449-5978
Web: www.rolf.org
Email: info@rolf.org

Australian Rolfing Association
PO Box 1511 Neutral Bay, NSW 2089
Australia
Ph: 61 (0)2 9953 5302
Fax: 61 (0)2 9908 3508
Web: www.rolfing.org.au
Email: info@rolfing.org.au

European Rolfing Assoc. e.V.
Kapuzinerstr, 25
D-80337 Munich
Germany
Ph: +49-89-54370940
Fax: +49-89-54370942
Web: rolfingeurope@compuserve.com
Email: www.rolfing.org

Brazilian Rolfing Assoc.
Alameda Casa Branca, 600
01408-000 Sao Paulo- SP
Brazil
Ph/fax: +55-11-3887-6070
Web: rolfing@rolfing.org.br
Email: www.rolfing.org.br

The Rolf Method of Structural Integration

Guild for Structural Integration
3107 28th St.
Boulder, CO 80301
United States
Ph: 800-447-0150 (toll free, US only)
Fax: 303-447-0108
Web: www.rolfguild.org
Email: gsi@rolfguild.org

Hellerwork

The Hellerwork Foundation
3435 M St
Eureka CA 95503
United States
Ph and Fax: 1-707 441 4949 or 1-800-392-3900
(in the US)
Web: www.hellerwork.com

Zentherapy®

International Zentherapy® Institute, Inc.
Melim Building, Suite 801
333 Queen Street
Honolulu, Hawaii 96813
Ph: (808) 528-2666
Fax: (808) 523-3052
Web: www.zentherapy.org
Email: Iziiorg@aol.com

Postural Integration

The International Council of Postural Integration
Trainers
Toekomststraat 99

B-9040 Ghent/St. Amandsberg
Belgium
Ph & fax: +32(0)92284911
Web: www.bodymindintegration.com
Email: icpit@posturalintegration.info

STRUCTURAL APPROACHES – MEMBERSHIP ORGANIZATIONS

International Association of Structural Integrators (IASI)
P.O. Box 8664
MISSOULA, MT 59807
Ph: 1-877-THE-IASI (1-877-843-4274) Toll-free US only
Web: www.theiasi.org

FUNCTIONAL APPROACHES – TRAINING AND MEMBERSHIP ORGANIZATIONS

Many countries have their own membership and training organizations. Only a few are shown here as first contacts.

The Feldenkrais Method

Feldenkrais Guild® of North America
3611 SW Hood Ave
Suite 100
Portland, OR 97239
United States
Ph: (503)221-6612 or (800)775-2118
Fax: (503)221-6616
Web: www.feldenkrais.com

Feldenkrais® Movement Institute
721 The Alameda
Berkeley, California 94707 USA
Ph: 800 342-3424
Fax 510 528-1332
Email: info@feldenkraisinstitute.org
Web: www.feldenkraisinstitute.org

Feldenkrais Guild UK
Email: enquiries@feldenkrais.co.uk
Ph: 07000 785506
Fax : 01224.861530
The Australian Feldenkrais Guild Inc.
Web: www.feldenkrais.org.au

The Alexander Technique

The Society of Teachers of the Alexander Technique (STAT)
1st Floor, Linton House
39-51 Highgate Road
London NW5 1RS
United Kingdom
Ph: 0845 230 7828
Fax: 020 7482 5435
Web: www.stat.org.uk

American Society for the Alexander Technique (AmSAT)
Ph: 800 473 0620

Australian Society of Teachers of the Alexander Technique (AUSTAT)
Ph: 1800 339 571
Web: www.alexandertechnique.org.au

The Trager Approach

Trager International
24800 Chagrin Blvd.
Suite 205
Beachwood, Ohio, 44122
United States.
Ph: USA 216-896-9383
Web: www.trager.com
Email: trager@trager.com

INDEX

Printed and bound by CPI Group (UK) Ltd, Croydon, CR0 4YY

03/10/2024

01040364-0012